Nutrition and Behavior of Uncommon Species

Guest Editors

LAURIE HESS, DVM, Dipl. ABVP–Avian
NATALIE ANTINOFF, DVM, Dipl. ABVP–Avian

VETERINARY CLINICS OF NORTH AMERICA: EXOTIC ANIMAL PRACTICE

www.vetexotic.theclinics.com

Consulting Editor
AGNES E. RUPLEY, DVM, Dipl. ABVP–Avian

May 2009 • Volume 12 • Number 2

SAUNDERS an imprint of ELSEVIER, Inc.

W.B. SAUNDERS COMPANY
A Division of Elsevier Inc.

1600 John F. Kennedy Boulevard • Suite 1800 • Philadelphia, Pennsylvania 19103-2899

http://www.vetexotic.theclinics.com

**VETERINARY CLINICS OF NORTH AMERICA: EXOTIC ANIMAL PRACTICE Volume 12, Number 2
May 2009 ISSN 1094-9194, ISBN-13: 978-1-4377-0558-4, ISBN-10: 1-4377-0558-8**

Editor: John Vassallo; j.vassallo@elsevier.com
Developmental Editor: Donald Mumford

Veterinary Clinics of North America: Exotic Animal Practice (ISSN 1094-9194) is published in January, May, and September by Elsevier, Inc.; Business and Editorial offices: 1600 John F. Kennedy Blvd., Suite 1800, Philadelphia, PA 19103-2899. Customer Service Office: 11830 Westline Industrial Drive, St. Louis, MO 63146. Subscription prices are $180.00 per year for US individuals, $323.00 per year for US institutions, $94.00 per year for US students and residents, $213.00 per year for Canadian individuals, $381.00 per year for Canadian institutions, $240.00 per year for international individuals, $381.00 per year for international institutions and $120.00 per year for Canadian and foreign students/residents. To receive student/resident rate, orders must be accompanied by name of affiliated institution, date of term, and the *signature* of program/residency coordinator on institution letterhead. Orders will be billed at individual rate until proof of status is received. Foreign air speed delivery is included in all *Clinics* subscription prices. All prices are subject to change without notice. **POSTMASTER:** Send address changes to *Veterinary Clinics of North America: Exotic Animal Practice*, 11830 Westline Industrial Drive, St. Louis, MO 63146. Customer Service (orders, claims, online, change of address): Elsevier Periodicals **Customer Service, 11830 Westline Industrial Drive, St. Louis, MO 63146. Tel: 1-800-654-2452 (U.S. and Canada); 314-453-7041 (outside U.S. and Canada). Fax: 314-523-5170. E-mail: journalscustomerservice-usa@elsevier.com (for print support); journalsonlinesupport-usa@elsevier (for online support).**

Reprints. For copies of 100 or more of articles in this publication, please contact the Commercial Reprints Department, Elsevier Inc., 360 Park Avenue South, New York, New York 10010-1710. Tel.: (212)-633-3813; Fax: (212)-633-1935; E-mail: reprints@elsevier.com.

Veterinary Clinics of North America: Exotic Animal Practice is covered in *MEDLINE/PubMed (Index Medicus)*.

Printed and bound by CPI Group (UK) Ltd, Croydon, CR0 4YY

Transferred to Digital Print 2011

Contributors

CONSULTING EDITOR

AGNES E. RUPLEY, DVM
Diplomate, American Board of Veterinary Practitioners–Avian Practice; and Director and
Chief Veterinarian, All Pets Medical Center, College Station, Texas

GUEST EDITORS

LAURIE HESS, DVM
Diplomate, American Board of Veterinary Practitioners–Avian Practice, Advanced Avian
and Exotics Vet, P.C., Fine Animal Hospital, Bedford Hills, New York

NATALIE ANTINOFF, DVM
Diplomate, American Board of Veterinary Practitioners–Avian Practice, Gulf Coast Avian
and Exotics, Gulf Coast Veterinary Specialists, Houston, Texas

AUTHORS

CHERYL S. ASA, PhD
Director, Research Department, Saint Louis Zoo, Saint Louis, Missouri

KAREN L. BAUMAN, BS
Laboratory Manager; and Association of Zoos and Aquariums Fennec Fox Species
Survival Plan Coordinator, Research Department, Saint Louis Zoo, Saint Louis, Missouri

JENNIFER CAMPBELL, PhD
Teaching Assistant Professor, Department of Biology, North Carolina State University,
Raleigh, North Carolina

JANET L. DEMPSEY, MS
Senior Nutritionist, Technical Services, Nestlé Purina PetCare Company, Checkerboard
Square, Saint Louis, Missouri

RYAN S. DE VOE, DVM, MSpVM
Diplomate, American College of Zoological Medicine; Diplomate, American Board of
Veterinary Practitioners—Avian Practice; and Senior Veterinarian, North Carolina
Zoological Park, Asheboro, North Carolina

ELLEN S. DIERENFELD, PhD, CNS
Manager, Sustainable Program Research, Novus International Inc., Saint Louis, Missouri

JERRY W. DRAGOO, PhD
Research Associate, Museum of Southwestern Biology, University of New Mexico,
Albuquerque, New Mexico

MARK S. EDWARDS, PhD
Associate Professor, Comparative Animal Nutrition, Animal Science Department,
California Polytechnic State University, San Luis Obispo, California

KERRIN GRANT, MS
ICU Assistant Supervisor/Nutritionist, The Wildlife Center, Espanola, New Mexico

SHERILYN J. HANNA
Owner, Exotic Endeavors, Camarillo, California

KATHARINE HOPE, DVM
Department of Animal Health, Smithsonian's National Zoological Park, Washington, DC

JOHN L. HOOGLAND, PhD
Professor of Biology, University of Maryland Center for Environmental Science,
Appalachian Laboratory, Frostburg, Maryland

DIANNE A. JAMES
President, Midwest Prairie Dog Shelter, Arcola, Indiana

KENNETH D. JONES, DVM
Private Practitioner, Jones Animal Hospital, Santa Monica, California

RANDALL E. JUNGE, MS, DVM
Diplomate, American College of Zoological Medicine; Director of Animal Health
and Nutrition, Saint Louis Zoo, Saint Louis, Missouri

DAVID S. KESSLER, BA
Biologist, Small Mammal Unit, Smithsonian's National Zoological Park, Washington, DC

SANTOSH P. LALL, PhD
Principal Research Officer and Group Leader, Institute for Marine Biosciences, National
Research Council of Canada, Halifax, Nova Scotia, Canada

SHANNON E. LIVINGSTON, MSc
Zoological Manager, Animal Nutrition Center, Disney's Animal Kingdom, Lake Buena
Vista, Florida

MICHAEL MASLANKA, MS
Department of Nutrition, Smithsonian's National Zoological Park, Washington, DC

DAVID L. McRUER, MSc, DVM
Director of Veterinary Services, Resident in Preventative Medicine, Wildlife Center
of Virginia, Waynesboro, Virginia

DEBORAH A. McWILLIAMS, MSc
Animal Nutritionist; Nutrition Advisor, American Association of Zoos and Aquariums
Rodent, Insectivore, and Lagomorph Taxon Advisory Group (AZA RIL-TAG); and Nutrition
Advisor, Canadian Association of Zoos and Aquariums Nutrition Advisory Group
(CAZA-NARG), Guelph, Ontario, Canada

JOSEPH A. SMITH, DVM
Veterinarian, Fort Wayne Children's Zoo, Fort Wayne, Indiana

SEAN M. TIBBETTS, MSc
Technical Officer, Institute for Marine Biosciences, National Research Council of Canada, Halifax, Nova Scotia, Canada

LYNDA WATSON
PMS Recycled Vermin, Lubbock, Texas

DOUGLAS P. WHITESIDE, DVM, DVSc
Diplomate, American College of Zoological Medicine; Staff Veterinarian, Calgary Zoo, Animal Health Care; Adjunct Associate Professor, Department of Ecosystem and Public Health, University of Calgary; and Faculty of Veterinary Medicine, Calgary, Alberta, Canada

CATHY V. WILLIAMS, DVM
Director of Animal Health, Duke Lemur Center, Duke University, Durham, North Carolina

KEVIN WRIGHT, DVM
Arizona Exotic Animal Hospital, Mesa, Arizona

Contents

Preface xiii

Laurie Hess and Natalie Antinoff

Considerations for Kinkajou Captive Diets 171

Kevin Wright and Mark S. Edwards

> Kinkajous are not suitable pets for most people, because the species takes considerable resources to accommodate their needs. They are often overlooked in zoo collections and in field research, because they are not considered threatened or endangered. The authors have presented an overview of the diets and enrichment methods that sustain reproduction, growth, and longevity in captive kinkajous. It is important, however, to recognize that kinkajous' nutritional needs are as poorly understood as almost everything else about their natural history.

Nutrition and Behavior of Coatis and Raccoons 187

Douglas P. Whiteside

> Raccoons and coatis are inquisitive members of the Procyonidae family, commonly found in zoos, treated in wildlife rehabilitation centers, and increasing in popularity as pets. Compared with other carnivores, both species have unique adaptations and behaviors associated with their omnivorous lifestyles. It is therefore important for clinicians to have an appreciation of their natural history, diet, and behavior to aid in the formulation of captive diets and feeding strategies to mitigate potential nutritional or behavioral pathologies.

Macropod Nutrition 197

Joseph A. Smith

> Macropods are herbivorous foregut-fermenters that have adapted to a wide variety of habitats. Anatomic adaptations such as dentition reflect differences in the diet consumed in the wild. Several key differences exist in anatomy and digestive physiology between macropods and other foregut-fermenters such as ruminants. The diet fed to macropods in captivity should be formulated with species-specific wild diets as a model. Hand-rearing orphaned macropods should be done with the unique physiology of macropod lactation in mind to ensure success. This article provides a summary of anatomic, physiologic, metabolic, and behavioral peculiarities of kangaroos and wallabies, with recommendations on captive management based on these traits.

Feeding Behavior and Nutrition of the Sugar Glider (*Petaurus breviceps*) 209

Ellen S. Dierenfeld

> Despite the sugar glider's popularity as a pet and a long-term history of captive management in zoologic institutions, little is known concerning

their specific nutritional requirements, apart from low basal energy and protein needs. Sugar gliders feed on plant and insect exudates—saps, gums, nectar, manna, honeydew, and lerp—as energy sources and rely on pollen and arthropods for dietary protein. Captive diets based on nutritionally balanced, commercially available products developed for other species, with added produce, have been fed successfully in zoo and private glider colonies, but these diets may not promote optimal gut function or feeding behaviors. Diets commonly fed by private owners were examined in feeding trials and were found to be highly digestible, but contained excess protein that was likely imbalanced in amino acids, as well as in calcium and phosphorus, because of improper supplementation. Suggestions are outlined for areas of relevant research to improve nutritional husbandry of sugar gliders.

Behavioral and Nutritional Aspects of the Virginian Opossum (*Didelphis virginiana*)   217

David L. McRuer and Kenneth D. Jones

Virginia opossums are widely distributed throughout the United States, except in the most arid regions, and wild individuals are commonly brought to practitioners for medical attention. Opossums' popularity as pets seems to be growing, and it is likely that pet opossums will be more common in veterinary practice. Clinicians must be aware of natural opossum behaviors so that thorough physical examination and diagnostic procedures can be performed on injured patients. For animals kept captive long-term or as pets, veterinarians must understand proper nutrition and nutritional disorders, such as secondary nutritional hyperparathyroidism, obesity, and dental disease, to properly treat this species.

Nutrition and Behavior of Degus (*Octodon degus*)   237

Mark S. Edwards

Octodon degus are herbivorous rodents that are adapted anatomically and behaviorally to utilize a fibrous diet with moderate-to-low levels of nonstructural carbohydrate. Captive degus should consume foods containing nutrients comparable to those consumed by free-ranging animals. The species is highly social, demonstrating a broad array of communication methods that make them appealing as a companion animal species. Controlled research studies with degus have produced a wealth of information that facilitates the care of this species in captivity.

Nutrition, Care, and Behavior of Captive Prairie Dogs   255

John L. Hoogland, Dianne A. James, and Lynda Watson

Prairie dogs are burrowing mammals that inhabit the grasslands of western North America. This article discusses the black-tailed prairie dog, the most common species and the one most likely to be found in zoos and private homes. The authors discuss several topics related to having prairie dogs as pets, such as why they make good pets, types of housing, diet, diseases, and injuries. The article concludes with information about where to obtain prairie dogs as pets.

Behavior, Nutrition, and Veterinary Care of Patagonian Cavies
(*Dolichotis patagonum*)   267

David S. Kessler, Katharine Hope, and Michael Maslanka

Patagonian cavies (*Dolichotis patagonum*) are large South American rodents well adapted for cursorial life (well adapted for running). They are monogamous but can live in groups of up to 70 individuals who maintain communal burrows. They are primarily herbivorous and may be maintained on commercially produced rodent or primate diets. Their long, thin legs and skittish nature make them difficult to restrain. Common medical problems include malocclusion of cheek teeth, gastrointestinal parasites, hypertrophic cardiomyopathy, and traumatic leg fractures.

Determinants for the Diet of Captive Agoutis (*Dasyprocta* spp.)   279

Deborah A. McWilliams

A critical factor affecting the dietary requirements of captive *Dasyprocta* species is their previous classification as a frugivore when there is evidence that supports classification as an omnivore. Other factors relevant to feeding captive *Dasyprocta* include the gastrointestinal tract anatomy, endogenous ascorbic acid, scatter-hoarding behavior, metabolic rate, apparent dietary requirements, life stage nutrition, diabetes, and dental caries and pathology. This article presents information currently available in the literature relevant to the dietary needs of captive *Dasyprocta* species.

Nutrition of Tree-dwelling Squirrels   287

Kerrin Grant

North American squirrels are categorized into one of three main groups based on physical characteristics, ecologic niche (including diet and food-hoarding strategies), and social structures. This article discusses wild diets, captive diets, hand-rearing infant squirrels, feeding regimens, and health issues of squirrels.

Nutrition and Behavior of Fennec Foxes (*Vulpes zerda*)   299

Janet L. Dempsey, Sherilyn J. Hanna, Cheryl S. Asa, and Karen L. Bauman

Fennec foxes make popular pets because of their small size, minimal odor, and highly social behaviors. They are kept in zoos for conservation and educational programs. The exotic animal practitioner is most likely to be presented with fennec foxes that are overweight because of inappropriate diets or excessive feeding. Clients attempting to hand-rear fennec foxes need advice about formula selection, amounts to feed, protocols for keeping pups warm, and weaning. This article provides information on social behavior, reproduction, and parental behavior, nutrition, and hand-rearing.

Nutrition and Behavior of Striped Skunks   313

Jerry W. Dragoo

Skunks are an integral part of the environment and a fascinating component of the earth's biodiversity. Their behavioral idiosyncrasies, made possible by their unique method of defense, make them entertaining to watch in the wild, and their beneficial habits far outweigh any potential negative attributes. Striped skunks can be a benefit in urban and agricultural areas because they prey on harmful and damaging insects and rodents that plague gardens and crops. The general public should be encouraged to live in harmony with skunks, as opposed to viewing them as nuisances. Keeping captive or pet skunks should be considered only after feeding, care, disease, and legal information has been investigated.

The Nutrition and Natural History of the Serval (*Felis serval*) and Caracal (*Caracal caracal*)   327

Shannon E. Livingston

There is little information regarding the specific nutrient and dietary needs of many species of exotic cats, including those kept sporadically as house pets, such as the serval and the caracal. The diets of exotic cats kept in captivity are usually based on the nutrient requirements of the domestic cat, although there is some evidence that different cat species may not metabolize certain nutrients in the same manner as domestic species. This article provides information on the natural diet and behavior of the serval and caracal and offers insight into some health issues that may arise in a domestic environment.

Feeding Behavior and Nutrition of the African Pygmy Hedgehog (*Atelerix albiventris*)   335

Ellen S. Dierenfeld

Despite their wide global distribution and popularity as pets, little is known concerning specific nutritional requirements of hedgehogs. They inhabit a wide variety of environments from desert to temperate forest, and they display flexible and opportunistic feeding behaviors. Natural diets include invertebrate and vertebrate prey, carrion, and plant material. Hedgehogs have enzymatic ability to digest chitin from insect exoskeletons as a dietary fiber source, but they do not seem to digest cellulose efficiently. Captive diets based on nutritionally balanced commercially available products containing moderate levels of protein (30%–50%, dry basis) and fat (10%–20%) are suitable for the omnivorous hedgehog.

Nutrition and Behavior of Lemurs   339

Randall E. Junge, Cathy V. Williams, and Jennifer Campbell

Attention to nutritional and behavioral factors is important for appropriate care of lemurs in captivity. Although only a few species are commonly held in captivity, differences between them are important. Knowledge of feeding ecology and natural diet guide nutrition guidelines, as well as management and prevention of common nutrition-related disorders, including obesity, diabetes, and iron-storage disease. Behavioral characteristics that influence captive management are related to social organization, reproductive behavior, territoriality, and infant care. Housing animals in appropriate social groupings in adequately complex environments reduces abnormal behaviors, and addition of enrichment activities and operant conditioning encourages normal behaviors.

Captive Invertebrate Nutrition 349

Ryan S. De Voe

The ability to maintain and propagate a species of animal in captivity is dependent on being able to provide adequate nutrition. Although the exact nutritional requirements of many invertebrate species are unknown, most commonly kept species are quite adaptable and seem to thrive on very basic diets. Veterinarians are often called upon to devise diets for captive invertebrates in research, display, and production facilities. A thorough knowledge of the natural history of the species is critical in developing dietary plans. This article focuses on terrestrial arthropods in the orders Insecta and Arachnida.

Nutrition, Feeding, and Behavior of Fish 361

Santosh P. Lall and Sean M. Tibbetts

Nutrition and feeding influence growth, reproduction, and health of fish and their response to physiologic and environmental stressors and pathogens. The basics of fish metabolism are similar to those of warm-blooded animals in that they involve food intake, digestion, absorption, and transport of nutrients to the various tissues. Fish, however, being the most primitive form of vertebrates, possess some distinguishing features which will be discussed. Unlike warm-blooded animals, which are homoeothermic, fish are poikilothermic, so their body temperature and metabolic rate depends on the water temperature and this has practical implications for the nutrition, feeding and health of fish. Several behavioral responses have been linked to methods of feeding, feeding habits, frequency of feeding, mechanisms of food detection, and food preferences. Fish are also unique among vertebrates in their ability to absorb minerals not only from their diets but also from water through their gills and skin.

Index 373

FORTHCOMING ISSUES

September 2009
Bacterial and Parasitic Diseases
Laura Wade, DVM,
Dipl. ABVP–Avian
Guest Editor

January 2010
Geriatric Medicine
Sharman M. Hoppes, DVM,
Dipl. ABVP–Avian Practice and
Patricia Gray, DVM, *Guest Editors*

RECENT ISSUES

January 2009
Cardiology
J. Jill Heatley, DVM, MS,
Dipl. ABVP–Avian, Dipl. ACZM
Guest Editor

September 2008
Hematology and Related Disorders
Tarah L. Hadley, DVM, Dipl. ABVP–Avian
Guest Editor

May 2008
Toxicology
Jerry LaBonde, MS, DVM
Guest Editor

RELATED INTEREST

Veterinary Clinics of North America: Small Animal Practice (Volume 39, Issue 2,
March 2009)
Veterinary Public Health
Rosalie T. Trevejo, DVM, PhD, MPVM, *Guest Editor*

THE CLINICS ARE NOW AVAILABLE ONLINE!

Access your subscription at:
www.theclinics.com

Preface

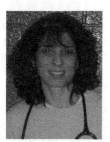
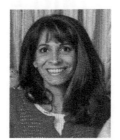

Laurie Hess, DVM, DABVP–Avian   Natalie Antinoff, DVM, DABVP–Avian
Guest Editors

"Of course, Mrs. Smith, the doctor can see your lemur when you bring your kinkajou and Patagonian cavy in next week for their check-ups," said the receptionist to the client on the telephone. As exotic animal veterinarians, we welcome telephone calls like this one that bring in new business; however, sometimes keeping up to date with all the unusual exotic animal species people now keep as pets can be daunting. It is hard enough to stay current with new treatments for the traditionally kept exotic pets, such as birds, rabbits, and guinea pigs, but it is even more challenging to stay on top of all the information out there on the exotic pets "du jour," such as small marsupials, primates, and invertebrates. There is little published information on many of these species, and most exotic animal practitioners have had little or no formal education on any of these species. Now, with the mass of information available on the Internet, exotic animal practitioners can search for information on the care of unusual exotic pets, but our results may be based on anecdotal information from breeders or hobbyists, without scientific foundation. Similarly, there is a wealth of information in zoos and accredited breeding and research facilities that is not readily available to veterinarians outside of these facilities, mainly because veterinarians, in general, do not know how to access this information. Practitioners attend conferences and read proceedings to try to amass a small file on these pets for reference, yet no single comprehensive volume has been printed that provides an overview of basic care (including nutrition, behavior, and common diseases) of these unusual animals.

The purpose of this issue was to put together a reference text containing information on many commonly kept unusual species an exotic animal veterinarian might encounter in practice. To do this, we sought the help of several experts, many of whom are not veterinarians but biologists, zoologists, and researchers who have spent significant portions of their careers studying these specific species. The emphasis is on nutrition and nutritional diseases, because so many of the problems we see are a result of inappropriate diet or feeding practices; however, additional information is provided for some species. By providing this text, we are not condoning ownership of these species; rather, we realize our obligation to provide proper and accurate care for these animals already in captive environments. We hope that by reading this issue, not only exotic pet practitioners but caretakers at zoos, wildlife facilities, rehabilitation centers,

Vet Clin Exot Anim 12 (2009) xiii–xiv
doi:10.1016/j.cvex.2009.02.001
1094-9194/09/$ – see front matter © 2009 Published by Elsevier Inc.   vetexotic.theclinics.com

seem to comprise their main diet, insects are a small but not insignificant portion. A population in Parque National Soberanía in Panama consumed almost exclusively fruits (90% as observed in feeding bouts, and 99% as observed via scat), with the remaining diet composed of nectar and leaves. They did not consume any insects or animal matter.[4–6] Fruit is the main water source (eg, preformed water) for wild kinkajous, and they often hang upside down while consuming water-rich fruits to avoid spilling a drop of juice (**Fig. 1**). Seeds often pass through the gastrointestinal tract undigested, which makes kinkajous excellent seed dispersers. They have 20-cm long tongues to collect nectar and pollen, and they are the known only carnivore that pollinates flowers (**Fig. 2**).

NUTRIENT AND ENERGY REQUIREMENTS

Nutrient requirements of kinkajous have not been studied clearly or defined under controlled conditions. To establish nutrient guidelines for practical feeding programs for exotic species such as kinkajous, we must evaluate gastrointestinal tract anatomy, types and nutrient content of foods consumed by free-ranging animals, and nutrient content of diets offered to animals in managed environments. A kinkajou's intestine is simple, without a cecum,[7] and it does not seem to have any grossly visible specialization for frugivory. Unfortunately, details of gastrointestinal tract anatomy and physiology are lacking, as is information on the nutrient content of free-ranging kinkajou diets. As a result, practical diets are extrapolated from the nutrient requirements of domestic dogs,[8] which are omnivorous distant relatives of kinkajous, and certain neotropical primates, which have similar foraging behaviors and food sources to kinkajous and are often found exploiting the same fruiting trees.[9]

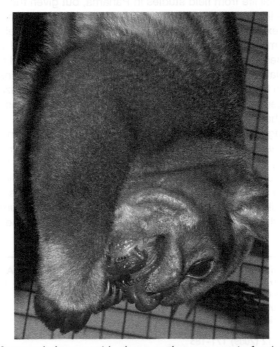

Fig. 1. Kinkajous frequently hang upside down as they eat certain foods, particularly juicy ones like grapes. (*Courtesy of* K. Wright, DVM, Mesa, AZ.)

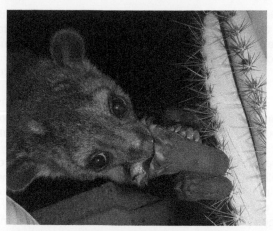

Fig. 2. Kinkajous pollinate many plant species as they forage for nectar. (*Courtesy of* K. Wright, DVM, Mesa, AZ.)

In the wild, fruit is considered a limiting food resource, especially for females. One study demonstrated a 2-month lag in body weight after low fruit production months.[10] Free-ranging kinkajous' activity budgets correlate with fruit abundance. When fruit is abundant, males eat less and rest more, whereas females eat less and travel more. This gender difference is hypothesized to be caused by differences between sexes in nutritional needs. Males presumably require a less nutrient-dense diet than pregnant females and are likely to rest and socialize when fruit is abundant. Females, by contrast, must forage more to find fruits with higher nutrient densities (eg, figs with calcium, protein) to support fetal development and nursing of offspring.[10,11]

A kinkajou needs approximately 50 kcal/d less than an equivalently sized mammal along the mouse-elephant (placental mammal) body curve because its basal metabolic rate is 30% to 34% lower.[6,12,13] A kinkajou diet created with daily kilocalories calculated from the metabolic rate formula for typical mammals provides too much food. As a result, kinkajous tend to be at greater risk for obesity when fed food quantities that are fed to other similarly sized mammals or when allowed to feed freely. A kinkajou's mean basal metabolic rate is approximately 0.316 mL O_2/g/h.[12] Foods need to be more nutrient dense (ie, amount of nutrient per kilocalorie consumed) to meet presumed nutritional needs without encouraging obesity. To prevent obesity and lessen the likelihood of diabetes mellitus, pancreatitis, arthritis, and cardiovascular diseases, especially in older kinkajous, caloric intake must be limited.

A kinkajou's body temperature ranges from nighttime active levels of 38.1 ± 0.4°C to daytime resting levels of 36.0 ± 0.6°C.[12] They cannot cool well through evaporation, and they show signs of heat stress when temperatures are higher than 33°C.[12,13] Their lowered metabolism also causes kinkajous to be less tolerant of cool temperatures. Kinkajous start to show heat-conserving postures and behaviors (eg, retreating to nest box, coiling with head buried between the thighs) when temperatures are below 15°C, and they show signs of hypothermic stress when temperatures drop to 5°C or less for more than a few hours (K. Wright, DVM, personal observation, 1993).

Kinkajous are extremely long-lived, with life spans commonly reaching two to four decades. Diets should be designed for life stages. A juvenile diet that supports growth and development should be fed for the first 12 to 18 months of life; an active adult diet should be fed into the second and possibly third decades (but discontinued when a female becomes reproductively senescent); a senior adult diet, with fewer calories and a shift in nutrients for reproductively senescent females and older males, should be fed after that. Given kinkajous' extreme longevity, geriatric diets that emphasize lower fat, increased levels of glucosamine and chondroitin, high-quality protein, and complex carbohydrates should be developed.

PRACTICAL DIETS

Diets offered to kinkajous in captivity, both in zoos and in private collections, tend to be overly complex and not representative of the species' natural diet in either ingredients or nutrients. In the authors' opinion, such diets are typically inadequate and potentially detrimental to health. A healthy and sound feeding program should be based on availability of nutritionally balanced foods. When consumed in appropriate quantities, these required foods are a source of consistent and reliable nutrition. The consumption of required foods safely allows caretakers to offer smaller amounts of nutritionally incomplete foods, such as commercial produce, insects, and other ingredients.

Fruit consumed by wild kinkajous has lower sugar, starch, and moisture content, higher protein and fiber content, and more concentrated minerals and vitamins than domestically available fruits.[14] Many captive diets include honey or other foods high in simple carbohydrates (ie, starch, sugar). The frequent occurrence of diabetes mellitus in kinkajous suggests that sugar-rich diets may contribute to the incidence of this disease (Mark S. Edwards, PhD, personal observation, 2008).

Captive diets often include raw meat, mice, and chicks, on the assumption that kinkajous catch and eat small animals in the wild. Kinkajous have developed salmonellosis and coliform enteritis and intestinal parasites, such as tapeworms, from consuming raw whole animals or raw meat.[15] Kinkajous do not apparently need these animal-based foods; in fact, field research shows that animal-based foods are a minor portion of the natural diet.[4,10] Free-ranging kinkajous consume plant protein via a variety of tropical fruits that they encounter over the year. There may be deficiencies of certain amino acids, fatty acids, or other nutrients in the fruit diet of free-ranging kinkajous that make consumption of relatively small amounts of animal prey necessary. Given these uncertainties and the probable inadequacy of domestic produce in meeting specific nutrient (ie, amino acids) needs, captive diets typically include animal protein with a balance of dietary essential amino acids (ie, those considered essential for domestic dogs).

A readily available basic diet capable of sustaining growth and reproduction over a 16-year period consists of 8 to 12 oz (227–340 g) of domestic dog kibble with 27% crude protein (eg, Purina Hi Pro, Nestlé Purina PetCare, St. Louis, MO; www.purina.com), 4 to 12 oz (113–340 g) of fresh fruit and/or vegetables, and 1 to 2 oz (28–57 g) of dried fruit. Fresh flowers (eg, hibiscus) and browse (eg, mulberry leaves and berries) may be eagerly eaten by some individuals. Favored fruits are bananas, apples, oranges, kiwi, melons, pears, and strawberries, but they must be given in moderation to prevent sugar overload. Cucumbers, sweet potatoes, corn, and snow peas are typically eaten eagerly. Sweet potato has a nutrient content similar to many wild fruits and is eagerly eaten raw or cooked. Various other seasonally fresh produce should be offered with care to avoid overfeeding any one item and potentially causing dietary deficiencies or imbalances. Figs are high in calcium and are eagerly eaten. Other favored dried fruits are raisins, dates, prunes, papaya, pineapple, and apricots, but overfeeding of these items must be avoided to prevent excess sugar ingestion.

Dog kibble is widely available and inexpensive and has been used long-term to support growth, reproduction, and aging. It seems to be an appropriate, practical, nutritionally complete food for kinkajous. With applied research and feeding trials, we will be able to more objectively define kinkajous' nutrient needs and how they respond to various foods. Kinkajous are often fed commercially available, extruded primate products as a part of their diet in place of dog kibble. These products may be fed to kinkajous because they are similar in nutrient content to dog kibble and meet the same nutrient needs provided by kibble. As long as caretakers keep in mind the nutrients that various foods provide, they can make dietary substitutions. Selected nutrient composition of foods included in kinkajou diets is given in **Table 1**.

By contrast, the types and quantities of foods included in a practical diet for a single adult kinkajou (BW = 2.89 kg) are provided in **Tables 2** and **3**. The calculated nutrient composition of that diet is compared with the estimated nutrient requirements of dogs (*Canis domesticus*).[8] (Note that values in **Table 2** are 30% less than typical placental mammal metabolic curve and are appropriate for most adult kinkajous. Values in **Table 3** follow the typical placental mammal metabolic curve and may be appropriate for pregnant and lactating kinkajous, growing kinkajous, and kinkajous recovering from severe illness with concomitant weight loss.) These tables provide only guidelines, and clinicians must adjust diet based on individual kinkajous' responses to diet (eg, changes in body condition score, body mass, and other health parameters). Data on the distribution of dry matter and energy of the major food components are provided in **Tables 4** and **5**.

Caution should be exercised in varying from these proven diets. One report provided husbandry and diet information for three male and three female kinkajous over a 2-year period with only a single birth reported.[16] The limited breeding in this study suggested suboptimal husbandry or subclinical disease. Kinkajous are prolific

Table 1
Selected nutrient composition of some foods offered to kinkajous (*Potos flavus*) in managed environments, expressed on a fresh weight and dry matter basis

	Dry Matter, %	Crude Protein, %	Crude Fat, %	Linoleic Acid, %	Crude Fiber, %	Ca, %	P, %	Vitamin A, IU/kg
Dog food,	92.0	27.4	16.3	1.75	2.7	1.32	1.02	18,500
original adult[a]	100	29.8	17.7	1.90	2.9	1.43	1.11	20,108
Puppy chow[b]	88.0	27.0	12.0	1.6	5.0	1.1	0.9	—
	100	30.7	13.6	1.8	5.7	1.3	1.0	—
HiPro dog food[b]	88.0	27.0	15.0	1.2	4.0	1	0.8	10,000
	100	30.7	17.0	1.4	4.5	1.1	0.9	11,364
KMR, canned liquid[c]	18.3	7.7	4.7	—	0.0	0.19	0.16	23,130
	100	42.1	25.6	—	0.0	1.04	0.87	126,393
KMR, powder[c]	97.3	43.0	29.5	—	0.0	1.01	0.89	110,700
	100	44.2	30.3	—	0.0	1.04	0.92	113,772
Leaf-eater food[d]	91.4	23.3	5.0	—	8.2	0.96	0.65	8000
	100.0	25.5	5.5	—	9.0	1.05	0.71	8753
Enfamil poly-Vi-Sol drops[e]	nd	—	—	—	—	—	—	1.5 million
	100	—	—	—	—	—	—	nd

[a] The Iams Company, Dayton, Ohio (www.iams.com).
[b] Nestlé Purina PetCare, St. Louis, Missouri (www.purina.com).
[c] Pet-Ag, Inc., Hampshire, Illinois (www.petag.com).
[d] Marion Zoologic Inc., Plymouth, Minnesota (www.marionzoological.com).
[e] Mead Johnson and Co., Evansville, Indiana.

Table 2
Examples of foods and quantities for feeding a single adult kinkajou (*Potos flavus*) (BW = 2.89 kg) from the Zoologic Society of San Diego and calculated nutrient composition of the offered diet as compared with estimated nutrient requirements of dogs (*Canis domesticus*)

	Food Type	Weight (g)	Schedule
1	Adult chunk dog food[a]	35	Daily
2	Leaf-eater food[a]	21	Daily
3	Roots, variable[b]	35	Daily
4	Vegetables, variable[c]	35	Daily
5	Fruits, variable[d]	35	Daily

Nutrient	Diet Concentration	Dog Requirement	Nutrient	Diet Concentration	Dog Requirement
Proximate			**Energy**		
Dry matter, %	40.3	nd	Metabolizable (ME), kJ/g	15.9	nd
Crude protein, %	24.7	10	**Fat-soluble vitamins**		
Lysine, %	1.2	0.68	Vitamin A, IU/kg	12,635	503
Crude fat, %	11.0	5.5	Beta-carotene, mg/kg	nd	nd
Linoleic acid, %	1.8	1.1	Vitamin D, IU/kg	1213	1380
Neutral detergent fiber (NDF), %	15.8	nd	Vitamin E, mg/kg	178	30
Acid detergent fiber (ADF), %	7.3	nd	Vitamin K, mg/kg	2.8	1.0
Carbohydrate (NDSC), %[e]	41.5	nd			
Minerals			**Water-soluble vitamins**		
Ash, %	7.0	nd	Thiamin, ppm	7.6	2.25
Calcium, %	1.1	0.3	Riboflavin, ppm	12.7	5.25
Phosphorus, %	0.8	0.3	Pyridoxine, ppm	2.6	1.5
Sodium, %	0.3	0.04	Niacin, ppm	47	15
Potassium, %	1.0	0.4	Biotin, ppb	303	nd
Magnesium, %	0.1	0.06	Choline, ppm	1342	1700
Iron, ppm	177	30	Pantothenic acid, ppm	26	15
Copper, ppm	36	6	Cyanocobalamin, ppb	89.5	35
Manganese, ppm	48.8	5.0	Vitamin C, ppm	673	
Selenium, ppm	0.29	0.35			
Zinc, ppm	129	60			

All nutrient concentrations, except dry matter, are expressed on a dry matter basis (DMB).
Abbreviation: nd, not determined.
   [a] Selected nutrient analysis provided in **Table 1**.
   [b] Variable roots may include, but are not limited to, beets, carrots, parsnips, sweet potatoes, turnips.
   [c] Variable vegetables may include, but are not limited to, broccoli, corn, green beans.
   [d] Variable fruits may include, but are not limited to, apples, bananas, grapes, melons, oranges, tomatoes.
   [e] NDSC (neutral detergent soluble carbohydrates) = 100 − crude protein,% + crude fat,% + neutral detergent fiber,% + ash,% (all DMB).
   M. Edwards, PhD, unpublished data, 2007.

on the dog kibble diet (described previously), and one pair on this diet produced a single offspring every 5 to 6 months for more than a decade (K. Wright, DVM, personal observations, 1993–2003).

Kinkajous are arboreal and have the tendency to ignore food that drops out of their hands during processing or eating. The food amounts noted previously are for

Table 3
Examples of foods and quantities for feeding a single adult kinkajou (*Potos flavus*) (BW = 2.89 kg) with special needs (ie, lactation, pregnancy, or illness) from the Zoologic Society of San Diego and calculated nutrient composition of the offered diet as compared with estimated nutrient requirements of dogs (*Canis domesticus*)

	Food Type	Weight (g)	Schedule
1	Adult chunk dog food[a]	50	Daily
2	Leaf-eater food[a]	30	Daily
3	Roots, variable[b]	50	Daily
4	Vegetables, variable[c]	50	Daily
5	Fruits, variable[d]	50	Daily

Nutrient	Diet Concentration	Dog Requirement	Nutrient	Diet Concentration	Dog Requirement
Proximate			**Energy**		
Dry matter, %	40.1	nd	Metabolizable (ME) kJ/g	3.81	nd
Crude protein, %	24.7	10	**Fat-soluble vitamins**		
Lysine, %	1.2	0.68	Vitamin A, IU/kg	12,635	503
Crude fat, %	11.0	5.5	Beta-carotene, mg/kg	nd	nd
Linoleic acid, %	1.8	1.1	Vitamin D, IU/kg	1213	1380
Neutral detergent fiber (NDF), %	15.8	nd	Vitamin E, mg/kg	178	30
Acid detergent fiber (ADF), %	7.3	nd	Vitamin K, mg/kg	2.8	1.0
Carbohydrate (NDSC), %[e]	41.5	nd			
Minerals			**Water-soluble vitamins**		
Ash, %	7.0	nd	Thiamin, ppm	7.6	2.25
Calcium, %	1.1	0.3	Riboflavin, ppm	12.7	5.25
Phosphorus, %	0.8	0.3	Pyridoxine, ppm	2.6	1.5
Sodium, %	0.3	0.04	Niacin, ppm	47	15
Potassium, %	1.0	0.4	Biotin, ppb	303	nd
Magnesium, %	0.1	0.06	Choline, ppm	1342	1700
Iron, ppm	177	30	Pantothenic acid, ppm	26	15
Copper, ppm	36	6	Cyanocobalamin, ppb	89.5	35
Manganese, ppm	48.8	5.0	Vitamin C, ppm	673	
Selenium, ppm	0.29	0.35			
Zinc, ppm	129	60			

All nutrient concentrations, except dry matter, are expressed on a dry matter basis (DMB).
Abbreviation: nd, not determined.
[a] Selected nutrient analysis provided in Table 1.
[b] Variable roots may include, but are not limited to, beets, carrots, parsnips, sweet potatoes, turnips.
[c] Variable vegetables may include, but are not limited to, broccoli, corn, green beans.
[d] Variable fruits may include, but are not limited to, apples, bananas, grapes, melons, oranges, tomatoes.
[e] NDSC (neutral detergent soluble carbohydrates) = 100 − crude protein, % + crude fat, % + neutral detergent fiber, % + ash, % (all DMB).
M. Edwards, PhD, unpublished data, 2007.

kinkajous kept in cages with wire bottoms that allow dropped food to fall out of reach to a cleaning tray below. For kinkajous kept on solid floors, a slightly smaller amount of food may be needed. To obtain optimum body condition, withholding dog kibble on intermittent days may be required. A reduction in food quantity or a fast day every

Table 4
Suggested distribution of mass, dry matter and dietary energy of foods and a diet for feeding adult kinkajous (*Potos flavus*)

Food Item	Amount g	Dry Matter %	Dry Matter g	Metabolizable Energy kJ per g (fresh weight)	Metabolizable Energy kJ	% Distribution
Dog food	35	91.98	32.2	16.98	594.3	57.75
High-fiber primate diet	21	91.40	19.2	11.67	245.1	23.81
Roots	35	12.21	4.3	1.81	63.4	6.16
Vegetables	35	16.07	5.6	1.16	40.6	3.95
Fruit	35	9.31	3.3	2.45	85.8	8.33
Total	161	—	64.5	—	1029.2	100

1 to 2 weeks, sometimes separated by as little as 48 hours, is tolerated well and simulates periods of reduced food availability when free-ranging kinkajous seek out new fruiting trees within their territories.

Food presentation is important to engage kinkajous by prolonging foraging and eating (see later discussion). By slowing the process of finding, grasping, and manipulating and ultimately consuming food morsels, a kinkajou has more time to develop satiety through a combination of stretch receptors in the stomach responding to the increasing volume of ingesta and chemosensory receptors throughout the body responding to elevated blood levels of glucose and fats. Careful feeding practices prevent gorging and overfeeding.

LIFE STAGE CONSIDERATIONS
Neonates and Juveniles

A single, or rarely two, offspring are born after a 112- to 118-day gestation period.[17] Neonatal kinkajous weigh 130 to 220 g, with twins weighing toward the lower end of this range (K. Wright, DVM, personal observations, 1993–2003). Pelage is gray with a dorsal black stripe, which changes to gold by weaning (**Figs. 3** and **4**). Variations in pelage coloration may be associated with subspecies. Eyes open at 7 to 25 days.[18] Juvenile kinkajous typically begin sampling solid foods at 6 to 7 weeks of

Table 5
Suggested distribution of mass, dry matter, and dietary energy of foods and a diet for feeding kinkajous (*Potos flavus*) with special needs (ie, lactation, pregnancy, or illness)

Food Item	Amount g	Dry Matter %	Dry Matter g	Metabolizable Energy kJ per g (fresh weight)	Metabolizable Energy kJ	% Distribution
Dog food	50	91.98	49.88	16.98	849	57.75
High-fiber primate diet	30	91.40	29.74	11.67	350	23.81
Roots	50	12.21	6.2	1.81	90.5	6.16
Vegetables	50	16.07	8.7	1.16	58.0	8.33
Fruit	50	9.31	5.1	2.45	122.5	3.95
Total	230	—	92.21	—	1470	

age[17] or earlier (K. Wright, personal observations, 1993–2003). Baby kinkajous should be left with the mother until at least partially weaned (8–9 weeks of age). Animals may hang using their prehensile tails at this age.[17]

Juveniles are often sold before they are fully weaned with the mistaken belief that this makes them better pets. In the authors' experience, weaned kinkajous that are allowed to live with their parents for at least 4 months make just as dependable pets as those removed from their parents at earlier ages and are less prone to developing behavioral vices, such as paw or tail sucking.

Although there are different hand-rearing diets published in older literature,[19,20] the readily available commercial product KMR (Kitten Milk Replacer, Pet-Ag, Inc., Hampshire, IL, www.petag.com) has been used as a wholesome diet for unweaned kinkajous. Moistened, banana-flavored rice baby cereal and crushed fresh banana can be used as initial solid food and quickly replaced by a moistened, dry dog food formulated for puppies. On a daily basis, incremental amounts of the moistened, dry dog food can be mixed with rice cereal/banana mixture. Dry extruded morsels typical of commercially available dog foods may not be eaten until 4 to 6 months of age, when adult teeth start erupting. Puppy kibble should be fed for the first year of life and then replaced with an adult dog food diet. Kinkajous that are kept on the cereal and banana mix too long before receiving dog kibble may develop mild metabolic bone disease manifested by an excessive plantigrade gait (angle of joint < 45°). Supplementing each feeding of the cereal and banana mixture with one to two drops of a children's pediatric vitamin (eg, Enfamil Poly-Vi-Sol, Mead Johnson and Co., Evansville, IN) and 1 mL of calcium glubionate (calcionate syrup, 1.8 g/5 mL, Rugby, Duluth, GA) per 1000 g of kinkajou bodyweight helps prevent this disorder. Caregivers always

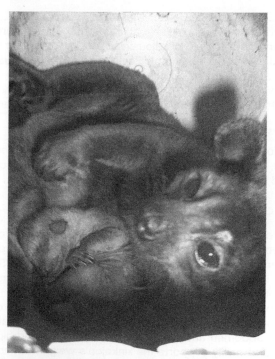

Fig. 3. Adult female with 7-day-old baby. (*Courtesy of* K. Wright, DVM, Mesa, AZ.)

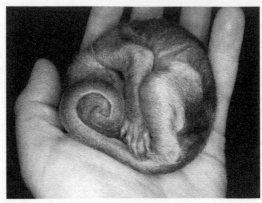

Fig. 4. Newborn kinkajou less than 24 hours old. (*Courtesy of* K. Wright, DVM, Mesa, AZ.)

should be aware of potential oversupplementation when adding vitamins to an already nutritionally complete food, such as dog kibble.

At weaning (60–100 days), a kinkajou readily follows larger moving objects, such as people and dogs. Most of them prefer to explore areas around where people are stationary and curl up to sleep in the crook of a human's arms or lap or other dark warm place. Hopping and running usually start by 12 weeks of age, and independent exploration, away from the leader, usually starts by 16 weeks of age. Mouthing and teething on the caregiver's fingers may start as early as 6 weeks of age. Dangerous aggression can build if this behavior is allowed to continue.

Adults

Body weights reported for free-ranging animals and from one population of captive kinkajous are provided in **Table 6**. Male kinkajous reach sexual maturity at 14 to 18 months. Females mature later, at 20 to 30 months. Females often rebreed during a postpartum estrus. In captivity, such females demonstrate an interbirth interval of 150 days and produce two offspring annually (K. Wright, DVM, personal observations, 1993–2003). This is in contrast to one offspring per year, which is typical for free-ranging females.[18]

Geriatric Kinkajous

In captivity, kinkajous typically live at least 15 to 20 years. Many living specimens are three decades old, however, and one specimen, Sugar Bear at the Honolulu Zoo, lived to be 41 years old (www.honoluluzoo.org/kinkajou.htm).

BODY CONDITION SCORES

Body condition scoring is an essential part of the health examination of domestic dogs and cats but is frequently overlooked with exotic pets. Using a score of 1 to 5, with 1 representing an emaciated kinkajou, 3 being a healthy weight, and 5 being an obese animal, clinicians should record body condition scores, in conjunction with body weight, on every physical examination.

A healthy kinkajou looks sleek from all sides, similar to a domestic cat (**Fig. 5**). From above, the ribs, abdomen, and hips are in a nearly straight line. A lateral view shows a slightly concave abdomen and clearly defined shoulders and hips. The tail coils readily, is strong, and easily supports the kinkajou's weight. Fat accumulates such that the abdomen becomes convex and eventually pendulous when viewed from

Table 6
Body weight of free-range and captive kinkajous (*Potus flavus*)

Status	Gender	Body weight Mean (kg)	Body weight Range (kg)	n	Location	Reference
Free range	B	3	—	—	French Guiana	7
	B	2	—	—	Mexico	21,22
	B	2.5	—	—	Surinam	17
	F	1.65	—	—	Surinam	23
	M	1.62	—	—	Surinam	23
	B	2.5	—	—	Venezuela	24
	B	—	1.4–4.6	—	not reported	a
Captive	M	3.59	1.90–4.75	3	San Diego, CA	a
	F	2.48	1.70–3.75	2	San Diego, CA	a

Abbreviations: B, both male and female; F, female; M, male; U, gender unreported.
^a M. Edwards, PhD, unpublished data, 2005.

the side, the shoulders disappear beneath fat, and the hips appear rounded, rather than angular (**Fig. 6**). The tail base becomes soft, and the tail cannot coil tightly. The kinkajou can support its own weight by a tail coiled around a hand but appears uncomfortable and cannot sustain an upside-down position for long. Fat accumulates around the neck and on the forehead, which causes the kinkajou's profile to appear slightly swollen and rounded. An emaciated kinkajou develops readily visible bony crests on its skull, the bones of the shoulders and ribs may be visible or easily palpable with slight digital pressure, and the hips appear sunken. The tail becomes listless and cannot coil to support the kinkajou's weight.

ENRICHMENT

Food presentation plays a significant role in engaging a kinkajou and is important in minimizing the development of abnormal behaviors and unhealthy body condition scores. Caregivers are encouraged to seek methods of enrichment that do not include

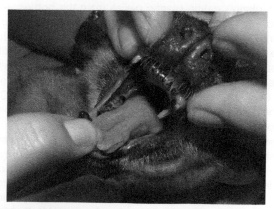

Fig. 5. The worn teeth of a kinkajou older than 20 years. The black staining varies with age and may be confused with tartar and calculus. (*Courtesy of* K. Wright, DVM, Mesa, AZ.)

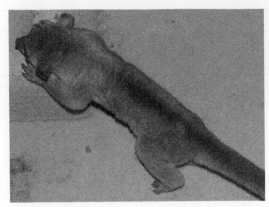

Fig. 6. This juvenile kinkajou has a body condition score of 3. (*Courtesy of* K. Wright, DVM, Mesa, AZ.)

food, such as training, olfactory stimuli, or new objects that stimulate scent marking. If food must be included in the enrichment plan, the authors promote the incorporation of novel methods for delivering the animal's nutritionally balanced diet rather than diluting the diet by adding nutritionally incomplete foods (eg, dried and fresh fruits, meat, and egg). Offering food in a covered bucket with feeding holes on its sides protects the food from soiling by the animal. It also makes foraging an essential part of feeding, because the kinkajou has to learn how to scoop food out of the bucket holes. Placing interfering objects, such as plastic balls (eg, Wiffle Ball, The Wiffle Ball Inc., Shelton, CT), or 4- to 6-cm hard rubber toys (eg, Ferret Treasure/Kong Ferret, Kong Company, Golden, CO), into the bucket along with kibble adds further challenge to the foraging experience. Another simple foraging container is a cube of wire (with 1- to 2-in gaps between the wire), so the kinkajou has to work to get the food out or try to eat it through the small openings in the cube's sides.

Additional enrichment may be provided easily by putting food treats inside 1- or 2-L soda bottles. These foods can be loaded in the bottle to be shaken out by the kinkajou, or if the animal is impatient, it may chew a hole in the bottle to more readily access the food. In more than 15 years of using this technique, caregivers have never noted a problem with a kinkajou eating plastic pieces from the bottles. A small amount of maple syrup can be put inside a bottle to keep the food pieces stuck to the insides of the bottle and make it more difficult for the animal to access the food. Paper towel holders, small boxes, and small hard plastic bottles are other readily available toys. Many kinkajous learn to unscrew bottle caps from soda bottles and may even open complicated locks. Polyvinylchloride (PVC) pipe toys can be made for hiding food, and a drip system in which a small amount of honey drips from a PVC pipe suspended above the cage, beyond the kinkajou's reach, keeps them focused for hours. Honey should be used sparingly to prevent diabetes mellitus.

Treats of cooked chicken or other meats are good training rewards. Sugary food may induce excitable behaviors that conflict with disciplined training. Feeding sugary food before or during playtime also may increase the risk of unpredictable or undesirable behaviors. Kinkajous may be trained to station, target, or perform other simple behaviors. Proper socialization requires at least 1 hour of combined free contact and training time daily. Providing daily training and appropriate behavioral enrichment helps prevent development of stereotypic and destructive behaviors.

NUTRITIONAL DISORDERS
Nutritional Secondary Hyperparathyroidism

This disorder results from diets that are calcium deficient, as a result of an absolute calcium deficiency, a relative calcium deficiency compared with phosphorus, or other factors, such as the presence in the diet of compounds that interfere with calcium uptake and absorption. This disease is common in hand-raised kinkajous and kinkajous that are fed fruit- and meat-rich diets. Clinical signs include a reluctance to move or hang by the tail, irritability (perhaps related to pain), shifting from an elevated plantigrade stance to one that collapses on the hocks, a hock angle < 45°, and deformities of the jaws and long bones (K. Wright, DVM, personal observation, 1995). Correction requires calcium supplementation, often with vitamin D_3, and providing a balanced diet. Pain management is essential for many cases.

Diabetes Mellitus

Despite adequate food intake, polydypsia, elevated blood glucose levels, glycosuria, and weight loss have been observed in several captive kinkajous (Mark S. Edwards, PhD, personal observation, 2008) with diabetes mellitus. Diet modification, including reducing meal size and intake of nonstructural carbohydrates and increasing feeding frequency, can be tried to manage early stages of disease. Fast days should not be part of the management of a kinkajou with diabetes. Prevention of disease, rather than management once it has occurred, is preferable.

Pancreatitis

Pancreatitis may be misdiagnosed if a clinician relies solely on blood amylase and lipase concentrations, because normal values of these enzymes are much higher in healthy kinkajous than in healthy dogs or cats. If these enzyme concentrations are correlated with elevated white blood cell counts, diarrhea, vomiting, and radiographic or ultrasonographic images consistent with pancreatitis, they are more reliable. One kinkajou has been on a diet that replaces dog kibble with a human liquid diet (Ensure, Abbot Laboratories, Abbott Park, IL, www.ensure.com) for several years after a presumed bout of pancreatitis. This kinkajou is also hypothyroid and is slightly overweight.

Obesity

Kinkajous' weights become alarmingly high if they are allowed to feed ad libitum (**Fig. 7**). One kinkajou actually reached a weight of 8.5 kg (D. Eshar, DVM, personal communication, 2008).

Dental Disease

Kinkajous need regular dental prophylaxis under general anesthesia as part of an annual or semiannual physical examination. Nutrient-poor diets or those that feature soft foods are associated with a higher incidence of tartar and gingivitis than nutritionally balanced diets that contain hard foods. Diets with hard foods, such as dog kibble and monkey biscuits, may wear down teeth over a kinkajou's long life (see **Fig. 4**).

FINAL THOUGHTS

Kinkajous are not suitable pets for most people, because the species takes considerable resources to accommodate their needs. They are often overlooked in zoo collections and in field research, because they are not considered threatened or endangered. The authors have presented an overview of the diets and enrichment

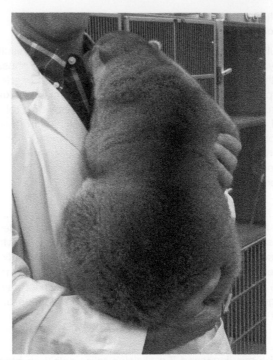

Fig. 7. This obese kinkajou has rolls of fat. It is approximately 200% heavier than it should be for a body condition score of 3. (*Courtesy of* D. Eshar, DVM, Philadelphia, PA.)

methods that sustain reproduction, growth, and longevity in captive kinkajous. It is important, however, to recognize that kinkajous' nutritional needs are as poorly understood as almost everything else about their natural history.

REFERENCES

1. Kays RW, Gittelman JL. Home range size and social behavior of kinkajous (*Potos flavus*) in the Republic of Panama. Biotropica 1995;27:530–4.
2. Kays RW, Gittelman JL, Wayned RK. Microsatellite analysis of kinkajou social organization. Mol Ecol 2000;9:743–51.
3. Kays RW, Gittelman JL. The social organization of the kinkajou *Potos flavus* (Procyonidae). J Zoo Soc London 2001;253:491–504.
4. Kays R. Social polyandry and promiscuous mating in a primate-like carnivore: the kinkajou (*Potos flavus*). In: Reichard UH, Boesch C, editors. Monogamy: mating strategies and partnerships in birds, humans and other mammals. Cambridge (MA): Cambridge University Press; 2003. p. 125–37.
5. Poglayen-Neuwall I. NonEn Zur fortpflanzungsbiologie und jugendentwicklung von *Potos flavus* (Schreber 1774). Der Zoologische Garten 1976;46:237–83 [as cited in Kays (2003)].
6. Ford LS, Hoffmann RS. Mammalian Species (Monograph). No. 321, Potos flavus. 1988. p. 1–9.
7. Charles-Dominique P, Atramentowicz M, Charles-Dominique M, et al. Les mammiferes frugivores arboricoles nocturnes d'une foret Guyanaise: inter-realtions plantes-animaux. Terre Vie 1981;35:341–435.

8. National Research Council (NRC). Nutrient requirements of dogs and cats. 10th edition. Washington, DC: National Academies Press; 2006.
9. Kays R. Kinkajou. In: MacDonald DW, editor. Encyclopedia of mammals. Oxford (MO): Oxford University Press; 2001. p. 92–3.
10. Kays RW. Food preferences of kinkajous (*Potos flavus*): a frugivorous carnivore. J Mammal 1999;80:589–99.
11. O'Brien TG, Kinnaird MF, Dierenfeld ES, et al. What's so special about figs? Nature 1998;126:1–15.
12. Müller EF, Kulzer E. Body temperature and oxygen uptake in the kinkajou (*Potos flavus*, Schreber), a nocturnal tropical carnivore. Arch Int Physiol Biochim 1977; 86:153–63.
13. Müller EF, Rost H. Respiratory frequency, total evaporative water loss and heart rate in the kinkajou (*Potos flavus*, Schreber). Z Säugetierk 1983;48:217–26 [as cited in Ford & Hoffman, 1988].
14. Edwards MS. Feeding the non-human primate. Presented at The North American Veterinary Conference. Orlando, FL, January 7–11, 2006.
15. Sheldon WG, Savage NL. Salmonellosis in a kinkajou. J Am Vet Med Assoc 1971; 159:624–5.
16. Pernalete JM. Management and reproduction of the Kinkajou *Potos flavus* at the Barquisimeto Zoo. Int Zoo Yearbook 1997;35:287–9.
17. Nowak RM, Paradiso JL. Walker's mammals of the world. 4th edition. Baltimore (MD): The Johns Hopkins University Press; 1983.
18. Nowak RM, Paradiso JL. Kinkajou. In: Nowak RM, editor. Walker's mammals of the world. 5th edition. Baltimore (MD): The Johns Hopkins University Press; 1991. p. 1103–4.
19. Clift CE. Notes on breeding and rearing a kinkajou *Potos flavus* at Syracuse Zoo. Int Zoo Yearbook 1967;7:126–7.
20. Bhatia CL, Desai JH. Growth and development of a hand-reared kinkajou *Potos flavus* at Delhi Zoo. Int Zoo Yearbook 1972;12:176–8.
21. Davis WB, Lukens PW. Mammals of the Mexican state of Guerrero, exclusive of Chiroptera and Rodentia. J Mammal 1958;39:347–67.
22. Eisenberg JF, Thorington RW. A preliminary analysis of a neotropical mammal fauna. Biotropica 1973;5:150–61.
23. Husson AM. The mammals of Suriname. London: Van Het Rijksmuseum van Natuurlijke Historie no 2; 1978.
24. Eisenberg JF, O'Connel MA, August PV. Density, productivity and distribution of mammals in two Venezuelan habitats. In: Eisenberg JF, editor. Vertebrate ecology in the northern neotropics. Washington, DC: Smithsonian Institution Press; 1979. p. 187–207.

Nutrition and Behavior of Coatis and Raccoons

Douglas P. Whiteside, DVM, DVSc, DACZM

KEYWORDS

- Coati • Raccoon • *Nasua* • *Procyon* • Nutrition • Behavior

Raccoons and coatis are inquisitive members of the Procyonidae family found within the order Carnivora. This New World family contains 15 species in 6 genera, with coatis and raccoons currently being linked together in the subfamily Procyoninae, although the taxonomy of the family is still under considerable debate.[1–3] Raccoons and coatis are commonly found in zoologic collections, are seen by wildlife rehabilitation centers, and with the increased availability of captive-bred animals afforded by the World Wide Web are increasing in popularity as pets. It is therefore important for clinicians to have an appreciation of their natural history, diet, and behavior to help formulate diets and feeding strategies in captivity to mitigate potential nutritional or behavioral pathologies.

The coati is sometimes referred to as a coatimundi, a misnomer that arose from the Brazilian vernacular "coati monde" used to denote solitary males. The genus name *Nasua* is derived from Latin for nose, whereas the common name is of Tupian Indian origin: *cua* meaning belt, and *tim* meaning nose, referring to sleeping position of the nose tucked onto the belly.[4,5] Four species of coatis are commonly recognized: the white-nosed coati (*Nasua narica*), the brown-nosed or South American coati (*Nasua nasua*), Wedel's coati (*Nasua wedeli*), and the mountain or Argentinian coati (*Nasuella olivacea*). Coati habitat is limited to some extent by seasonal environmental temperatures, but nonetheless they have a widespread geographic range extending from southern Arizona, New Mexico, and Texas southward through Mexico and Central America. There are also populations on distinct islands, such as Panama's Barro Colorado Island (*N narica*), and throughout the neotropical forests of Colombia and Venezuela through to Uruguay, Brazil, and Northern Argentina (*N nasua*), where they are often the most abundant carnivore species.[3–7]

Three species of raccoon are most frequently recognized: the common raccoon (*Procyon lotor*) with numerous subspecies, the crab-eating raccoon (*P cancrivorous*), and the Tres Marias raccoon (*P insularis*).[3,8] The common name for the raccoon is derived from the Algonquin word "arukan" which means "he who washes," whereas the scientific name for the genus (*Procyon*) comes from the Latin for "before dog." Raccoons are among the most widely distributed carnivores in the New World. The common raccoon (*P lotor*) is found transcontinentally from southern Canada to

Calgary Zoo Animal Health Centre, 1625 Centre Avenue East, Calgary, Alberta, Canada T2E 8K2
E-mail address: dougw@calgaryzoo.ab.ca

Vet Clin Exot Anim 12 (2009) 187–195
doi:10.1016/j.cvex.2009.01.002
1094-9194/09/$ – see front matter © 2009 Elsevier Inc. All rights reserved.

Panama, on islands off the Atlantic and Pacific coasts, with translocations in North America finding them as north as two Alaskan islands, whereas crab-eating raccoons have a range that extends from southern Central America to northern Argentina.[8–10]

Although both genders of raccoons are generally considered to be solitary and nocturnal in nature, female coatis are social, diurnal procyonids. Adult male coatis are solitary and extend their diurnal activity into the evening hours, postulated to be associated with a higher metabolic demand.[11] Females are philopatric with matri-line-based dominance hierarchies. Females coatis and juvenile males (<2 years of age) travel in groups known as bands with up to 30 individuals and exhibit cooperative foraging, nursing, grooming, vigilance, and aggressive antipredator behavior.[6–8,12–14]

BODY WEIGHT

Adult male coati tend to be approximately one-third heavier than females on average, whereas adult male raccoons average 17% heavier than their female conspecifics.[14] There is considerable geographic variation in adult raccoon weights, with the more northern raccoons being heavier than their southern counterparts. In addition, adult raccoon weights tend to fluctuate seasonally with an increase during autumn, peaking in January, and declining in the spring.[8,15] Fat stores can increase by 30% in northern climates in anticipation of decreased caloric availability.[16] Average weights and ranges are summarized in **Table 1**.

FUNCTIONAL ANATOMY, PHYSIOLOGY, AND BEHAVIOR RELATED TO FEEDING

Raccoons and coatis are considered opportunistic omnivores, but lack any special-ized adaptations to their digestive tracts and do not possess a cecum. Their dental formula is 3/3 (I), 1/1 (C), 4/4 (P), 2/2 (M) for a total of 40 teeth, with teeth generally smaller but canines sharper in coatis compared with raccoons. In both species the carnassial blades are reduced in height, reflective of a more omnivorous lifestyle as seen with members of the Ursid family.[4,5,8] The ratio of length of intestinal tract of raccoons to body length is smaller than in the cat or dog, but similar to mink.[17] Fluid and particulate matter pass through the raccoon's gastrointestinal tract at a rate greater than in the dog, or even the omnivorous pig, with a mean retention time less than 24 hours.[18] These factors are compensated, however, by an extremely efficient digestive tract that can procure approximately 85% to 90% of the energy from their diets.[19] In addition, female raccoons can significantly increase the mass of their gastrointestinal tract when lactating.[20]

Coati rely heavily on smell and tactile sensitivity of the nose to discover their inver-tebrate prey and dig holes to capture subterranean prey. They have the longest claws

Table 1
Average weight and weight ranges for adult coatis and raccoons

Species	Average Weight (kg)		Average Weight Range (kg)	
	Male	Female	Male	Female
Common raccoon (*P lotor*)	6.76	5.94	5.8–21.6	4.8–8.6
Crab-eating raccoon (*P cancrivorus*)	8.81		7.5–10.2	
White-nosed coati (*N narica*)	5.9	3.7	3.7–6.8	3.1–4.8
Brown-nosed coati (*N nasua*)	4.6	4.1	2.7–6.5	2.9–4.3

Data from Refs.[1,4,5,8,15,54,57]

and snout of the procyonids. Their forepaws are used to dig holes and shred dead logs in search of hidden animal prey, to pry open enrichment devices, and to tear open fleshy fruits or hold down larger food items. The rostral surface of their rhinarium is densely innervated by sensory receptors, their nose is highly mobile, and their facial vibrissae are better developed than other procyonids. Coatis have an enlarged sensory cortex region for receiving the afferent projections from the rhinarium and from vibrissae located just proximal to the carpal pad, and the arteries that supply the olfactory apparatus are of larger caliber compared with raccoons. When drinking, coatis curl their snouts above the water. They have color vision that evolved for feeding on brightly colored fruit. Their long, slender, non-prehensile tail is often held vertically erect while foraging and aids in balance when navigating the arboreal terrain, and they stake their food claims by eliciting snorting sounds with an erect tail.[4,5,21]

Coatis can stand bipedally for short periods of time, allowing the foraging coati to rise up on its hind feet to investigate the surface of a leaf above its head or an object or commotion at some distance. Unlike raccoons, they do not place food to the mouth with their forepaws or hold food cupped between the two paws or grasped in a single paw. They use their forepaws to bring fruit toward their mouth to grasp it. If offered food in a closed hand, coatis use their nose and claws to pry it open.[4,5,21]

A well-known coati feeding behavior is the rapid rolling of invertebrate prey on the ground using alternating movements of the forepaws, which quickly dispatches invertebrates with potentially harmful stings or bites, removes undesirable exoskeletal projections, such as spines or urticarial hairs, and depletes arthropods of their defensive secretions.[4,22,23] The behavior is also elicited by benzoquinones from millipedes and possibly other insects that make up a significant portion of the invertebrate prey; for behavioral enrichment, wood doweling and paper strips sprayed with benzoquinones and toluquinone elicit a similar response.[23] Vertebrate prey is typically pinned under the forepaws and bitten through the skull. Owing to their social nature, both intra- and interspecific grooming with ingestion of ectoparasites has been reported.[24,25] Captive coatis often show little interest in many live prey items enthusiastically eaten in the wild; however, they take common captive invertebrate foods, such as mealworms and crickets.[26]

Raccoons use their forepaws to locate and handle animal prey and other dietary items. A notable behavior is the incessant patting motions made with the forepaws even when their visual attention is directed elsewhere. The feet of the raccoon each bear five digits with no webbing between the digits, a feature unusual among carnivores. Although coatis have little fine control of digital movements, raccoons possess exquisite fine control of their forefeet.[24] They have a well-developed somatic sensorimotor area of the cerebral cortex devoted to the forepaws and tactile acuity is evidenced by the density and diversity of cutaneous nerve ending organs in their forepaw. Balancing easily on their hind feet, they can hold small items between two flattened forepaws and raise small food items to their mouths. Although the digits are capable of flexion, extension, and extreme abduction, there is little grasping ability that involves opposition of the first and fifth digits. When presented with a closed hand containing a food item, they pat the outside of the hand first and then try to wedge a forepaw into a space between the fingers.[8,24]

Raccoons are probably best known for their food-dousing behavior, sometimes dipping their food in water and grasping it and rubbing it in a way that makes them look like they are washing it. They also douse nonfood items.[27] Similar to coatis, raccoons also carry out rolling behavior, although this is often performed in water. The rolling behavior seems to enable raccoons to feed on toxic amphibians irrespective of prey size, because it is sufficient to stimulate noxious and toxic secretions and eventually reduces the amount of secretion by the prey item, thus limiting the prey's defensive capabilities. In addition, because some of their prey items have less palatable or toxic parts, raccoons often bite only the palatable parts, such as the abdomen, viscera, or limbs, off their prey to avoid the less palatable area; this behavior is influenced by experiential learning.[28-30]

NEONATAL NUTRITION AND DEVELOPMENT

After a gestation period of 70 to 77 days, coati kits nurse for 3 to 5 weeks in the nest before emerging and initiating the weaning process.[31] Captive litters range from 1 to 7 kits with 3 to 4 being most common. Coati kits weigh between 78 and 140 g at birth, reaching 214 g by 10 days, and 500 g by 40 days of age. They are born without teeth; the incisors erupt around 15 days of age, the canines by 27 days, and the milk dentition is complete around 2 months of age. By 3 months deciduous dentition of incisors, canines, and premolars are present, whereas adult canines erupt around 9 months of age.[4,5]

The lactation demands placed on female raccoons are significantly higher than on female coatis. Raccoon kits are born after a gestation period of 63 to 65 days (range 54–70 days). Litter size ranges from 2 to 5 kits. They usually nurse for 7 to 12 weeks and are completely weaned by 16 weeks.[8,32] Between 6 and 7 weeks of age they begin to emerge from the nesting area for short periods of time and start to eat solid food around 9 weeks. At birth, raccoons weigh 60 to 75 g and have average weight gains of 118 to 132 g per week up to 6 weeks of age, 23 to 27 g per week from 7 to 9 weeks of age, and 168 to 245 g per week between 10 and 16 weeks. Most have reached 1 kg by 9 weeks of age. Rapid growth continues during the first 6 months of age with a four- to sixfold increase in weight.[15] Their eyes open around 23 days of age (range, 18–30 days).[32] Their deciduous incisors and canines erupt around 1 month of age and their deciduous premolars by 1.5 months of age, with their permanent incisors and molars coming in between 2 and 2.5 months of age and adult canines by 3.5 months of age.[33]

The protein, fat, carbohydrates, and solids content for coati (N narica, N nasua) and raccoon (P lotor) milk has been studied and is summarized in **Table 2**. Chemical analysis of coati milk reveals that free lactose is approximately 30% of the total free milk oligosaccharides, which is lower than most eutherian species but still greater than bears and marsupials. Two novel pentasaccharides were discovered, suggesting that there is considerable interspecific variation in milk oligosaccharide levels even within the family Carnivora. The oligosaccharide profile for raccoons has not yet been documented.[34-36]

For both species, commercial milk replacement formulas have been used with good success. For raccoons kits, a 1:2 ratio of KMR kitten milk replacer (Pet Ag, Hampshire, IL)

Table 2
Analyses of coati (*Nasua narica, Nasua nasua*) and common raccoon (*Procyon lotor*) milk on as-fed basis

Species	Protein (%)	Fat (%)	Carbohydrate (%)	Total Solids (%)
White-nosed coati (*N narica*)	12.3	8.9	2.2	24.4
Brown-nosed coati (*N nasua*)	7.4	14.9	6.4	34.9
Raccoon	4.9–6.11	3.9–4.19	4.7	16.2

Data from Refs.[34-36]

mixed with water most closely approximates their natural milk, whereas for coatis, a combination of Zoologic milk powders (23/30 and 30/55, Pet Ag) that contain lower levels of lactose and have a higher fat content are most suitable. Both species consume approximately 3.5% to 5% of body weight per feeding and should be fed every 3 to 4 hours for the first 6 weeks. A mash composed of milk-supplement powder, high-protein baby cereal, and soaked cat or dog food is used when weaning.[37]

ADULT NUTRITION
Coati

Although animals in each genus are adapted to a terrestrial and arboreal lifestyle, the foraging is predominately done on the ground and much of their inactive time is spent in trees. In the wild, coatis spend approximately 90% of the daytime foraging for food, with 91% to 99% of that activity on the ground, depending on whether it is the wet or dry season. Resting makes up the remainder of their daily activity budget, and they sleep at night. Animal-based prey is discovered by scent.[31] Coati are omnivorous with arthropods, such as beetles, millipedes, spiders, snails, caterpillars and small crabs making up approximately 44% to 60% of their diet. They also consume a wide variety of fruit (35%–55% of diet), with more than 53 species of ingested fruit described, including palm (*Scheelea* and *Astrocaryum* sp), Almendro (*Dipteryx* sp), fig (*Ficus* sp), and century plant (*Agave palmeri*).[31,38,39] Vertebrate prey (caecilians, frogs, small lizards and snakes, small birds and rodents, reptile and bird eggs) contribute less than 10% of the diet, and often make up less than 1% of their natural diet.[6,9,13,31,38,40]

Most captive diets for coati are centrally based around dog and cat food supplemented with fruits and vegetables, and prey items, such as insects, mice, and day-old chicks. Omnivore chow and New World primate chow are sometimes used, with commercial exotic feline or carnivore diets, such as the horse meat–based Nebraska (North Platte, NE) or Toronto Zoo carnivore diets (Milliken Meats, Scarborough, Ontario, Canada) less frequently making up portions of the diet. Energy requirements for coatis can be determined with the formula: basal metabolic rate (BMR) (kcal) = 0.49 (body weight in grams)$^{0.738}$. Depending on activity level, this may be increased by a factor of 1.2 to 1.5. For female coatis, the greatest energy demands on resources are associated with reproduction, because the litter weighs 20% to 30% of the female's postpartum weight and over 3 to 5 weeks of nursing the litter increases to 45% to 60% of her weight. At this time foraging decreases to less than 2 hours a day, so energy requirements increase by a factor of 2 to 2.5.[31,41–43]

Obesity is a common problem in captive coatis due to relative inactivity and higher caloric intake compared with their wild counterparts. Stereotypies, such as tail chewing, have been observed in coatis that do not have suitable foraging and mental and physical stimulation opportunities in captivity. As with other carnivore species, metabolic bone disease is a potential nutritional pathology in coatis associated with imbalanced diets (low calcium, improper calcium-to-phosphorus ratio, inadequate dietary vitamin D, hypervitaminosis A).[44] Iron storage disease is a recently recognized captive nutritional disease, with 10 cases of moderate to marked hepatic iron deposition noted in a retrospective pathology study of 13 coatis. The authors attributed the iron deposition to captive diets, usually dog- and cat-food based, which contain more heme iron compared with the wild diet.[45] Based on these findings, diets that contain less iron, such as commercial insectivore and primate diets, may be more suitable.

21. McClearn D. Locomotion, posture and feeding behaviour of kinkajous, coatis and raccoons. J Mammal 1992;73(2):245–61.
22. Ingles LG. Observation on behaviour of the coatimundi. J Mammal 1957;38(2): 263–4.
23. Weldon PJ, Cranmore CF, Chatfield JA. Prey-rolling behaviour of coatis (*Nasua* spp.) is elicited by benzoquinones from millipedes. Naturwissenschaften 2006; 93(1):14–6.
24. McClearn D. The rise and fall of mutualism? Coatis, tapirs and ticks on Barro Colorado Island, Panama. Biotropica 1992;24(2):220–2.
25. Overall KL. Coatis, tapirs and ticks: a case of mammalian interspecific grooming. Biotropica 1980;12(2):158.
26. Smith HJ. Behavior of the coati (*Nasua narica*) in captivity. Carnivore 1980;2: 88–136.
27. Lyall-Watson M. A critical re-examination of food "washing" behaviour in the raccoon (*Procyon Lotor* Linn). Proc Zoolog Soc London 1963;141:371–93.
28. Mochida K, Matsui K. Counter-defense techniques to mitigate prey toxicity in raccoons (*Procyon lotor*). Mammal Study 2007;32:135–8.
29. Schaaf RT, Garton JS. Raccoon predation on the American toad, *Bufo americanus*. Herpetologica 1970;26:334–5.
30. Wright JW. Predation on the Colorado River toad, *Bufo alvarius*. Herpetologica 1966;22:127–8.
31. Russell JK. Timing of reproduction by coatis (*Nasua narica*) in relation to fluctuations in food resources. In: Leight EG, Rand AS, Windsor DM, editors. The ecology of a tropical forest. Washington, DC: Smithsonian Institution Press; 1982. p. 413–31.
32. Montgomery GG. Weaning of captive raccoons. J Wildl Manage 1969;33(1): 154–9.
33. Montgomery GG. Tooth eruption in preweaned raccoons. J Wildl Manage 1964; 28(3):582–4.
34. Ben Shaul DM. The composition of the milk of wild animals. Int Zoo Yearbk 1962; 4:333–42.
35. Oftedal OT. Milk composition, milk yield and energy output at peak lactation: a comparative review. Symp Zool Soc Lond 1984;51:33–85.
36. Urashima T, Yamamoto M, Nakamura T, et al. Chemical characterisation of the oligosaccharides in a sample of milk of a white-nosed coati, *Nasua narica* (Procyonidae: Carnivora). Comp Biochem Physiol A Mol Integr Physiol 1999;123(2):187–93.
37. DeGhetto D, Papageorgiou S, Convy J. Raccoons. In: Gage LJ, editor. Hand-rearing wild and domestic mammals. Ames (IA): Iowa State Press; 2002. p. 191–206.
38. Alves-Costa CP, Eterovick PC. Seed dispersal services by coatis (*Nasua nasua*, Procyonidae) and their redundancy with other frugivores in southeastern Brazil. Acta Oecol 2007;32(1):77–92.
39. McColgin ME, Brown EJ, Bickford SM, et al. Use of century plants (*Agave palmeri*) by coatis (*Nasua narica*). Southwest Nat 2003;48(4):722–5.
40. Jonsen WL, Nijboer J. Animal mass and metabolic rates. In: Zoo animal nutrition—Tables and guidelines. 1st edition. Amsterdam (Holland): European Zoo Nutrition Centre; 2003. p. 26–37.
41. Nagy KA. Field metabolic rate and food requirement scaling in mammals and birds. Ecol Monogr 1987;57(2):112–28.
42. White CR, Seymour RS. Allometric scaling of mammalian metabolism. J Exp Biol 2005;208:1611–9.

43. Ullrey DE. Metabolic bone disease. In: Fowler ME, Miller RE, editors. Zoo and wildlife medicine. 5th edition. St. Louis (MO): Elsevier Science; 2003. p. 749–56.
44. Clauss M, Hänichen T, Hummel J, et al. Excessive iron storage in captive omnivores? The case of the coati (*Nasua* spp.). In: Fidgett A, Clauss M, Eulenberger K, et al, editors. Zoo animal nutrition. vol 3. Fürth: Filander Verlag; 2006. p. 91–9.
45. McFadden KW, Sambrotto RN, Medellín RA, et al. Feeding habits of endangered pygmy raccoons (*Procyon pygmaeus*) based on stable isotope and fecal analyses. J Mammal 2006;87(3):501–9.
46. Baker RH, Newman CC, Wilke F. Food habits of the raccoon in eastern Texas. J Wildl Manage 1945;9(1):45–8.
47. Barton BT, Roth JD. Raccoon removal on sea turtle nesting beaches. J Wildl Manage 2007;71(4):1234–7.
48. Carrillo E, Wong G, Rodríguez MA. Feeding habits of raccoon (*Procyon lotor*) (Carnivora: Procyonidae) in a coastal tropical wet forest of Costa Rica. Rev Biol Trop 2001;49(3–4):1193–7.
49. Dorney RS. Ecology of marsh raccoons. J Wildl Manage 1954;18(2):217–25.
50. Greenwood RJ. Nocturnal activity and foraging of Prairie raccoons (*Procyon lotor*) in North Dakota. Am Midl Nat 1982;107(2):238–43.
51. Schoonover LJ, Marshall WH. Food habits of the raccoon (Procyon lotor hirtus) in north-central Minnesota. J Mammal 1951;32(4):422–8.
52. Tester JR. Fall food habits of the raccoon in the south Platte Valley of northeastern Colorado. J Mammal 1953;34(4):498–518.
53. Dos Santos M, De Fatima M, Hartz SM. The food habits of *Procyon cancrivorus* (Carnivora, Procyonidae) in the Lami Biological Reserve, Porto Algre, Southern Brazil. Mammalia 1999;63(4):525–30.
54. Mugaas JN, Seidensticker J, Mahlke-Johnson K. Metabolic adaptation to climate and distribution of the raccoon *Procyon lotor* and other procyonidae. Smithson Contrib Zool 1993;542:1–38.
55. Hamir AN, Kunkle RA, Miller JM, et al. Age related lesions in laboratory-confined raccoons (*Procyon lotor*) inoculated with the agent of chronic wasting disease of mule deer. J Vet Diagn Invest 2007;19:680–6.
56. Hull RL, Westermark GT, Westermark P, et al. Islet amyloid: a critical entity in the pathogenesis of type 2 diabetes. J Clin Endocrinol Metab 2004;89(8):629–43.
57. Redford KH, Eisenberg JF. Order Carnivora (Fissipedia). In: Redford KH, Eisenberg JF, editors. Mammals of the neotropics: the southern cone, vol. 2. Chicago: University of Chicago Press; 1992. p. 144–78.

Macropod Nutrition

Joseph A. Smith, DVM

KEYWORDS

• Macropod • Kangaroo • Wallaby • Joey • Nutrition

Macropods are marsupials belonging to the family Macropodidae and are commonly referred to as kangaroos and wallabies. Macropods are frequently kept in zoologic parks and are becoming increasingly more popular as pets and in hobby exhibits. The most common species maintained in captivity in North America are the red kangaroo (*Macropus rufus*), the Eastern gray kangaroo (*M. giganteus*), the Western gray kangaroo (*M. fuliginosus*), the red-necked/Bennett's wallaby (*M. rufogriseus*), the Tammar wallaby (*M. eugenii*), and the common wallaroo (*M. robustus*). Other species, such as the Parma wallaby (*M. parma*), yellow-footed rock wallaby (*Petrogale xanthopus*), and tree-kangaroos (*Dendrolagus* spp), are also kept in zoos but are nearly absent in private collections.

Macropods are all herbivorous, but they have evolved to adapt to a wide variety of habitats and associated vegetation. Macropods can be loosely grouped into three main classifications based on dietary preference: (1) primary browsers, (2) primary grazers, and (3) an intermediate browser/grazer grade.[1] In reality, dietary preference is more of a spectrum ranging from exclusive browsers to exclusive grazers. In general, the larger species tend to be primarily grazers, whereas the smaller species are primarily browsers. A summary of the dietary classification of various macropods is provided in **Table 1**.[2]

All macropods are foregut fermenters, with most digestion occurring in the stomach by microbial flora. This method of digestion is less dependent on the quality of dietary nitrogen and has the added advantage of being able to degrade plant cell walls to produce energy and provide access to the plant cellular contents. In general, this method allows macropods to use poorer quality forages when compared with other herbivores with different digestive strategies. Macropod nutrition is fairly well studied, and an excellent comprehensive review has been published.[3,4]

ANATOMY AND PHYSIOLOGY
Dentition

Macropods belong to the order Diprotodontia, members of which are characterized by the presence of two large procumbent (horizontally arranged) mandibular incisors. The maxillary incisors are much smaller and are found in three pairs. Macropods use their incisors for prehension of food. Mandibular canines are absent, and maxillary canines

Fort Wayne Children's Zoo, 3411 Sherman Boulevard, Fort Wayne, IN 46808, USA
E-mail address: vet@kidszoo.org

Vet Clin Exot Anim 12 (2009) 197–208
doi:10.1016/j.cvex.2009.01.010
1094-9194/09/$ – see front matter © 2009 Elsevier Inc. All rights reserved.

vetexotic.theclinics.com

Table 1
Dietary characteristics of macropod species mentioned in the text

Common Name	Scientific Name	Average Adult Weight (kg)	Diet Classification	Wild Diet
Tree-kangaroo	*Dendrolagus* spp	3.7–15.0	Browser	Leaves, fruit, flowers, grass
Dorcopsis	*Dorcopsis* spp and *Dorcopsulus* spp	1.5–11.5	Browser	Leaves, flowers, fruit
Hare-wallaby	*Lagorchestes* spp	0.8–4.6	Intermediate	Forbs, green grass, seed heads, fruit
Tammar wallaby	*Macropus eugenii*	4–10	Intermediate	Short grass, forbs
Parma wallaby	*Macropus parma*	3.2–5.9	Intermediate	Short grass, forbs
Bennett's wallaby	*Macropus rufogriseus*	11–27	Intermediate	Short grass, forbs, bushes
Common wallaroo	*Macropus robustus*	15–21	Grazer	Grass, forbs
Red kangaroo	*Macropus rufus*	26–85	Grazer	Grass, forbs
Western gray kangaroo	*Macropus fuliginosus*	22–54	Grazer	Grass, sedges, shrubs, forbs
Eastern gray kangaroo	*Macropus giganteus*	26–66	Grazer	Grass
Nailtail wallaby	*Onychogalea* spp	4–9	Grazer	Forbs, green grass, fallen leaves
Rock-wallaby	*Petrogale* spp	0.9–7.5	Browser	Forbs, young grass, leaves, woody shrubs, ferns
Quokka	*Setonix brachyurus*	2.5–5.0	Browser	Forbs, shrubs, sedges, grass
Pademelon	*Thylogale* spp	1.8–12.0	Browser	Ferns, fallen leaves, short grass, fruit
Swamp wallaby	*Wallabia bicolor*	10–20	Browser	Sedges, forbs, shrubs, grass, ferns, fungi, seeds

Data from Sanson GD. Morphological adaptations of teeth to diets and feeding in the Macropodoidea. In: Grigg G, Jarman P, Hume I, editors. Kangaroos, wallabies, and rat-kangaroos. Sydney: Surrey Beatty; 1989. p. 151–68; Dawson TJ. Diets of macropodoid marsupials: general patterns and environmental influences. In: Grigg G, Jarman P, Hume I, editors. Kangaroos, wallabies, and rat-kangaroos. Sydney: Surrey Beatty; 1989. p. 129–42.

are rare, which results in a relatively long diastema. In adults, a single premolar and four molars are found in each arcade, all of which are used for mastication. Molar progression, a specialized adaptation of some macropods whereby older molars migrate rostrally, and molar eruption can be used along with species-specific data charts to estimate the age of macropods.[5] The three different grades of macropods based on dietary preference (ie, grazers, browsers, and intermediates) exhibit dental adaptations that are specific to their preferred food source.

In macropods that are primarily browsers, the first maxillary incisors are larger than the others and occlude the mandibular incisors over a relatively small area to allow for precise prehension of specific plant species or plant parts. The premolars are permanent and larger than those of grazers, and they act as an anchor to prevent the molar progression seen in grazers. The dental arcade is relatively flat, allowing all molars (which remain permanent) to reach occlusion at the same time resulting in a crushing action.

Species in the intermediate browser/grazer grade still have large first maxillary incisors, but the third maxillary incisors are slightly wider to allow for more surface area during occlusion to allow cropping of larger quantities of vegetation. The premolar is smaller and therefore less effective at preventing molar progression, which occurs in most species in this grade. Molars possess crushing and shearing abilities, which makes them adaptable but less efficient at either task.

The Nabarlek (*Petrogale concinna*) is a member of the intermediate grade with adaptations more like the grazers. This is because the *Marsilea* spp ferns, which comprise a large part of its diet, are high in silicates and cause excessive dental wear. Adaptations include a markedly reduced premolar, a highly curved dental arcade, and well-developed molar progression. The Nabarlek is the only marsupial with an unlimited number of molars, with new molars produced as older ones are shed when worn.[1] The banded hare-wallaby (*Lagostrophus fasciatus*) is also an aberrant member of the intermediate grade. It has a small premolar with resultant molar progression, but its dental arcade is flat. Instead of older molars being shed, they are retained, which results in a progressively shortening diastema.[1]

Macropods that are primarily grazers have adaptations, including harder enamel, that are targeted at preventing dental wear caused by the higher levels of silicates in the grasses they eat.[6] The first maxillary incisors are relatively small, whereas the third maxillary incisors are wide, which increases the occlusive contact with the mandibular incisors and allows for cropping of larger quantities of forage. The premolar is vestigial and allows for molar progression. The dental arcade is highly curved, resulting in an average of only two molars in occlusion at any given time. As molars are worn, molar progression allows newer, more caudal molars to enter into occlusion while worn ones move rostrally and are eventually shed. Morphology of individual molars of grazers allows for reduced surface contact between teeth, which results in efficient shearing forces during mastication, as opposed to the crushing forces of browsers, which result in more wear.

Salivary Glands

Macropods possess three main groups of salivary glands. The parotid glands are the largest, followed by the mandibular glands, with the sublingual glands being the smallest.[7] The composition of saliva from each group of glands is different. Parotid saliva is high in sodium, calcium, phosphate, and bicarbonate. Phosphate and bicarbonate are important in buffering the short-chain fatty acids produced in the forestomach by fermentation.[8,9] Phosphates from saliva also serve as a source of phosphorus for bacteria in the forestomach. In contrast, mandibular gland saliva is low in phosphate and bicarbonate, making it less useful as a buffer. Instead, it is composed of a hypotonic solution of sodium chloride and potassium chloride, which results in less electrolyte loss when this saliva is spread onto the forearms in a unique adaptation that allows for evaporative cooling during times of hyperthermia or stress.[10]

Esophagus

The esophagus is lined by stratified epithelium with no glands. Except in tree-kanga-roos, the macropod esophagus has a well-keratinized epithelial layer. The morphology of the macropod esophagus has been classified into four main types.[11] Type I has a smooth lining and is found in the browsing and intermediate grade groups: rock-wallabies (*Petrogale* spp), tree-kangaroos, pademelons (*Thylogale* spp), nailtail wallabies (*Onychogalea* spp), hare-wallabies (*Lagorchestes* spp), dorcopsis (*Dorcopsis* spp and *Dorcopsulus* spp), and the Quokka (*Setonix brachyurus*). The Type II esophagus has a smooth lining with large irregular longitudinal folds. This type is found in the large grazing species within the genus *Macropus*. The Type III esophagus is lined with finger-like papillae and is found in smaller wallabies within the genus *Macropus* and in swamp wallabies (*Wallabia bicolor*). The Type IV esophagus has longitu-dinal folds cranial to the diaphragm and papillae caudal to the diaphragm and is found in Bennett's wallabies. Esophageal nematode species with specialized confor-mations adapted to keep them anchored near the esophageal lining have been described.[12] Esophageal bacterial flora also have adaptations such as extracellular coats and capsules for attaching to the surface epithelium, on which they only colonize the superficial layers.[13]

Stomach

The stomach of macropods can be divided into two main regions: the forestomach and the hindstomach. The forestomach is an expansion of the cardiac region of the stomach and is the primary site of fermentation. The forestomach can be divided into sacciform and tubiform regions, which are separated by a ventral fold (**Fig. 1**). In general, the smaller species have relatively larger sacciform regions compared with larger macropods. Exceptions include the hare-wallabies, which have a more tu-biform forestomach. Histologically, the forestomach contains regions of squamous epithelium and cardiac glandular mucosa. The amount and location of each tissue type varies widely with species. The cardiac mucosa has mucin-secreting glands and little enzymatic activity. Three taenia are present in the forestomach, resulting in numerous haustrations, the pattern of which varies with species.

The hindstomach is the site of digestive enzyme production. The gastric glandular region appears rugose and reddish in color. Histologically it is a typical gastric epithe-lium. Pyloric glands similar to the mucin-secreting glands in the cardiac glandular mucosa are also present. A gastric sulcus that connects the esophagus and the hind-stomach exists in some species, but the morphology can vary. In pouch young, proteolytic activity exists throughout the stomach, so the presence of a sulcus is prob-ably of little benefit in this age group.[14] The sulcus may be an adaptation that benefits joeys-at-foot (ie, those that are out of the pouch and beginning to eat solid foods but still nursing periodically). The sulcus also may aid digestion in adult macropods by moving more liquid products of fermentation caudally toward the hindstomach.[15]

Two types of contractions have been described in macropod stomachs.[15] The first type is localized contractions that function to aid mixing of digesta. The second type is a sequential wave of contractions that propulses digesta caudally. Unlike the rumen, which acts like a large fermentation vat in which ingesta is mixed throughout, the for-estomach of macropods mixes ingesta within localized pockets with an overall tubular flow of ingesta caudally.

The fauna and flora of the macropod forestomach is diverse. In wild macropods, the biomass of helminths has been described as larger than that of microbes.[3] Helminth fauna consists of anoplocephalid cestodes, strongyloids, trichostrongyloids,

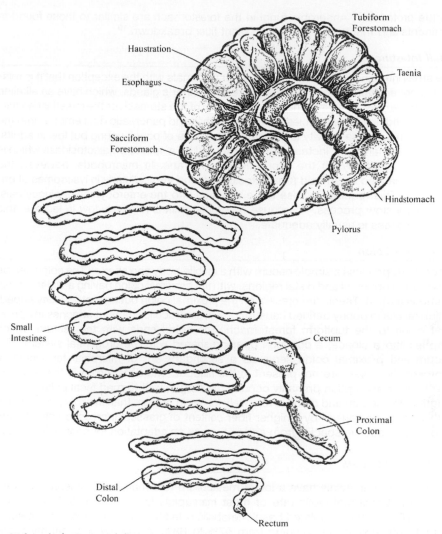

Tubiform
Forestomach

Haustration

Taenia

Esophagus

Sacciform
Forestomach

Hindstomach

Pylorus

Small
Intestines

Cecum

Proximal
Colon

Distal
Colon

Rectum

Fig.1. A typical macropod digestive tract using the Eastern gray kangaroo (*Macropus gigan-teus*) as a model. (*Drawing by* V.L. Piebenga.)

metastrongyloids, oxyurids, and filaroid nematodes.[16] Of the strongyloids alone, 40 genera and 171 species have been described, with many more still undescribed. The pathogenicity of specific helminth species has not been well researched. The bacterial flora of the macropod forestomach is morphologically similar to that of sheep, with similar bacterial densities. The flora is predominantly gram negative, but gram-positive rods become more dominant in regions with lower pH.[17] The bacterial flora should be considered when selecting route of administration and class of antimicrobials and other drugs. General rules used for ruminants can serve as guidelines for prudent drug use until more pharmacokinetic research is done in macropods. Forestomach ciliates are mostly holotrichs with a few spirotrichs. The morphology of the forestomach protozoa is distinct from those of domestic species. A new family of entodiniomorph protozoa (Macropodiniidae) has been proposed to describe these unique protozoa.[18] Anaerobic fungi in the forestomach are similar to those found in ruminants and function to assist with plant fiber breakdown.[19]

Small Intestine

The small intestine is typical of that of other mammals with the exception that it is relatively shorter than that of other herbivores.[3] Brunner's glands, which have an alkaline secretion, empty either into the pyloric mucosa of the stomach or the intestinal epithelium, depending on the species.[20] A common bile and pancreatic duct empties into the duodenum. Lactase activity is high in the intestines of pouch young but low in adults. In eutherian mammals, lactase activity is caused by a neutral β-galactosidase which is found extracellularly on the microvillous membrane. In macropods, however, the activity is caused by an acid β-galactosidase found intracellularly in lysosomes of enterocytes. This requires lactose to be taken up into the enterocytes via pinocytosis, a relatively slow process.[21] Because macropod milk is relatively low in lactose, this slower process is usually adequate.

Cecum and Colon

Macropods possess a simple cecum with a mobile body and apex.[22] The colon can be divided into proximal and distal regions, with the proximal colon having a wider luminal diameter (**Fig. 1**). Taenia are present on the proximal colon but are not well developed, which results in poorly defined haustrations. A gastrocolic ligament attaches the proximal colon to the tubiform forestomach. The colon ends with the rectum, which empties into a cloaca, a common opening shared with the urogenital system. The cecum and proximal colon serve as a secondary site of microbial fermentation. Protozoa, however, are not present in the hindgut. The distal colon is the region in which water absorption primarily occurs, resulting in well-formed fecal pellets.[23] The length of the cecum and colon is relatively longer in grazers than in browsers,[24] which is thought to be caused by a higher fiber content of grasses. Increased colon length also may be seen in species from arid regions as an adaptation for conserving water.

ENERGY METABOLISM

On average, marsupials have a lower metabolism rate than their eutherian counterparts. The basal metabolic rate of most marsupials falls between 65% and 74% (mean, 70%) of the calculated basal metabolic rate for a eutherian mammal of equal weight, with macropods ranging from 57% to 88%.[25] This lower basal metabolic rate results in lower average body temperatures and an overall decreased caloric requirement when compared with eutherians. The maintenance energy requirement for marsupials is usually 150% to 250% of the basal metabolic rate, with larger marsupials having a maintenance energy requirement in the lower end of the range.[25]

The primary source of energy for macropods is short-chain fatty acids produced by microbes through fermentation. Most short-chain fatty acids are produced and absorbed in the forestomach, with production and absorption highest in the sacciform region.[17] The cecum and proximal colon also serve as a secondary site of microbial fermentation. Short-chain fatty acids can lower the forestomach pH from approximately 8.0 in a fasting animal to approximately 5.0 in a recently fed animal. The types and proportions of short-chain fatty acids are similar to those produced in the rumen of domestic species. Like in ruminants, large proportions of acetic acid are converted to butyric acid, the principle short-chain fatty acids used by the forestomach epithelium for energy. Byproducts of this reaction are ketone bodies, especially acetoacetate, which can be further oxidized by other tissues. Unlike ruminants, however, in which this ketogenic activity occurs throughout the squamous epithelial lining of the rumen, ketogenic activity in macropods is restricted to the cardiac glandular mucosa.[26]

Microbial fermentation also results in production of ammonia, which serves as the primary nitrogen source for microbial protein synthesis. The ability of microbes to break down proteins, other microbes, and nonprotein nitrogen sources into ammonia allows macropods to use different nitrogen sources of varying quality. During periods of nitrogen shortage when ingesting a low-protein diet, macropods are able to recycle endogenously produced urea into the gut to be used as a nitrogen source instead of excreting it in the urine.[27] Gases produced by forestomach fermentation are primarily carbon dioxide and hydrogen. Methane is also produced, especially during active eating, but at lower levels compared with ruminants.[3]

Soluble sugars are rapidly digested and absorbed in the sacciform forestomach. This process results in little disaccharidase activity in the small intestines, because few digestible carbohydrates ever reach this location before they are broken down by microbes and absorbed. Similar to sheep, there is minimal glucose uptake into the liver. Instead, the liver continuously produces and releases glucose into the blood through gluconeogenesis, which occurs postprandially and during fasting. Macropods exhibit considerable tolerance to hypoglycemia induced by intravenous injections of insulin[28,29]; however, they are much less tolerant of hyperglycemia.[29]

The tubular flow of ingesta through the macropod forestomach results in a shorter retention time. One disadvantage to this system is that digestibility of the ingesta is lower compared with ruminants of similar size. An advantage of this system is that dietary fiber continues to move through the forestomach regardless of fiber length and size. In ruminants, the rumen retains fiber particles until they are degraded to a certain size, which prolongs digestion and results in greater rumen fill and decreased dietary intake. High-fiber diets can limit food intake in ruminants. On the other hand, dietary intake in macropods depends less on fiber content. Smaller macropods (with larger sacciform forestomachs) are more affected by dietary fiber than the larger grazing macropods.

BEHAVIOR

Most macropods are either nocturnal or crepuscular and rest during the hottest part of the day. In captivity, however, they also may be active during the day, especially during periods of mild weather. The smaller species tend to be more solitary, whereas the larger, grazing species are more gregarious and form groups called mobs. The formation of groups while feeding is an adaptation to better protect the macropods from predators. These feeding groups may even be formed from different species.[30] In captivity, many macropod species are kept in small groups, including mixed species mobs. Keeping a gregarious species in isolation may result in anxiety and stress.

Macropods prehend food with their incisors. The forelimbs also may be used for manipulation of food items. Macropods differ from ruminants in the way they process food items during mastication. Although ruminants loosely chew their food before swallowing, macropods chew their food thoroughly upon ingestion. Ruminants later regurgitate the coarse ingesta in coordination with rumen contractions for remastication and reswallowing (rumination). Macropods do occasionally regurgitate, remasticate, and reswallow food, a processed called merycism. This process is not true rumination because it is not integrated with forestomach contractions. Merycism is not performed as frequently as rumination is in ruminants because the process is not necessary for further breakdown of ingesta. The act of merycism has been described differently for different species, but it can involve a rather violent heaving action that may be confused with hiccups or choke. The frequency of merycism may depend on diet, with high-starch diets increasing the frequency.[15] Starches are easily fermentable and rapidly reduce the pH of the forestomach. It is believed that merycism is an adaptation that helps to stimulate saliva production, which in turn buffers the ingesta in the forestomach and raises the pH. A second behavior that consists of rhythmic jaw movements several hours after feeding is also thought to be a method of stimulating saliva production in response to a low forestomach pH.[17] This behavior does not involve regurgitation or mastication.

Some macropods have developed adaptations that allow them to survive extreme conditions. Tammar wallabies on the Abrolhos Islands have evolved physiologic adaptations that allow them to drink seawater during summers when fresh water is scarce. In contrast, Eastern gray kangaroos are adapted to low-sodium environments. The common wallaroo has physiologic adaptations that allow it to survive arid regions where forages are low in protein and high in fiber. The red kangaroo's solution to surviving the same arid regions is to be more mobile and travel great distances to graze where forage quality is highest. The installation of wells and dams for livestock (primarily sheep) by European settlers in Australia has allowed some macropods to survive in areas where populations were previously limited by drought. Similar to camels and burros, macropods have the ability to conserve their plasma volume when subjected to moderate to severe dehydration.[31] The forest-dwelling species, such as Parma wallabies and pademelons, have higher protein and energy requirements and are less able to adapt to extreme conditions.

CAPTIVE DIET

In captivity, macropods should be given a diet that best approximates the forage consumed by wild members of a given species. Access to high-quality grass pasture is recommended, especially for grazing species. Nontoxic browse items also can be offered to provide variety and mimic natural behaviors. For many species, providing fresh limbs with leaves and bark allows macropods to consume the leaves and strip the bark, which also provides behavioral enrichment.

Basic captive diets mimic those fed to ungulates. Items are given in lower quantities on a per weight basis, however, because of lower metabolism rates of macropods. If overfed, some species (especially smaller ones) are predisposed to obesity. Good quality grass hay is recommended ad libitum for all species, especially if not kept on a grass pasture. Quality is important because coarse, sharp, or abrasive food items (eg, oat awns, stalky hay, hay contaminated with thorny plants) can cause oral trauma and provide an avenue for secondary bacterial infections that lead to soft tissue infections, dental lesions, and osteomyelitis (commonly but controversially referred to as "lumpy jaw"). Food items should not be too soft either (eg, bread), because soft foods do not adequately toughen the oral mucosa or wear the teeth to allow molar progression. Macropods are susceptible to toxoplasmosis from ingesting food items contaminated with infected cat feces. Contamination of hay from barn cats at the hay storage location has been implicated as the source of toxoplasmosis outbreaks in several zoologic collections. It is recommended that food items be fed elevated from the ground (eg, in a hay rack, elevated bowl, or trough feeder) to prevent contamination with feces and reduce the transmission of parasites. Food containers should be cleaned daily and regularly disinfected. To reduce food competition and aggression, multiple feeding areas are recommended when macropods are kept in a group.

Pelleted rations are also recommended in moderation. Several commercially available pellets formulated specifically for macropods are available. Vegetables can be offered in small amounts, and fruits can be used only as an occasional treat. These produce items must be restricted to a small proportion of the diet, however, because they contain higher levels of simple sugars and carbohydrates and are easily fermentable, possibly leading to gastrointestinal and dental problems. Sweet feed mixes should not be used for the same reasons. The smaller, forest-dwelling species that are primarily browsers are more tolerant of larger amounts of produce in their diet than the grazing species. Items such as bread, peanut butter, jam, and other sweet treats may be helpful in getting a macropod to take medications, but they should not be a regular part of the diet. Salt blocks are recommended for the species commonly kept in captivity as a source of electrolytes and minerals. Fresh, clean water should be offered daily to all macropods. Although some species are drought-tolerant, captive diets usually contain less moisture than wild forages, which increases the captive animal's need for water intake.

Vitamin E is an antioxidant required by macropods to prevent myopathy, or white muscle disease. Hind limb weakness that progressed to paralysis, muscle wasting, and death was described in captive Quokkas fed a commercial sheep pellet.[32] Smaller enclosure sizes were found to increase the requirement of vitamin E because of the additional stress of overcrowding. Myopathy was prevented with vitamin E supplementation regardless of enclosure size, however.[33] In most species of animals, selenium can be used as an antioxidant substitute in the place of vitamin E to prevent myopathy, but selenium supplementation alone was found to be ineffective in preventing myopathy in Quokkas and Tammar wallabies.[4,34] Vitamin E supplementation is recommended for all macropods. The amount of supplementation required will vary based on the vitamin E content of the diet ingredients. Feeding large amounts of varied natural browse may reduce the need for vitamin E supplementation.

NUTRITION OF JOEYS

Macropods have a short gestation period, with most growth and development occurring postpartum while the joey is in the pouch attached to the mammary gland. Initially, the joey is permanently attached to the teat, but later it develops the ability to detach and reattach at will. Unlike that of eutherians, marsupial milk composition changes dramatically over the course of lactation to accommodate changing nutritional requirements of the developing joey. Early in lactation, the milk is low in total solids, lipids, and proteins and the carbohydrate fraction is relatively higher and composed of oligosaccharides.[35] Later in lactation, the milk composition increases in lipids and proteins, and the oligosaccharides are replaced by low levels of monosaccharides.[35] Macropods possess four teats, although only one develops for each joey. As a survival strategy, some macropods have the capability of having three joeys at one time, each in a different stage of development. One joey can be out of the pouch but still nursing (joey-at-foot) while another is developing in the pouch (pouch joey) and a third is waiting in utero as a result of embryonic diapause. This occurrence can result in teats in four different stages of lactation: one undergoing regression from a previous joey, one for the joey-at-foot, one for the pouch joey, and one undeveloped teat for the joey yet to be born. The two teats that are actively lactating simultaneously produce milk of different compositions that are appropriate for each joey's stage of development.

The need for hand-rearing can occur as a result of health issues or death of the dam or if the dam throws the joey from the pouch as a result of stress. Artificial rearing of macropod joeys can be challenging, with joeys in early stages of pouch development having a low success rate. As a joey ages, however, the success rate dramatically increases. Because milk composition changes over time, so too must that of the artificial milk replacers. A commercial product (Wombaroo, Perfect Pets Inc., Belleville, MI) has been developed specifically for macropods. The feeding amounts, frequency, and type of formula should be fed according to the product's species-specific recommendations for the age of the joey. Body measurements, and not weight, should be used along with species-specific growth charts to determine the joey's age. The weight of the joey can be decreased by dehydration and a history of suboptimal nutrition, which might result in an underestimate of age when this variable is used alone. Artificial milk replacers designed for other species and whole milk from other species should not be used, because they often contain higher levels of oligosaccharides (eg, lactose, sucrose). Because of the previously described slower mechanism for digestion of these oligosaccharides in macropods, their use can result in severe problems, such as osmotic diarrhea, gastrointestinal bacterial overgrowth, and cataracts. More detailed information on hand-rearing macropods is available.[36]

SUMMARY

Although often compared with ruminants, macropods exhibit many unique differences in the way they acquire, process, and digest food. These differences and an overall lower metabolic rate affect the way macropods should be fed in captivity. Differing diets in the wild have resulted in different anatomic variations that also must be considered. The unique developmental process of marsupials has significant effects on the nutrition of growing joeys, which must be taken into account during artificial hand-rearing.

REFERENCES

1. Sanson GD. Morphological adaptations of teeth to diets and feeding in the Macropodoidea. In: Grigg G, Jarman P, Hume I, editors. Kangaroos, wallabies, and rat-kangaroos. Sydney: Surrey Beatty; 1989. p. 151–68.
2. Dawson TJ. Diets of macropodoid marsupials: general patterns and environmental influences. In: Grigg G, Jarman P, Hume I, editors. Kangaroos, wallabies, and rat-kangaroos. Sydney: Bearry; 1989. p. 129–42.
3. Hume ID. Foregut fermenters: kangaroos and wallabies. In: Marsupial nutrition. New York: Cambridge University Press; 1999. p. 205–60.
4. Hume ID. Nutritional ecology of kangaroos and wallabies. In: Marsupial nutrition. New York: Cambridge University Press; 1999. p. 261–314.
5. Jackson SM. Macropods. In: Jackson SM, editor. Australian mammals: biology and captive management. Collingwood (Australia): CSIRO Publishing; 2003. p. 245–96.
6. Palamara J, Phakey PP, Rachinger WA, et al. On the nature of the opaque and translucent enamel regions of some Macropodinae (Macropus giganteus, Wallabia bicolor and Peradorcus concinna). Cell Tissue Res 1984;238:329–37.
7. Forbes DK, Tribe DE. Salivary glands of kangaroos. Aust J Zool 1969;17:765–75.
8. Beal AM. Electrolyte composition of parotid saliva from sodium-replete red kangaroos (Macropus rufus). J Exp Biol 1984;111:225–37.
9. Beal AM. Differences in salivary flow and composition among kangaroo species: implications for digestive efficiency. In: Grigg G, Jarman P, Hume I, editors. Kangaroos, wallabies, and rat-kangaroos. Sydney: Surrey Beatty; 1989. p. 189–95.
10. Beal AM. Effects of flow rate, duration of stimulation and mineralocorticoids on the electrolyte concentrations of mandibular saliva from the red kangaroo (Macropus rufus). J Exp Biol 1986;126:315 30.

11. Obendorf DL. The macropodid oesophagus: I. Gross anatomical, light microscopic, scanning and transmission electron microscopic observations of its mucosa. Aust J Zool 1984;32:415–35.

12. Obendorf DL. The macropodid oesophagus: III. Observations on the nematode parasites. Aust J Zool 1984;32:437–45.

13. Obendorf DL. The macropodid oesophagus: II. Morphological studies of its adherent bacteria using light and electron microscopy. Aust J Zool 1984;37: 99–116.

14. Griffiths M, Barton AA. The ontogeny of the stomach in the pouch young of the red kangaroo. CSIRO Wildlife Research 1966;11:169–85.

15. Dellow DW. Physiology of digestion in the macropodine marsupials [doctoral Thesis]. Armidale: University of New England; 1979.

16. Beveridge I, Spratt DM. The helminth fauna of Australasian marsupials: origins and evolutionary biology. Adv Parasitol 1996;37:135–254.

17. Moir RJ, Somers M, Waring H. Studies on marsupial nutrition: I. Ruminant-like digestion in a herbivorous marsupial Setonix brachyurus (Quoy and Gaimard). Aust J Biol Sci 1956;9:293–304.

18. Dehority BA. A new family of entodiniomorph protozoa from the marsupial forestomach, with descriptions of a new genus and five new species. J Eukaryot Microbiol 1996;43:285–95.

19. Dellow DW, Hume ID, Clarke RTJ, et al. Microbial activity in the forestomach of free-living macropodid marsupials: comparisons with laboratory studies. Aust J Zool 1988;36:383–95.

20. Krause WJ. The distribution of Brunner's glands in 55 marsupial species native to the Australian region. Acta Anat 1972;82:17–33.

21. Messer M, Crisp EA, Czolij R. Lactose digestion in suckling macropodids. In: Grigg G, Jarman P, Hume I, editors. Kangaroos, wallabies, and rat-kangaroos. Sydney: Surrey Beatty; 1989. p. 217–21.

22. Richardson KC, Wyburn RS. The structure and radiographic analysis of the alimentary tract of the tammar wallaby, Macropus eugenii (Marsupialia): II. The intestines. Aust J Zool 1980;28:499–509.

23. Stevens CE, Hume ID. Comparative physiology of the vertebrate digestive system. 2nd edition. Cambridge (UK): Cambridge University Press; 1995.

24. Osawa R, Woodall PF. A comparative study of macroscopic and microscopic dimensions of the intestine in five macropods (Marsupialia: Macropodidae): II. Relationship with feeding habits and fibre content of the diet. Aust J Zool 1992; 40:99–113.

25. Hume ID. Metabolic rates and nutrient requirements. In: Marsupial nutrition. New York: Cambridge University Press; 1999. p. 1–34.

26. Henning SJ, Hird FJR. Concentrations and metabolism of volatile fatty acids in the fermentative organs of two species of kangaroo and the guinea-pig. Br J Nutr 1970;24:145–55.

27. Lintern S. Aspects of nitrogen metabolism in the Kangaroo Island wallaby—Protemnodon eugenii (Desmarest) [doctoral thesis]. Adelaide (Australia): University of Adelaide; 1970.

28. Barker JM. The metabolism of carbohydrate and volatile fatty acids in the marsupial, Setonix brachyurus. Q J Exp Physiol 1961;46:54–68.

29. Griffiths M, McIntosh DL, Leckie RMC. The effects of cortisone on nitrogen balance and glucose metabolism in diabetic and normal kangaroos, sheep and rabbits. J Endocrinol 1969;44:1–12.

reproduction. During autumn and winter, gliders spent most time consuming gum, sap, honeydew, and manna (a sweet mucilaginous secretion produced by plants in response to insect damage). Saps and gums were consumed year round and formed the staple diet.

In other studies of other glider colonies,[4,6] primary feeding activity focused on consuming *Banksia* and *Eucalyptus* flowers for nectar (energy) and pollen (protein) for much of the year, even when insects were abundant. Only in autumn did pollen incidence in feces decrease; pollen feeding directly correlated with flowering seasons, and gliders may be an important native pollinator. Sap and arthropods were important foods when flowers were not available. Gliders have been reported to strip the wings and legs off insects before consumption and to forage for insects on the ground.

Gum sites consist of holes made by insects into which gum accumulates; gliders often enlarge these holes using their incisors. Gliders also use incisors to strip bark and create sap-feeding sites by gouging into the phloem (nutrient transport) columns. Such behaviors may be important for maintaining tooth and gum health and should be encouraged, using natural materials such as nontoxic tree branch materials (ie, various branches with either smooth or rough bark). Gliders lick honeydew from branches and beneath bark and harvest manna from new leaves and flower buds through close examination, smelling, and licking. Cage furnishings that allow these natural feeding behaviors and food presentation can provide important environmental enrichment.

NATIVE DIETARY CONSTITUENTS

Plant exudates consumed by free-ranging sugar gliders include nectar, sap, manna, and gums. Additionally, sugar gliders consume insect exudates, such as honeydew and lerp, excess sugars excreted by sap-eating insects on the surface of leaves and small branches. All exudates that have been measured contain low protein content (<1% dry weight[7,8]). Nectars and saps comprise simple sugar solutions that, in general, also contain low concentrations of vitamins and minerals; manna is derived from sap in response to insect damage on tree branches and leaves. Gums are complex carbohydrates: plant polysaccharides that form gels in water. Gums, produced by trees in response to insect and mechanical damage, are refractive to digestive enzymes but fermentable by microbial populations.[9] Gums produced by some Australian *acacia* sp are chemically similar to those found in African *Acacia senegal* trees used for commercial production of gum arabic.[7] Gum acacia has been shown to contain 1% (dry weight) calcium and offsets the lack of calcium in arthropods eaten by the Senegal bush baby.[10] In this respect, it would be valuable to know if mineral content of gums is similar between African and Australian acacias, such that gum arabic might provide a suitable, available substitute feed for gliders. Phloem-feeding insects, such as aphids, scale insects, and psyllids, consume large quantities of sap to meet their nitrogen (protein) requirements and excrete honeydew or lerp on the surface of leaves and small branches. Clearly, the abundance of some of these food sources for sugar gliders is dependent on fluctuating insect populations, as well as on seasonal flow of saps.

Arthropods important as protein sources in sugar glider diets include moths, spiders, and scarabaeid beetles.[3,4] Information on specific nutrient composition of these native arthropods is not available. Nonetheless, most feeder insects that have been analyzed are deficient in calcium relative to phosphorus[10,11] and in specific amino acids.[11] Arachnid invertebrates (spiders) may be an exception, as they contain elevated levels of taurine, a sulfur-containing amino acid.[12]

Pollen is also a source of dietary protein for sugar gliders; 34% of *Eucalyptus* pollen grains in feces were empty, as compared with 66% to 71% from *Banksia* pollen,[4,5] with the contents presumably digested in the small intestine, rather than in the stomach.

DIGESTIVE PHYSIOLOGY

Anatomically, sugar gliders, unlike other arboreal possums but similar to other mammalian gumivores,[7] have an enlarged cecum well-suited for microbial fermentation of complex dietary carbohydrates, such as gums. However, this assumption has not yet been investigated experimentally.

Basal metabolic rate measured in 128-g (g) captive sugar gliders is reported at 209 $kJ\ kg^{-0.75}$ per day^{-1}, or about 45 kJ per day^{-1} (11 kcal per day^{-1}).[13] Field metabolic rate has also been measured in sugar gliders at about 153 kJ per day^{-1} (approximately 37 kcal) for a 112-g female and 192 kJ per day^{-1} (approximately 46 kcal) for a 135-g male,[14] about four-times basal metabolic rate. Normal captive activity energy requirements might thus be calculated at around two-times basal metabolic rate, or between 76.5 kJ and 96 kJ per day^{-1} (18 kcal–23 kcal) for animals averaging approximately 124 g, although some studies suggest higher energy expenditures than this theoretical minimum.[7] A recent feeding trial comparing three diets in young, growing males averaging 96 g found animals consumed 100.1 kJ to 147 kJ (24 kcal–35 kcal) per day^{-1}.[2] Sugar gliders do not hibernate but can display shallow daily torpor periods, with a drop in body temperature from about 35°C, to 11°C to 28°C for several hours, accompanied by decreases in metabolic rate to 10% to 60% of basal metabolism, mainly in response to food restriction.[15]

Sugar gliders fed honey-pollen diets containing 1.0%, 3.1%, or 6.5% protein, on a dry basis, had maintenance nitrogen requirements determined at 87 $mg\ kg^{-0.75}$ per day^{-1}, or about 248-mg crude protein for a 100-g animal.[16] Gliders displayed low nitrogen losses in both feces and urine, which may be related to low metabolic rates, overall, or to efficient use of a potentially limited resource. Based on these laboratory studies, free-ranging males are likely able to meet minimal protein requirements with diets comprised of exudates alone, but females must supplement with pollen or arthropods to meet demands of reproduction. Amino acid balance in pollens and native insects feeding on natural vegetation may also be superior to amino acid balance in commercial products and in cultured insects used as substitute foods; thus, this difference should be investigated.[7,11]

In feeding trials conducted with common mixed diets containing 19% to 26% crude protein (dry basis), 96-g growing gliders consumed 1,330-mg to 2,270-mg protein per day (with approximately 70% digestibility). Although most animals gained weight during the 60-day trial period, differences were apparent across dietary treatments, and two of nine animals (on the same diet) actually lost weight, suggesting amino acid balance may have varied considerably across diets.[2] Gliders may have consumed excess protein to meet specific amino acid requirements; unfortunately, amino acids were not measured, and further investigations are needed.

Sugar gliders do not require particularly high-protein diets, and excessive protein may, in fact, be detrimental to overall health; refining amino acid balance and overall level is critical for understanding and providing optimal protein nutrition. In this respect, use of a properly balanced dry or canned commercial product that also includes vitamins and minerals essential for other omnivorous species (ie, dogs or primates) is superior to protein sources comprised of unsupplemented animal products, such as meat, eggs, and insects.

5-g other fruit
5-g sweet potato
1-g mealworm (or other invertebrates, such as grasshoppers, moths, fly pupae, crickets; optional)

Such a diet provides 126 kJ energy, 21% crude protein (1,750 mg), 0.77% calcium, 0.64% phosphorus, vitamin D 1.1 IU/g with this particular (dry generic) cat food.

Another adequate sample diet,[18] blended into a slurry, contains:

12-g chopped, mixed fruit (any type, <10% citrus)
2.5-g cooked, chopped vegetables
10-g peach or apricot nectar
5.5-g ground, dry, low-iron bird diet
1-g mealworm (or other invertebrates, as above; optional)

This diet provides 159 kJ energy, 17% crude protein (1,550 mg), 0.61% calcium, 0.44% phosphorus, and vitamin D 0.9 IU/kg.

From a crude-protein perspective, dry dog, avian, or primate foods lower in protein (approximately 15%–25% dry basis) than cat foods (approximately 30%–45% protein) could be used to meet the protein requirements of sugar gliders. Fruits and vegetables can be frozen and thawed; however, canned fruits packed in syrup or processed baby foods ideally should not be used. Fresh produce is preferred, particularly fruits and vegetables that contain more calcium than phosphorus (ie, berries, citrus, figs, papaya, or flower blossoms). Minimize use of fruits with inverse Ca:P ratios (ie, grapes, bananas, apples, pears, melon). Information on mineral balance can be found on the United States Department of Agriculture Nutrient Database (http://www.nal.usda.gov/fnic/foodcomp/search). Feeder insects should be healthy and maintained on a gut-loaded diet before feeding to gliders. Treat items also must be carefully controlled to prevent obesity. Three grams (one-half teaspoon) of unsupplemented applesauce, for example, provides up to 7% of daily calculated energy needs for a 130-g sugar glider; such treats should be factored in as part of the daily total dietary produce allotment.

Fresh water should always be available and changed at least daily; gliders can drink from sipper bottles. The use of nutritionally balanced nectar products for liquid feeding is preferred over the use of diluted fruit juices, fruit nectars, or electrolyte solutions. Caloric contributions of liquid feeds must also be factored into daily energy calculations. In addition, gliders should be weighed and body condition assessed regularly.

AREAS FOR FURTHER INVESTIGATION

To complete an understanding of sugar glider's dietary needs, several areas still need to be investigated:

Mineral content of native Acacia gums consumed by gliders should be quantified.
Methods and products to increase gum feeding by captive gliders must be developed to enhance digestive function, as well as to highlight natural behaviors.
Sugar glider's ability to ferment soluble fiber (gum) should be investigated. Their gastrointestinal tract anatomy suggests that they have a large capacity to harbor beneficial microbial populations, and their feeding ecology is heavily dependent on ingestion of plant gums to meet energy needs.
Limiting amino acids in captive sugar glider diets should be identified, and balance in commercial products should be adjusted to optimize protein nutrition.

Vitamin D metabolism should be examined in detail through controlled feeding studies.

Incidence and health implications of hemosiderosis should be surveyed in captive sugar glider populations.

REFERENCES

1. Ness RD, Booth R. Sugar gliders. In: Quesenberry KE, Carpenter JW, editors. Ferrets, Rabbits, and Rodents Clinical Medicine and Surgery. 2nd edition. Saint Louis (MO): Elsevier Inc; 2004. p. 330–8.
2. Dierenfeld ES, Thomas D, Ives R. Comparison of commonly used diets on intake, digestion, growth, and health in captive sugar gliders (*Petaurus breviceps*). J Exotic Mammal Medicine and Surgery 2006;15(3):218–24.
3. Smith AP. Diet and feeding strategies of the marsupial sugar glider in temperate Australia. J Anim Ecol 1982;51:149–66.
4. Howard J. Diet of *Petaurus breviceps* (Marsupialia:Petauridae) in a mosaic of coastal woodland and heath. Aust Mammal 1989;12:15–21.
5. Van Tets IG, Whelan RJ. *Banksia* pollen in the diet of Australian mammals. Ecography 1997;20:499–505.
6. Quin DG. Population ecology of the squirrel glider (*Petaurus norfolcensis*) and the sugar glider (*P. breviceps*) (Marsupialia: Petauridae) at Limeburners Creek, on the central north coast of New South Wales. Wildl Res 1995;22:471–505.
7. Hume ID. Omnivorous marsupials. In: Marsupial Nutrition. Cambridge: Cambridge Press; 1999. p. 76–124.
8. Lindenmeyer DB, Boyle S, Burgman MA, et al. The sugar and nitrogen content of the gums of Acacia species in the mountain ash and alpine ash forests of central Victoria and its potential implications for exudivorous arboreal marsupials. Australian Journal of Ecology 1994;19:169–77.
9. Van Soest PJ. Carbohydrates. In: Nutritional Ecology of the Ruminant. 2nd edition. Ithaca\London: Cornell University Press; 1994. p. 156–77.
10. Bearder SK, Martin RD. *Acacia* gum and its use by bush babies, *Galago senegalensis* (Primates: Lorisidae). Int J Primatol 1980;1(2):103–28.
11. Finke MD. Complete nutrient composition of commercially raised invertebrates used as food for insectivores. Z Biol 2002;21(3):169–85.
12. Ramsay SL, Houston DC. Amino acid composition of some woodland arthropods and its implications for breeding tits and other passerines. Ibis 2003;145(2):227–32.
13. Dawson TJ, Hulbert AJ. Standard metabolism, body temperature, and surface areas of Australian marsupials. Am J Phys 1970;218:1233–8.
14. Nagy KA, Suckling GC. Field energetics and water balance of sugar gliders, *Petaurus breviceps* (Marsupialia: Petauridae). Aust J Zool 1985;33:683–91.
15. Fleming MR. Thermoregulation and torpor in the sugar glider, *Petaurus breviceps* (Marsupialia: Petauridae). Aust J Zool 1980;28:521–34.
16. Smith AP, Green SW. Nitrogen requirements of the sugar glider (*Petaurus breviceps*), an omnivorous marsupial, on a honey-pollen diet. Physiol Zool 1987;60:82–92.
17. Booth RJ. General husbandry and medical care of sugar gliders. In: Bonagura JD, editor. Kirk's Current Veterinary Therapy XIII. Philadelphia: WB Saunders; 2000. p. 1157–63.
18. Pye GW, Carpenter JW. A guide to medicine and surgery in sugar gliders. Vet Med 1999;94(10):891–905.

captive opossums, these species cannot be treated successfully without familiarizing oneself with normal opossum behaviors. Regardless of how healthy wild opossums may initially appear, many have pre-existing problems that require a complete examination to diagnose. Like other wild animals, opossums mask their illnesses with defensive posturing and appear unhealthy only when their energy reserves fail and they can no longer compensate. Clinicians who are unfamiliar with normal opossum behavior are likely to mistake these defensive actions for good health and miss medical problems. Unless veterinarians can recognize normal behavior and correct underlying problems, many sick captive opossums continue to deteriorate.[1]

Evaluating captive opossums Evaluating a captive opossum's condition begins by obtaining an accurate history and determining the circumstances under which the opossum was found. Healthy opossums often arrive in feral cat traps (**Fig. 1**), and many are injured or deceased. Many good Samaritans arrive at the clinic with infants taken off an injured or deceased jill. These are critical cases, and treatment, ongoing care, and prognosis often depend on the accuracy and extent of the history obtained.

When presented with a captive opossum, the practitioner must determine the client's intentions for the animal, which will guide the practitioner's advice to the client. Many veterinarians work closely with wildlife rehabilitators to try to release these animals back into the wild. These animals should have minimal interaction with humans to avoid habituation. Opossums that have become habituated to people can be used in educational settings. Owners of these captive animals are often knowledgeable regarding opossum husbandry and natural history; captivity-induced medical problems are rare in this group. Finally, well-meaning citizens who find injured opossums often wish to obtain medical treatment to eventually release the animals back into the wild or keep the animals as captive pets. This group of opossums frequently develops problems associated with poor nutrition.

Behavioral response of trapped captive opossums Healthy captive opossums are often fearful, defensive, and difficult to handle. The degree of their behavioral response depends on the circumstance of their capture, severity of injury, and degree of illness.

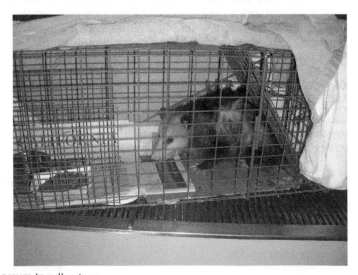

Fig. 1. Opossum in a live trap.

When approached, a trapped opossum lowers its lip, pulls its lips back, and begins to drool. It hisses, spits, growls, opens its mouth as wide as possible, and bares its teeth, expanding its palatine pouches while attempting to frighten you away. If unsuccessful, the opossum increases the intensity of its hissing and growling and then strikes and snaps. When caught, opossums continue to growl with open mouths, defecate, urinate, and express their anal scent glands. Opossums do not use their claws as weapons, but they are sharp and can scratch when they struggle to get away.

Opossums can deliver a painful bite, so handlers should be cautious. Although more resistant to rabies then other mammals, they are not immune. In California, there have been five confirmed cases of rabies in opossums in the last 10 years.[2] Opossums likely contract rabies by eating dead bats. All opossum bites are reportable to state public health agencies, and protection of all individuals exposed to potentially rabid animals is paramount.

Restraining captive opossums Always use gloves or a towel when attempting to restrain a captive opossum. The restraint method used depends on the size, age, and condition of the opossum. Even when using gloves, the restrainer can use a towel not only to distract the opossum from biting the handler by covering its head but also to add an extra layer of protection against flea bites. Opossums carry the cat flea, *Ctenocephalides felis*, which is known to transmit murine typhus, *Rickettsia typhi*.[3] Whenever handling any wildlife, anyone coming in contact with the animal should wear protective latex/vinyl gloves and thoroughly wash his or her hands. Once restrained, an opossum may give up and relax, clasping its paws together as in a prayer-like pose. All age groups may demonstrate this pose, which does not mean the opossum has given up. It still bites if given the chance.

To examine an infant opossum, place a towel over its head and wrap it around its body. With the opossum wrapped in a towel, hold the animal vertically and extend the tail downward, allowing the body to hang. This gives the animal a sense of security and it struggles less.[4] Juvenile and adult opossums can be restrained on a flat surface by holding a towel over their heads with one hand while grasping the base of their tail with the other hand. This manner of restraint makes the animals feel more secure, so they are less apt to cling to surrounding surfaces or attempt to escape. They can be grabbed around their neck with gloved hands to control their head while avoiding their teeth. Holding them by the scruff of their neck (as one would a cat) is difficult, however, because the neck is short and there is limited skin in this region. Although the opossum is restrained by the tail, it may be turned over for a cursory examination of the head, mouth, and body. Move slowly, because opossums are sensitive to sudden movements, loud noises, and bright lights. Be quiet and handle them gently and securely. When an opossum is restrained excessively, it struggles to try to get away; sometimes, less restraint is better.

If a captive opossum is too uncooperative or fractious, it should be anesthetized with an inhalant anesthetic agent for a complete examination and any diagnostic or therapeutic procedures (**Fig. 2**).

Examining captive opossums On initial examination, determine the opossum's gender, check for presence of young in the pouch if it is a female, and record weight and temperature. Injured opossums found on roadsides often are hyperthermic and should be treated immediately. The average body temperature of Virginia opossums is approximately 35.2°C. Estimate the patient's age based on size and weight. The Virginia opossum moves to the pouch after only 13 days' gestation, at which point it weighs only several grams and is approximately the size of a bumblebee. The infant's eyes open between 9 and 11 weeks of age, while they are still suckling and weigh

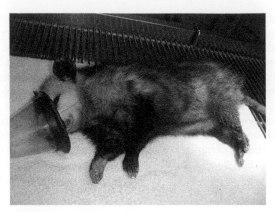

Fig. 2. Anesthetized opossum.

approximately 55 to 75 g. Juvenile opossums live on their own when they weigh approximately 400 to 500 g and are approximately 15 weeks of age. They should be checked for external parasites, wounds, abscesses, cuts, and injuries. Juvenile and adult opossums are often covered with fleas, ticks, and dirt. Scars and abrasions on the head from past trauma are common, as are torn ears, broken and chipped teeth, and sores or scabs on the feet, tail, and nose.

Appearance of a healthy opossum A healthy opossum has clear, bright eyes, intact, shiny, white teeth, a slightly pink gum line, and clean ear canals. Its anus should be dry, clean, and closed, with no signs of diarrhea or anal prolapse. The hair coat should be smooth and cool to the touch. The lungs and heart should auscult clearly and steadily. The kidneys and liver are not palpable. The spine should be smooth and free of deviations, and the tail, joints, and hands should be flexible and grip well.[1]

Captive opossums in trauma situations should be initially stabilized, which includes supporting fractures, cleaning abscesses, preventing blood loss, and treating all wounds. These patients should be treated for shock, administered fluids, given antibiotics, and supported thermodynamically by adjusting the surrounding temperature. Once animals are stabilized, diagnostic tests, including blood and urine samples, radiographs, and fecal examination, may be conducted. All opossums also should be treated for internal and external parasites.[5]

Housing captive opossums Two or more juvenile or adult captive opossums should not be housed together in the same enclosure if they have not grown up together. Wild opossums are solitary animals by nature, and fighting ensues if they are housed in close quarters. Opossums raised together from infancy may get along. Observations of captive opossums kept in large outdoor enclosures show that some females may form stable, noncombative hierarchical social relationships. Extreme antagonistic behavior has been observed between males. When males and females are housed together, females are more dominant.[6]

Cannibalism has been reported in captive opossums. This behavior has been attributed to poor husbandry, overcrowding, stress, improper diet, mixing different sized animals, mixing litters, and placing sick or injured opossums in cages with healthy opossums. Placing different sized infants on a surrogate mother also may lead to injured ears, bite wounds, and missing toes. Hand-raised females that are accustomed to other opossums have been known to take on and nurse infants of different sizes from other litters.[1,6,7]

Healthy opossums from different litters that weigh less than 400 g each but are approximately the same weight can be housed together. Housing these opossums together reinforces normal wild behavior. Habituated opossums quickly lose their ability to discriminate between friend and foe and their natural survival instinct to find food in the wild. Captive opossums must be returned to the wild as soon as possible. Providing proper long-term care is not practical, unless they are being housed in established educational or zoologic facilities operated by trained staff. Preparing correct diets, monitoring appetite and health, and providing appropriate enclosures for different life stages is an involved and time-consuming process. Individuals considering long-term opossum management must be made aware of these requirements and the repercussions to the animal's health if these needs are not met.

Behavioral response to confinement Wild opossums do not exhibit typical wild behaviors in a hospital setting and do not adjust well to being confined. These patients can be sensitive to the sights, smells, and sounds of normal hospital activity and, as a result, can become stressed and have delayed recovery from injury. In the hospital, the opossum's cage must be secure to prevent escape. Opossums are nocturnal animals that become active in the early morning, exploring their cages and looking for ways to break out.[8] They can squeeze through bars, turn handles and latches, climb anything, and hide everywhere.

When housed in a cage, opossums must be provided with fresh food and water daily. Every morning, their bowls must be checked to see how much and what kind of food has been eaten. Being nocturnal, opossums sleep up to 16 hours a day and likely are not active during peak hospital working hours. Captive opossums spend most of their time hiding in a den box or sleeping under a towel or blanket. Captive opossums should be kept in a quiet, dark location away from dogs or cats. Caged opossums demand regular and consistent daily monitoring. Captive opossums may not eat when brought to the hospital, although most healthy captive animals begin eating in a few days. If an opossum does not begin to eat within 72 hours of hospitalization, look for an underlying problem; a healthy opossum lives to eat!

Case management of captive opossums Marsupial case management and treatment follow standard protocols for nonmarsupial companion mammals. Most practitioners who work with opossums associate management of this species with that of management of cats. Allometric scaling techniques show that opossums have lower basal metabolic rates when compared with placental mammals, however; they require lower medication dosing regimens.[9,10] Opossums may appear normal despite an underlying illness, or they may have clinical symptoms that take time to manifest. Clinical signs may wax and wane from day to day, so continued monitoring is imperative.

BEHAVIORAL MANIFESTATIONS OF DISEASE

Trauma is the most common problem in opossums that present to veterinary practices. Common signs include paralysis, paresis, fractures, labored breathing, shock, and bleeding. Pacing, hyperactivity, and pawing at the mouth are often associated with head injuries. Immediate care is required in most cases, and maintenance of body temperature and cardiovascular support is essential. Radiographs should be performed in every trauma case after stabilization, unless life-threatening injuries that require immediate diagnosis are suspected. If the opossum cannot eat after being stabilized, a pharyngostomy tube may be placed for nutritional support.[11]

Abandoned infants are commonly seen and require immediate attention and supportive care. These patients need to be kept warm and rehydrated and should be fed frequently to provide the greatest chance for survival. A young opossum that weighs less than 100 g is truly an orphan, not a victim of kidnapping by well-meaning individuals, as is common in many other wildlife species. For these orphans, care must be provided.

If an opossum does not eat after 72 hours in the hospital, underlying medical conditions must be sought. Anorexia is always a sign for concern. Check for broken teeth, fractured jaws, and other signs of head trauma. Look for indications of abdominal or back pain, bruising, ruptured bladder, or anemia. Perform a fecal examination, and treat intestinal parasites. Obtain radiographs to diagnose intestinal blockage, intestinal stasis, or other signs of internal trauma. Complete blood cell counts, serum biochemistry analysis results, and urinalysis results should be collected as part of a minimal database to investigate ongoing problems. Provide nutritional and fluid support while diagnostic test results are pending and until causes for anorexia can be addressed. If the opossum is anemic, an injection of iron dextran and vitamin supplements, such as Hi Vites (EVSCO Pharmaceuticals, Buena, NJ) or Liqui-Tinic 4X (PRN Pharmacal, Pensacola, FL), can be administered. In general, blood transfusions in opossums are impractical.

Weakness, staggering, falling over, and circling are all signs of neurologic disease. Neurologic signs may be temporary or permanent and may be static or progressive. Concussion from head trauma, migrating parasites, muscle myopathy, spinal myelopathy, and chronic nutritional deficiency can result in generalized weakness and should be considered as differential diagnoses for neurologic disease. A standard neurologic examination to assess proprioception, motor function, and superficial and deep pain can be conducted on opossums as in companion animals. Assess for the ability to grasp, hang, and climb and check for circling, pacing, and stereotypic behavior. Atonic bladder, along with concurrent bladder infections, is commonly found with spinal damage.

Labored and open-mouthed breathing, flail chest, and cyanotic mucous membranes are signs of trauma or underlying respiratory disease. Many opossums develop verminous pneumonia and protozoal lung disease in the wild and may present to practitioners with end-stage infection. Inhaling noxious substances and particulate matter also can lead to lung disease. Fungal, bacterial, and mycoplasmal infections can cause serious lung damage.[4,5] If radiographic changes are present, tracheal and bronchial lavage should be performed to obtain cultures for a more accurate diagnosis. Puncture wounds, fractured ribs, and flail chest occur commonly from cat and dog bites. Radiographs should be taken, antibiotics should be administered, and oxygen supplementation and nebulization should be considered.

Parenteral fluids should be given in cases of shock, dehydration, and cardiovascular collapse. Cardiovascular signs include pale mucous membranes, low core body temperature, and cold extremities. Determine the state of dehydration by checking the degree of skin tenting over the shoulder region. Warm a hypothermic opossum by placing it on a warm water heating pad or forced air heating device. Administer fluids via the lateral or ventral tail vein. If catheterization is not possible, give fluids subcutaneously or use an intraosseous catheter. Tube feeding with warm blended food can be administered for support.

Skin disease is common but usually not life-threatening, unless it reflects internal circulatory problems. Opossums can develop chronic, nonhealing abscesses that can take longer than 3 months to heal. These wounds may get progressively worse no matter what the treatment regimen, and euthanasia may be the only option in the end. Dermal septic necrosis and "crusty ear syndrome" have been described.[1] These skin conditions can be caused by systemic yeast or bacterial infections or the development of peripheral microabscesses that affect capillary filling. Anemia from severe ectoparasitic infection is common and must be treated with appropriate antiparasitic drugs and supportive care.

Opossums also may present with gastrointestinal problems resulting from trauma-induced nerve damage, foreign body ingestion with obstruction, dietary mismanagement, or endoparasites. A prolapsed rectum is also common in this species and is usually associated with chronic diarrhea, constipation, or trauma. Surgical repair can be performed, but prolapses often reoccur. In all cases of gastrointestinal problems, a complete nutritional history should be obtained and a standard evaluation that includes radiographs, fecal examination, and treatment for helminths should be performed.

Pain Response and Treatment

Opossums are tough animals, and in the wild they can withstand considerable abuse and pain. Recovered opossum skeletons have showed healed bone fractures that equivalent-sized placental mammals could never have survived. Opossums are generally more stoic than other mammals when it comes to experiencing pain. Opossums exhibit different kinds of pain responses.[12]

Acute pain

This is a reflexive, instinctive, and immediate response to an acute injury, and it is the response most easily observed. Opossums show a startle response that includes a quick squeal or cry and a quick snap while they move away from their source of discomfort.[13] Opossums in pain may become aggressive and attack when approached. When faced with anticipation of overwhelming pain, they appear fearful, crouch and become immobile, and freeze or "play dead."

Chronic pain

Chronic pain is more subtle and is most often manifested by anorexia, sitting or sleeping in a hunched position, pacing, and crawling in circles. This response is more difficult to evaluate.

Postoperative pain

This response in opossums depends on the type of surgery and the resultant pain elicited. Pain is best evaluated postoperatively when the opossum is awake and aware of its surroundings. Opossums seem to respond favorably to most analgesics. An array of pain responses has been observed, from stoic calmness, to chewing or pawing at the surgical site, to aggressive behavior that makes postoperative care difficult. Nonsteroidal anti-inflammatory medications, such as meloxicam (Metacam, Boehringer Ingelheim, St. Joseph, MO), are commonly used for mild pain and inflammation, whereas narcotics such as butorphanol tartrate (Equanol, Vedco, St. Joseph, MO) and buprenorphine hydrochloride (Buprenex, Reckitt Benckiser Pharmaceuticals, Inc., Hull, England) can be used to control more severe pain.[13]

Euthanasia

When an injured or ill captive opossum comes to the hospital, the goal is to reintroduce it back into the wild as soon as possible. The longer it remains in the hospital, the more it loses its instinct for survival upon release. Some captive opossums regain their health quickly, whereas others never seem to completely recover; injuries may be too great or the illness too severe. Evaluating quality of life may be a subjective decision, and being familiar with normal opossum behavior may help the clinician with this

Spaying and neutering pet opossums

Spaying female opossums prevents endometritis and a Cushing's-like syndrome associated with partially paralyzed, unspayed opossums (**Fig. 4**). This syndrome is often associated with urine retention, urinary tract infections, and obesity. Nonreleasable females should be spayed and not bred.[1,3] Neutering male opossums is neither desirable nor necessary. An unneutered male opossum does not become aggressive with age or develop body odor. Neutering a paralyzed opossum prevents trauma caused by increased genital contact with the ground, and neutering may reduce anxiety around intact females. Castrated opossums stop vocalizing and instead respond with lip smacking noises.

Diseases of pet opossums

Secondary nutritional hyperparathyroidism, obesity, and dental disease are the most common nutritional disorders in pet opossums. Obesity occurs in opossums because of lack of exercise and overfeeding.

NUTRITIONAL CONSIDERATIONS IN THE MANAGEMENT AND TREATMENT OF CAPTIVE AND HOSPITALIZED VIRGINIA OPOSSUMS
Oral and Gastrointestinal Morphology

The gastrointestinal morphology of the Virginia opossum is consistent with that of many other mammalian omnivores. The dental formula is 5/4, 1/1, 3/3, 4/4, and the salivary glands include large mandibular and smaller parotid and sublingual glands. The distal esophagus has raised, transverse rugae and is comprised of smooth muscle fibers. The opossum's distal esophagus, pylorus, and ileocecal junction have been studied extensively, because the smooth muscle arrangements in these areas closely resembles that of humans.[15]

Virginia opossums have a simple, globular stomach; most of the gastric mucosa is comprised of fundic glands. Pyloric glands and a narrow ridge of cardiac glands exist near the esophageal-gastric border.[16] Like most placental mammals (also known as Eutherian mammals), opossums have enteroendocrine cells lining portions of their gastrointestinal tract. These cells, in addition to endocrine cells in the pancreas, aid in secreting peptides that control various digestive functions such as gastric acid secretion, pancreatic secretion of electrolytes and enzymes, and contraction of the gall bladder.[17] In the stomach, 90% of the enteroendocrine cells are located in the pyloric region and secrete a variety of hormones, such as gastrin, gastric-inhibitory peptide, secretin, cholecystokinin, and pancreozymin.[18]

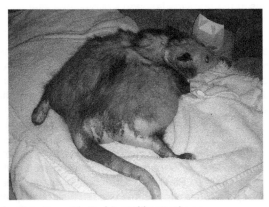

Fig. 4. Obese female opossum with Cushing's-like syndrome.

In opossums, the Brunner's glands secrete their products into mucosal depressions located on the duodenal wall. Virginia opossums possess a cecum that is simple, conical, and approximately 20% to 40% of the total body length. Distal to the cecum, the colon is mobile because of its simple, loose mesenteric attachment.[19] A more detailed summary of the Virginia opossum's gastrointestinal anatomy is available for interested readers.[15]

General Diet Information

Many captive diets exist for the Virginia opossum, and the veterinarian or wildlife rehabilitator must take care in choosing which one to use. Many diets are designed for laboratory research opossums or are deficient in nutrients essential for growing or adult opossums to thrive. Captive diet information (see later discussion) has been developed and used successfully at the Wildlife Center of Virginia to rehabilitate and release wild opossums. A summary of the feeding schedule for Virginia opossums can be found in **Table 1**. Alternative reliable diet information can be found by contacting the National Opossum Society.[20]

Table 1
Feeding schedule for the growing Virginia opossum (*Didelphis virginiana*)

Approximate Weight (g)	Physical Characteristics	Amount per Feeding (mL)	No. Feedings per Day
< 10	Body is pink and nested; oral membrane present over mouth	.25–.50	Round the clock; difficult to rehabilitate
10–20	Eyes closed; skin turning gray; fur beginning to grow in	.50	5+
21–30	Eyes closed; fur is smooth and sleek	.50–1	4
31–54	Eyes closed or just opened; oral membrane is completely gone	1.25–2 (begin to offer mash)	3
55–74	Eyes open; fully furred; look like opossums; approximately 9–11 wk old	2.5–3.5 (add soft foods and dish of fresh water)	2
75–100	Beginning to run around; eating on its own	4–5 (introduce small mouse pieces)	1
101–200	Climbing, active, and using tail	Juvenile meal (see menu) and a mouse	None
200+	Aggressive defense behavior; becoming more nocturnal; eating whole mice	Gradually change to adult meal over a 2-wk transition period	None
500	Aggressive, nocturnal	Release	

Opossums are born after 12 to 13 days' gestation. The naked young climb to the pouch, where they attach for 60 days. Eyes begin to open around 63 days after birth, and weaning begins around 87 to 104 days after birth. Because the actual birth date is often unknown, feeding is often based the animal's weight.

Neonatal Opossum Nutrition

Lactation in the average female opossum lasts for 15 weeks.[21] The nutrient composition of the milk changes over the course of lactation. When rearing captive infant Virginian opossums, caretakers should try to replicate the type, amount, and relative percentage of nutrients found in the jill's milk. The milk is initially comprised of 9% total solids, peaking at 34% at week 11. There is then a decrease to 27% at week 13, which is maintained until the end of lactation.[22] Carbohydrate, protein, and fat content of the milk fluctuates at different times in the lactation cycle. Hexose seems to be the most abundant carbohydrate in opossum milk; it reaches a peak concentration of 7% at week 7.[22] Although opossums are frequently reported as being lactose intolerant, the jill's milk contains lactose. Lactose concentrations are higher during the initial weeks of lactation and taper off to almost undetectable amounts by week 15.[23]

The total protein concentration of opossum milk mirrors that of the total solids, peaking at 10% at week 11 of lactation. The milk fat concentration is stable at 8% up to week 9; it increases to 17% at week 11 and then declines to 11% by week 13 of lactation.[22] Magnesium, sodium, and potassium concentrations in milk remain constant throughout lactation (mean concentrations of 9.2 ± 1.2 mmol, 41 ± 4 mmol, and 35 ± 11 mmol, respectively). Calcium concentration increases from 13 mmol during the beginning of lactation to 100 mmol by week 7 and remains at this level until week 10.[22] The estimated energy content of milk at the beginning of lactation is just over 500 kJ per 100 mL and then peaks at week 11 to 966 kJ per 100 mL. This increase in energy concentration coincides with significant growth periods in young joeys.[22]

Until their eyes are open, joeys can be tube fed formula that consists of two parts Esbilac powder (PetAg, Inc., Hampshire, IL), one part Zoologic Milk Matrix 30/55 powder (PetAg, Inc., Hampshire, IL), four parts warm water, and a half teaspoon of dicalcium phosphate (28:18.5) powder (UPCO, St. Joseph, MO). After joeys have opened their eyes, the formula should be changed to one part Esbilac powder, two parts warm water, and a half teaspoon of calcium/phosphorus powder. Tube feeding young opossums is the fastest and surest way to ensure that milk is delivered into the stomach. Animals that weigh less than 20 g can be fed through 2.8- to 3.5-Fr tubes, whereas opossums that weigh 20 to 100 g may be fed through 5.0-Fr tubes. A tube whose length equals the distance from the opossum's nose to just proximal to the sternum should be passed gently down the esophagus. Care must be taken not to administer too much formula because of the risk of aspiration. If aspiration occurs, the opossum should be treated with appropriate antibiotics (broad spectrum and good systemic penetration into respiratory tissues) for a minimum of 5 days. Other methods of feeding infant opossums, such as syringe or pipette feeding, may be used successfully but tend to be more time intensive, especially when large numbers of animals must be fed.

The volume of formula per feeding and the number of feedings per day depend on the animal's age and size. A retrospective analysis from archived Wildlife Center of Virginia records indicated that the success rate of rearing orphaned young opossums decreases significantly if joeys weigh less than 24 g on admission. These smaller animals require round-the-clock feeding and often have concurrent bacterial infections from suckling on contaminated milk from dead jills. Unless orphaned opossums are removed from their mothers immediately after they are killed, they should be treated with antibiotics upon entering the hospital to decrease the likelihood of developing bacterial infections.

Juvenile Opossum Nutrition

Weaning commences in juvenile wild opossums at 12 weeks' postpartum, when joeys weigh approximately 165 g;[24] however, joeys that weigh as little as 100 g can be weaned successfully. A juvenile mash that consists of 2 tbsp of infant opossum tube feeding formula (recipe listed above), 1 tbsp of baby rice cereal, and 2 tbsp high-quality puppy kibble can be introduced when the opossum weighs 31 to 54 g and can be given concurrently with tube feeding. This soft appetizing diet encourages young opossums to sample solid food and can be given until they weigh 100 g. When joeys weigh 55 to 75 g, they can be fed small pieces of soft food and offered fresh water in a separate bowl. When the joeys weigh 75 to 100 g, they can be offered small pieces of cut-up mice.

When they weigh more than 100 g, joeys require only a juvenile opossum diet that can be prepared in bulk if several joeys are being fed. The daily juvenile diet consists of approximately 4 tbsp soaked puppy chow, 1 tbsp meat-based baby food, 2 tbsp canned puppy food, 1 tbsp cat chow, several small chunks of soft vegetables (ie, broccoli, carrots, cauliflower, sweet potato, squash), one to two pieces of fruit just large enough for the opossum to handle and manipulate, and one fifth of a dead mouse cut up with the bones included. Only high-quality meat, non–soy-based dog and cat food should be offered. This juvenile diet may be given until the opossums weigh approximately 200 g, at which point they should be switched to an adult diet.

Adult Opossum Nutrition

The Virginia opossum is an omnivore.[25] Dietary studies of wild adult opossums indicate that opossums eat a variety of insects, small vertebrates, fruits, nuts, seeds, and vegetation that vary geographically and seasonally. In a study of opossums in New York, analysis of the stomach contents of 187 road-killed Virginia opossums showed that the average opossum diet consists of 18% fruit, 17.2% amphibians, 14.2% mammals, 13.4% insects, 6.6% grass, 5.4% worms, 5.3% reptiles, 5% birds, 4.8% carrion, and 6.7% other items.[26] Another study showed that stomach contents of road-killed opossums in Portland, Oregon consist of 27% mammals, 11% leaf litter, 10% fruits, seeds, and bulbs, 10% gastropods, 9% garbage, 9% earthworms, 9% pet food, 8% grass and green leaves, 3% insects, 3% birds, and 1% unidentified animal tissue.[27] Both studies examined stomach rather than fecal content because fecal analysis reveals food items that readily pass through the gastrointestinal system and may not account for more digestible food items. One study showed that of 39 food items typically found in opossums' diets in eastern Texas, 36 appeared in the stomach contents, whereas only 10 could be identified in fecal contents.[28]

Like infant and juvenile diets, many adult diet variations exist, and maintaining the proper Ca:P ratio and avoiding high fat meals should be a priority. A well-balanced diet includes 6 tbsp of dry, high-quality cat food, a half cup of small vegetable chunks, two to three small pieces of fruit, 7 tbsp of high-quality, canned dog food, several earthworms, one hard-boiled egg with shell, and one whole mouse (approximately 30 g). This diet can be given once a day with unlimited amounts of fresh water.

Vitamins

If given an appropriately balanced diet, healthy opossums do not need vitamin supplementation. When appropriate diets are given, vitamin deficiencies are uncommon, and the risk of health problems associated with oversupplementation can be avoided. Vitamin D deficiencies are uncommon in opossums because they, like other crepuscular mammals, are highly efficient at producing vitamin D_3 (cholecalciferol, the active

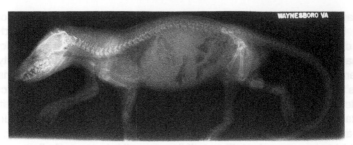

Fig. 6. Radiographic lesions typical of secondary nutritional hyperparathyroidism in a growing juvenile opossum, including decreased cortical opacity (especially in digits), enlarged, nonmineralized physes in carpal and tarsal joints, and degenerative changes in elbow and stifle joints.

is essential, because opossums with metabolic bone disease are commonly fed high-protein, low-calcium meals, infant milk formulas, or excessive fruits and vegetables. Although calcium supplementation is often required in treatment of metabolic bone disease, Ca:P ratios vary between sources, and supplements must be selected carefully. For example, calcium gluconate administration may be appropriate for animals that exhibit signs of hypocalcemic tetany; however, the calcium concentration in calcium gluconate is not high enough to overcome clinical signs and radiographic changes associated with long-term effects of dietary Ca:P imbalance. Appropriate supplements may be chosen from a review of relative Ca:P content of various supplements.[29] Calcitonin may be administered to severely affected animals; however, it should be given only if plasma calcium concentrations are within reference ranges. Calcitonin decreases circulating plasma calcium levels by inhibiting PTH-induced osteoclastic activity. Calcitonin also decreases serum calcium and phosphorus levels, however, and if adequate calcium is not supplemented when calcitonin is administered, further hypocalcemia may occur.[33]

Obesity

Obesity is a common problem in adult Virginia opossums. Obesity can lead to cardiac, hepatic, and pancreatic disease[33] and often shortens their lifespan. Signs of obesity

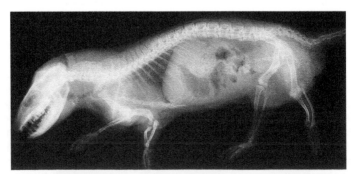

Fig. 7. Radiographic findings of chronic secondary nutritional hyperparathyroidism in an adult opossum. This animal was on a poor diet deficient in calcium during neonatal and juvenile growth phases but managed to survive. Note persistent degenerative changes in elbows and stifles, folding fractures in long bones and caudal vertebrae, and decreased cortical opacity in digits. Most other bones are well calcified at this time.

include weight gain and fat deposition throughout the body; fat deposits are most noticeable in the tail and around the eyes. Buphthalmia may occur secondary to fat deposition in the retrobulbar fat pads. In general, obesity is caused by a lack of exercise and a diet too high in fat and protein. The clinician must control body weight and still provide a nutritious, balanced diet. The metabolic rate in marsupials is 30% that of similar sized placental mammals.[34] To avoid obesity, captive opossums should be fed portions based on metabolism rather than size.[35]

The number of calories in the diet should be reduced at the end of the juvenile growth phase—approximately 9 months of age. At this time, the proportion of cat or dog chow in the diet should be reduced so that by 1 year of age, only 45 to 60 mL are given per day.[32] If the opossum is still gaining weight, cat or dog senior or weight-control formula should be used to lower the dietary fat and total kilocalories. In addition to caloric restriction, exercise is also important for weight maintenance of captive opossums. They should be provided with a large enclosure with vertical space to allow climbing. Opossums can be trained to walk on leashes attached to a body harness and run in exercise wheels. The Opossum Society of the United States has published instructions on how to build an exercise wheel appropriate for opossums.[36]

Dental Disease

Virginia opossums commonly have broken teeth and periodontal disease from collisions with vehicles. With car accidents, if opossums survive the impact, wounds may make them more susceptible to development of systemic infection, such as endocarditis, a common cause of opossum death. In captivity, periodontal disease is often seen in marsupial omnivores as a result of sugary, moist diets.[37] To prevent

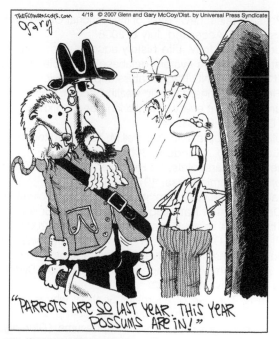

Fig. 8. Opossums are in. (THE FLYING MCCOYS © 2007 Glenn and Gary McCoy. Distributed by Universal Press Syndicate. Reprinted with permission. All rights reserved.)

dental disease in opossums, regular brushing and prophylactic cleaning is essential.[38]

SUMMARY

Virginia opossums are widely distributed throughout the United States, except in the most arid regions, and wild individuals are commonly brought to practitioners for medical attention. It has been estimated that there are 100,000 or more opossums in the state of California (W. Sakai, personal communication, 2008). Opossums' popularity as pets seems to be growing, and it is likely that pet opossums will be more common in veterinary practice (**Fig. 8**). Clinicians must be aware of natural opossum behaviors so that thorough physical examination and diagnostic procedures can be performed on injured patients. For animals kept captive long-term or as pets, veterinarians must understand proper nutrition and nutritional disorders, such as secondary nutritional hyperparathyroidism, obesity, and dental disease, to properly treat this species.

ACKNOWLEDGMENTS

The authors wish to acknowledge the wildlife rehabilitators of the Wildlife Center of Virginia, particularly Amanda Nicholson and Dani Stumbo, for their assistance in reviewing the nutritional information in this article. The authors also thank Dr. William Krause and the late Dr. Anita Henness for their pioneering work and inspiration.

REFERENCES

1. Henness A. Possum tales: newsletter of the National Opossum Society. Available at: www.opossum.org. Accessed July 6, 2008.
2. Mayer K, Laudenslayer Jr W. Life history accounts and range maps: California wildlife habitat relationships system database. Available at: http://www.cdph.ca.gov/HEALTHINFO/DISCOND/Pages/rabies.aspx. Version 8.1 2005. California Dept Public Health, Veterinary Public Health Section; Accessed July 29, 2008.
3. Johnson-Delaney C. What every veterinarian needs to know about Virginia opossums. Exotic DVM 2005;6(6):38–43.
4. Carboni D, Tully T. Marsupials. In: Mitchell M, Tully T, editors. Manual of exotic pet practice. St. Louis (MO): Saunders; 2008. p. 304–19.
5. Potkay S. Disease of marsupials. In: Hunsaker D II, editor. The biology of marsupials. New York: Academic Press; 1977. p. 415–96.
6. Krause W, Krause W. The opossum: its amazing story. Columbia (MO): University of Missouri, Department of Pathology and Anatomical Sciences; 2006.
7. Scardina J. The tonight show. [Episode 3551]. June, 5 2008; season 16.
8. Hunsaker D II, Shupe D. Behavior of new world marsupials. In: Hunsaker D II, editor. The biology of marsupials. New York: Academic Press; 1977. p. 279–344.
9. Hainsworth F. Animal physiology: adaptations in function. Sydney: Addison-Wesley Publishing Company, Inc.; 1982.
10. Schmidt-Nielsen K. The use of allometry. Scaling: why is animal size so important? New York: Cambridge University Press; 1984. p. 21–9.
11. Neff T. Use of pharyngostomy tubes in opossums (*Didelphis virginiana*). In: Selected papers of the seventeenth annual symposium of the National Wildlife Rehabilitation Association. St. Cloud (MN):1999. p. 43–7.

12. Bays T, Lightfoot T, Mayer J. Exotic pet behavior, birds, reptiles, and small mammals. St. Louis (MO): Saunders; 2006.
13. O'Dell S. Pain-induced aggression in animals: snake, opossum, turtle, ferret, rat, raccoon, and pigeon. Psychol Today 1967;1(1):28–33.
14. Tyndale-Biscoe H. Opossums of the Americas: cousins from a distant time. Life of marsupials. Collingwood, Australia: CSIRO Publishing; 2005. p. 103–38.
15. Hume I. Omnivorous marsupials: marsupial nutrition. Cambridge: Cambridge University Press; 1999. p. 76–123.
16. Bensley R. The cardiac glands of mammals. Am J Anat 1902;2(1):105–56.
17. Stevens C, Hume I. Comparative physiology of the vertebrate digestive system. 2nd edition. Cambridge (United Kingdom): Cambridge University Press; 1995.
18. Krause W, Yamada J, Cutts J. Quantitative distribution of enteroendocrine cells in the gastrointestinal tract of the adult opossum, *Didelphis virginiana*. J Anat 1985; 140(4):591–605.
19. Owens R. Comparative anatomy and physiology of vertebrates. London: Longans and Co.; 1868.
20. The National Opossum Society. 2008. Available at: www.opossum.org. Accessed July 7, 2008.
21. Harder J. Reproductive biology of South American marsupials. In: Hamlett W, editor. Reproductive biology of South American vertebrates. New York: Springer-Verlag; 1992. p. 211–28.
22. Green B, Krause W, Newgrain K. Milk composition in the North American opossum (*Didelphis virginia*). Comp Biochem Physiol 1996;113B(3):619–23.
23. Bergman H, Housley C. Chemical analyses of American opossum (*Didelphis virginiana*) milk. Comp Biochem Physiol 1968;25:213–8.
24. Cutts J, Krause W, Leeson C. General observations on the growth and development of the young pouch opossum, *Didelphis virginiana*. Biol Neonate 1978;33: 264–72.
25. Hunsaker D. The biology of marsupials. New York: Academic Press; 1977.
26. Hamilton W Jr. The food of the opossum in New York State. J Wildl Manage 1951; 15:258–64.
27. Hopkins D, Forbes R. Dietary patterns of the Virginia opossum in an urban environment. The Murrelet 1980;61(1):20–30.
28. Wood J. Food habits of furbearers in the upland post oak region of Texas. J Mammal 1954;35:406–14.
29. Fowler M. Metabolic bone disease. In: Fowler M, editor. Zoo and wild animal medicine. 2nd edition. Philadelphia: WB Saunders Company; 1986. p. 69–90.
30. Binkley N, Krueger D. Hypervitaminosis A and bone. Nutr Rev 2000;58(5): 138–44.
31. Wisner E, Konde L. Diseases of the immature skeleton. In: Thrall D, editor. Textbook of veterinary diagnostic radiology. 4th edition. Philadelphia: WB Saunders Company; 2002. p. 146–60.
32. Hughlett J. The Virginia opossum, *Didelphis virginiana*, orphan care handbook. Baltimore (MD): The National Opossum Society; 2005.
33. Ness R, Booth R. Sugar gliders. In: Quesenberry K, Carpenter J, editors. Ferrets, rabbits, and rodents clinical medicine and surgery. 2nd edition. St. Louis (MO): Saunders; 2004. p. 330–8.
34. Hume I, Barboza P. Monotremes and marsupials: designing artificial diets for captive marsupials. In: Fowler M, editor. Zoo and wild animal medicine: current therapy. 3rd edition. Philadelphia: WB Saunders; 1993. p. 281–8.

35. Gamble K. Marsupial care and husbandry. Vet Clin Exotic An Pract 2004;7(2): 283–98.

36. Opossum Society of the United States. 2003. Available at: www.opossumsocietyus. org. Accessed July 7, 2008.

37. Booth R. General husbandry and medical care of sugar gliders. In: Bonagura J, editor. Kirk's current veterinary therapy XIII: small animal practice. Philadelphia: WB Saunders; 2000. p. 1157–63.

38. Johnson-Delaney C. Common procedures in hedgehogs, prairie dogs, exotic rodents, and companion marsupials. Vet Clin Exotic An Pract 2006;9(2):415–35.

Nutrition and Behavior of Degus (*Octodon degus*)

Mark S. Edwards, PhD

KEYWORDS

- *Octodon degus* • Degu • Nutrition • Diet
- Behavior • Management

DESCRIPTION

Three extant species in the genus *Octodon* are each commonly described as degus.[1] *Octodon degus* (degu or trumpet-tailed rat) is a caviomorph rodent inhabiting subtropical to temperate savanna and scrub environments of the western slopes of northern and central Chile.[1–4] *Octodon degus* are semifossorial, diurnal, and live in colonial or familial groups of 5 to 10 animals.[2,5]

Considered an agricultural pest in some regions of its natural range,[2] *O. degus* adapts well to most laboratory conditions for research on reproduction, diabetes mellitus, and cataract development.[1,4] Objective information regarding husbandry, nutrition, and behavior, generated from their documented care under controlled research conditions, can be applied to care of degus kept as companion animals or in other managed environments.

Gastrointestinal Tract

Ocotdon degus are herbivorous, with microbial fermentation of ingesta occurring in a large, haustrated cecum after gastric and autoenzymatic digestion. Other species with similar adaptations for postgastric fermentation of digesta by symbiotic microorganisms include guinea pigs (*Cavia porcellus*), hamsters (*Mesocricetus auratus*), and voles (*Microtus townsendii*).[6]

The species dental formula is i 1/1, c 0/0, p 1/1, m 3/3, total = 20.[7] Incisor enamel is pale orange.[3] Premolars and molars, which are flat-crowned and hypsodont, have deeply infolded margins in the mid-region resembling a figure-eight, thus leading to the family and genus name.[1,3,7] Continually growing teeth are maintained in proper condition by chewing various substrates, including fibrous foods, nontoxic wood,

Comparative Animal Nutrition, Animal Science Department, California Polytechnic State University, 1 Grand Avenue, 010-0147, San Luis Obispo, CA 93407-0255, USA
E-mail address: msedward@calpoly.edu

Vet Clin Exot Anim 12 (2009) 237–253
doi:10.1016/j.cvex.2009.01.003
1094-9194/09/$ – see front matter © 2009 Published by Elsevier Inc.

vetexotic.theclinics.com

soil during digging, and commercially available rodent tooth conditioners (eg, pumice stone blocks).[8-10]

The stomach is simple (eg, lacking off-sets or chambers) and glandular.[11] The small intestine, the primary site of nutrient absorption, is not described in current literature. The cecum has longitudinal muscular bands (taeniae), separated by diverticulations (haustra).[11] Such cecal structures create fermentation chambers in which digesta are digested by symbiotic microbial organisms (alloenzymatic digestion).[6,11] Fermentive digestion is beneficial, as it allows the host to use structural carbohydrates for energy, amino acids, water-soluble vitamins, and vitamin K produced by gut microbes. Carbon dioxide and methane are both end-products of fermentive digestion the host animal cannot absorb. Methane is produced by microoganisms in the degu hindgut at a rate of 2-nmol per gram feces per hour.[12]

The colon of *O. degus* lacks the haustra seen in the cecum.[11] Colonic absorption of water from digesta, driven by an osmotic gradient associated with transepithelial sodium chloride transport and mediated by water channels like aquaporin-1, results in a high degree of fecal dehydration.[13]

When consuming *ad libitum* quantities of an experimental diet (**Table 1**), degus had a total gastrointestinal tract transit time (eg, first appearance of an indigestible marker in feces) of 5.1 hours for particulate digesta and 5.2 hours for fluid.[14] In the same study, total tract mean retention time was 15.5 hours for particulates and 19.4 hours for fluid.[14] When *ad libitum* food was offered, higher dry matter intake resulted in longer mean retention time.[15] Degus, like guinea pigs, do not selectively retain liquid digesta in the hindgut, as compared to particulate digesta.[14]

Ocotdon degus are coprophagic (eg, re-ingest feces). One study reported 38% of feces produced in 24 hours were re-ingested, with 87% of this activity at night.[16] This behavior is normal and commonly practiced by herbivores with hindgut fermentation, as an adaptation to recover nutrients not initially absorbed from the feces. Coprophagy occurs in juveniles as young as 3 days of age and may inoculate the hindgut with beneficial bacteria.[17]

Feeding Ecology

Octodon degus is fundamentally herbivorous, ingesting mainly herbaceous foliage (60.0% by volume).[18,19] Seasonally, seeds of shrubs, rather than herbaceous plants, become a significant part of the diet.[18,19] Free-ranging degus consumed significantly higher amounts of new leaves than mature leaves of three plant species.[20] This preference may be because young plants contain more moisture and protein and less structural carbohydrate than mature plants of the same species. Free-ranging degus preferred to eat low-fiber, high-protein plants when allowed to choose among five different plant species.[21]

When offered *ad libitum* quantities of an experimental diet (see **Table 1**), degus consumed a lower, although not statistically different, absolute amount than two other rodent species, and they lost weight.[14] When offered *ad libitum* quantities of experimental diets, adult degus ingested (dry matter intake or DMI) 10.2 g to 15.1 g per day or 57.8 g to 94.2 g per body weight (BW_{kg}) per day (**Table 2**). DMI of growing *O. degus* was 56.1 g to 67.5 g per day, or 323.5 g to 355.1 g per BW_{kg} per day (see **Table 2**). Intake was not influenced by changes in food availability. Animals offered food for only 5 hours or 11 hours during a 24-hour period consumed as much as those with 24-hour access to the same diet.[16]

Dry matter digestibility of an alfalfa-based, high-fiber diet was 53%.[16] Across a wide range of plant-based diets, similar levels of dry matter digestibility (51.6%–69.9%) have been reported (see **Table 2**).

NUTRIENT AND ENERGY REQUIREMENTS
Energy

Basal metabolic rate (BMR), the amount of energy expended while at rest, in a thermo-neutral zone in a postabsorptive state of *O. degus* is 0.839 to 0.930 mL O_2 per BW_g per hour (approximately 82.06–90.96 kJ per day).[11,22,23] Daily energy expenditure (DEE) ranged seasonally from 125.0 to 155.9 kJ per day.[24] Compared to BMR (kJ per day) measured for the seasons, DEE was 1.6 to 2.2 times higher.[24] A generalized formula to predict average daily metabolic rate (kJ per day) in rodents, 358.53 $(BW_{kg}^{0.54})$, produces values comparable to measurements described above.[25] For example, an adult degu weighing 175 g, is estimated to require 139.9 kJ per day [358.53 $(0.175^{0.54})$].

Dietary energy is derived from carbohydrates, lipids, and proteins. When measured as part of controlled feeding studies, daily digestible energy intake (DEI) of animals at maintenance ranged from 181.0 to 250.8 kJ (1,091–1,565 kJ per BW_{kg}) (see **Table 2**). Similar measurements taken during growth ranged from 636.0 to 746.1 kJ (3,668–3990 kJ per BW_{kg}) (see **Table 2**).[26] Energy intake during growth is typically two to three times that of maintenance.[25]

A practical diet used to support a nonreproductive colony of female degus provided 336.5 kJ per animal per day (**Tables 3** and **4**). This dietary energy level is higher than required for DEI at maintenance and the body weight of these animals is on the upper end of the range reported (**Table 5**).

Structural Carbohydrates (Fiber)

Plant fiber is a significant dietary component of *O. degus*. *Octodon* was classified among herbivores consuming more than 200 g crude fiber per kg DM.[11] Degus' gastro-intestinal tracts are structurally adapted to promote symbiotic microbial digestion of plant fiber (eg, cellulose, hemicellulose); their behavior (eg, coprophagy) also increases their ability to utilize this abundant food source. Grasses consumed by free-ranging degu at Quebrada del a Plata contained 61.1% neutral detergent fiber (NDF) during the dry season (summer) and 37.3% NDF during the wet season (fall–winter).[26] Apparent digestibility of an experimental diet with 30.5% NDF and 17.4% acid deter-gent fiber or ADF (dry matter basis or DMB) was 47.1% and 34.9%, respectively.

Two commercially available rodent diets (Prolab RMH 2000 Diet, 5P06, PMI Nutrition International, Saint Louis, Missouri; Laboratory Rodent Diet, 5001, PMI Nutrition International, Saint Louis, Missouri) (see **Table 1**), with moderate levels of structural carbohydrate (12.3% NDF with 4.4% ADF, and 15.6% NDF with 6.7% ADF, respec-tively) successfully support degus in all life stages.[4] Another practical diet used to support a colony of nonreproductive female degus contained 49.3% NDF and 31.7% ADF (DMB) (see **Table 3**).

Nonstructural Carbohydrates (Sugars, Starch)

Plant parts consumed by free-ranging degus are naturally lower in nonstructural carbohydrates, such as sugars and starch. Over-consumption of foods containing high levels of these carbohydrates could be detrimental to microbial organisms in the hindgut, as well as to the host animal. Elevated consumption of nonstructural carbohydrates has been implicated in the onset of clinical disease, including obesity, diabetes mellitus, and related illnesses, although the specific threshold at which detri-mental effects occur has not been quantified.

Although sugar and starch concentrations of animal foods are not often reported by manufacturers, they are collectively represented in neutral detergent soluble

Table 1
Selected nutrient composition of foods used in feeding *Octodon degus*[a,b]

Description	Dry Matter, %	Gross Energy, kJ/g	Crude Protein, %	Lysine, %	Crude Fat (EE), %	Linoleic Acid, %	Crude Fiber, %	ND Fiber, %	AD Fiber, %	NFE, %	NDSC, %	Ash, %	Source
High-fiber herbivore, (ADF-25) pellet	90.0	—	14.3	0.56	3.0	1.5	21.0	39.1	25.5	43.4	25.3	8.3	f
	100	—	15.9	0.62	3.3	1.7	23.3	43.4	28.3	48.2	28.2	9.2	
Rodent diet, 5001[c]	89.1	14.06	23.9	1.41	5.0	1.22	5.1	15.6	6.7	48.7	37.6	7.0	4
	100	15.62	26.8	1.58	5.6	1.37	5.7	17.5	7.5	54.7	42.2	7.9	
Rat chow, 5012[c]	89.0	17.32	23.2	1.35	5.0	2.25	3.8	13.1	4.9	51.2	41.1	6.6	39
	100	19.91	26.1	1.52	5.6	2.53	4.2	14.7	5.5	57.5	46.2	7.4	
Prolab[c] RMH2000, 5P06	89.6	17.87	19.9	1.03	9.6	4.93	3.2	12.3	4.4	50.8	41.3	6.5	4
	100	19.86	22.2	1.15	10.7	5.50	3.6	13.7	4.9	56.7	46.1	7.3	
Rabbit food pellet	90.6	18.40	20.0	—	3.0	—	16.5	37.8	19.8	40.3	19.0	10.8	5
	100	20.30	22.1	—	3.3	—	18.2	41.7	21.9	44.5	21.0	11.9	
Alfalfa food pellet	90.8	17.80	12.4	—	1.5	—	29.7	45.1	34.6	39.0	23.5	8.2	5
	100	19.60	13.7	—	1.7	—	32.7	49.7	38.1	43.0	25.9	9.0	
Experimental diet	99.5	—	17.8	—	7.9	—	13.7	30.3	17.3	52.5	35.9	7.6	14
	100	—	17.9	—	7.9	—	13.8	30.5	17.4	52.8	36.1	7.6	
Low-fiber diet[d]	90	15.26	17.5	—	—	—	—	31.5	—	—	—	—	46
	100	16.96	19.4	—	—	—	—	35.0	—	—	—	—	
Medium-fiber diet[d]	90	15.15	11.3	—	—	—	—	42.3	—	—	—	—	46
	100	16.83	12.5	—	—	—	—	47.0	—	—	—	—	
High-fiber diet[d]	90	14.99	7.7	—	—	—	—	51.3	—	—	—	—	46
	100	16.66	8.5	—	—	—	—	57.0	—	—	—	—	

	%DMB										Ref
High fiber–high, tannic acid diet[d]	90	16.20	13.3	—	—	46.7	28.8	—	—	—	26
	100	18.00	14.8	—	—	51.9	32.0	—	—	—	
Low fiber–low, tannic acid diet[d]	90	16.13	13.0	—	—	38.4	18.3	—	—	—	26
	100	17.92	14.4	—	—	42.7	20.3	—	—	—	
Low fiber–high, tannic acid diet[d]	90	16.16	14.6	—	—	39.2	18.5	—	—	—	26
	100	17.95	16.2	—	—	43.6	20.5	—	—	—	
High fiber–low, tannic acid diet[d]	90	16.25	14.8	—	—	46.4	27.5	—	—	—	26
	100	18.05	16.4	—	—	51.5	30.6	—	—	—	
Alfalfa pellets[d]	90	—	12.3	1.5	29.5	44.7	34.3	—	—	—	16
	100	—	13.7	1.7	32.8	49.7	38.1	—	—	—	
Commercial rabbit, pellet	90.6	16.7	18.1	2.7	14.9	34.2	17.9	45.0	25.7	9.8	33
	100	18.4	20.0	3.0	16.5	37.8	19.8	49.7	28.4	10.8	
Milk, O. degus	26.9	4.0	4.4	17.3	—	—	—	3.1[e]	—	2.7	33
	100	14.9	16.4	64.3	—	—	—	11.5[e]	—	10.0	

Abbreviations: AD, acid detergent; ADF, acid detergent fiber; DMB, dry matter basis; ND, neutral detergent; NDSC, neutral detergent soluble carbohydrates; NFE, nitrogen-free extract

a NFE,% (DMB) = 100,%–crude protein,%–crude fat,%–crude fiber–ash,% (all DMB).
b NDSC,% (DMB) = 100,%–crude protein,%–crude fat,%–neutral detergent fiber,%–ash,% (all DMB).
c Manufactured by PMI Nutrition International, Saint Louis, Missouri.
d Estimated dry matter content based on personal communication with author.
e Lactose, measured by anthrona method.
f Mark S. Edwards, PhD, Smithsonian National Zoological Park, unpublished data, 2007.

Table 2
Body weight, dry matter intake, digestible energy intake, and apparent digestibility of dry matter, gross energy, and neutral detergent fiber demonstrated by *Octodon degus* fed several experimental diets

Gender	BW, g	Diet Type[a]	DMI, g	DMI, g per BWkg	DEI, kJ	DEI, kJ per BWkg	Digestibility DM, %	GE, %	NDF, %	Source
B	177.0	Experimental cubed diet	10.23	57.8	—	—	69.9	—	47.1	14
M	175.6	Low fiber, 35% NDF	13.4	76.5	221.5	1261	63.3	62.1	38.1	46
M	165.9	Medium fiber, 47% NDF	10.8	65.1	181.0	1091	54.9	56.4	34.9	46
M	160.3	High fiber, 57% NDF	15.1	94.2	250.8	1565	49.7	46.8	33.1	46
U	192.7	High fiber–high tannic acid	67.5	350.3	708.0	3674	57.3	58.9	—	26
U	187.0	Low fiber–low tannic acid	66.4	355.1	746.1	3990	62.9	62.2	—	26
U	173.4	Low fiber–high tannic acid	56.1	323.5	636.0	3668	65.1	63.5	—	26
U	176.8	High fiber–low tannic acid	60.4	341.5	670.0	3790	61.7	61.7	—	26
U	170.4	Alfalfa pellet, 24-h availability	15.08	88.5	—	—	51.6	—	—	16

Abbreviations: B, both male and female; DEI, digestible energy intake; DM, dry matter; F, female; GE, gross energy; M, male; NDF, neutral detergent fiber; U, gender unreported.
[a] Nutrient composition of each diet type provided in **Table 1**.

carbohydrates (NDSC) or nitrogen-free extract (NFE) (see footnote, **Table 1**). Two commercial rodent diets containing 54.7% to 56.7% NDSC and 42.2% to 46.1% NFE supported *Octodon* in a laboratory environment without clinical signs associated with excessive intake of nonstructural carbohydrates.[4] Another practical diet used to support a colony of nonreproductive female degus contained 26.3% NDSC (DMB) (see **Table 3**).

Protein

Octodon degus require dietary essential amino acids, including lysine, which are collectively included in the analytical measurement, crude protein. Diets used to support laboratory colonies of *Octodon* contained 1.15% to 1.58% lysine and 54.7% to 56.7% crude protein (DMB) (see **Table 1**).[4] A practical diet used to support a colony of nonreproductive female degus contained 0.58% lysine and 13.5% crude protein (DMB) (see **Table 3**).

Lipids

A commercial rodent diet (Prolab RMH 2000 Diet 5P06, PMI Nutrition International, Saint Louis, Missouri), containing 10.7% crude fat and 5.5% linoleic acid (DMB) (see **Table 1**) improved weight gain and health in lactating females and pups when compared to a similar diet (Laboratory Rodent Diet 5001, PMI Nutrition International, Saint Louis, Missouri) containing 5.6% crude fat and 1.37% linoleic acid (DMB) (see **Table 1**).[4] To avoid obesity, degus should be switched at 3 months of age from a higher fat diet to a lower fat diet.[4] Another practical diet used successfully to support a colony of nonreproductive female degus contained 3.0% crude fat and 1.1% linoleic acid (DMB) (see **Table 3**).

Minerals

Little information on the mineral requirements of *Octodon* is published. Commercial diets formulated for other rodent species sustain *Octodon* through all life stages. The mineral composition of a practical diet used to support a colony of nonreproductive female degus is listed in **Table 3**. Until data specific to degus are available, dietary guidelines for macro- and trace-minerals should be based on those described for rats (see **Table 3**).[27]

Vitamins

Concentrations of fat- and water-soluble vitamins provided in natural-ingredient diets formulated for other rodent species (eg, rats, mice) appear adequate for degus (see **Table 3**). Controlled studies to determine vitamin requirements of degus, with the exception of ascorbic acid (vitamin C) (see below), have not yet been reported. Fat- and water-soluble vitamin content of a practical diet used to support a colony of nonreproductive female degus is listed in **Table 3**. The ascorbic acid in this diet originated from produce (eg, greens, roots), not the pelleted portion, forages, or supplements.

Despite their taxonomic relatedness and similarities in diet and gastrointestinal tract physiology to guinea pigs, degus do not have a dietary requirement for ascorbic acid.[28] The activity of L-gulonolactone oxidase,[29] the hepatic enzyme required for *de novo* ascorbic acid synthesis from substrate precursors, was quantified in 20 male and 19 female degus, at 2.3 µmole per gram per hour and 3.5 µmole per gram per hour, respectively.[30] This level of enzyme activity supports the degu's lack of

Table 3

Example foods and quantities (as-fed basis) for feeding a single adult degu (*Octodon degus*) from the Smithsonian National Zoological Park (Washington, DC), calculated nutrient composition of the offered diet, and estimated nutrient requirements of rats (*Rattus norvegicus*)

Item	Food Type	Weight, g	Schedule
1	High fiber herbivore (ADF-25) pellet[a]	25	Daily
2	Greens, variable[b]	10	Daily
3	Roots, variable[c]	10	Daily
4	Mixed grass hay[d]	11	Daily

Nutrient	Diet conc.	Rat reqt.
Proximate		
DM, %	64.41	nd
Crude protein, %	13.52	5.6
Lysine, %	0.58	0.12
Crude fat, %	3.03	5.6
Linoleic acid, %	1.10	0.7
NDF, %	49.30	nd
ADF, %	31.68	nd
Carbohydrate (NDSC), %[e]	26.26	nd
Minerals		
Ash, %	7.89	nd
Calcium, %	0.85	0.56
Phosphorus, %	0.51	0.33
Sodium, %	0.22	0.06

Nutrient	Diet conc.	Rat reqt.
Energy		
Metabolizable, kJ/g	9.33	nd
Fat soluble vitamins		
Vitamin A, IU/kg	4,505	2,556
Beta-carotene, mg/kg	69.6	1.3
Vitamin D, IU/kg	832	1,111
Vitamin E, mg/kg	271	20
Vitamin K, mg/kg	5.5	1.1
Water soluble vitamins		
Thiamin, ppm	8.9	4.4
Riboflavin, ppm	8.1	3.3
Pyridoxine, ppm	1.4	6.7
Niacin, ppm	73	17
Biotin, ppb	374	222

Nutrient			Nutrient		
Potassium, %	1.57	0.40	Choline, ppm	797	833
Magnesium, %	0.25	0.06	Pantothenic acid, ppm	25	11
Iron, ppm	269	39	Cyanocobalamin, ppb	15.9	55.6
Copper, ppm	16.7	5.6	Vitamin C, ppm	358.5	0.0
Manganese, ppm	152.2	11.1	—	—	—
Selenium, ppm	0.29	0.17	—	—	—
Zinc, ppm	116.6	13.3	—	—	—

All nutrient concentrations, except dry matter, expressed on a dry matter basis.[27,37]

Abbreviations: DM, dry matter; nd, not determined.

[a] High-fiber (ADF-25) herbivore pellet contains 15.9% crude protein, 3.3% crude fat, 28.3% acid detergent fiber (DMB) (see Table 1).

[b] Variable greens may include, but are not limited to, kale, collard greens, romaine lettuce, dandelion greens.

[c] Variable roots may include, but are not limited to, beets, carrot, parsnip, sweet potato, turnip.

[d] Mixed grass hay includes multiple cool-season grass species, including, but not limited to, orchard grass (*Dactylis glomerata*), brome (*Bromus inermis*), or timothy (*Phleum pratense*).

[e] NDSC, % = 100 − (crude protein,% + crude fat, % + neutral detergent fiber, % + ash, %) (all on DM basis).

Table 4
Distribution of mass, dry matter, and metabolizable energy of foods and diet for feeding a single adult degu (*Octodon degus*) from the Smithsonian National Zoological Park (Washington, DC)[a]

Food Item	Amount, g	Dry Matter, %	g	Metabolizable Energy, kJ per g (Fresh Weight)	kJ	% Distribution
Concentrate	25.0	92.00	23.0	8.79	219.8	65.3
Greens	10.0	15.54	1.6	2.09	20.9	6.2
Roots	10.0	12.21	1.2	1.80	18.0	5.4
Forage	11.0	93.60	10.3	7.07	77.8	23.1
Total	56.0	—	36.1	—	336.5	100

[a] Details of diet provided in **Table 2**.

a dietary requirement of ascorbic acid.[30] When degus were maintained on a diet with either a low (< 1 mg per day) or high (100 mg per day) level of ascorbic acid, there was no difference between L-gulonolactone oxidase activity; however, there was a significant increase in liver concentrations of ascorbate between the two treatments.[30] From an applied perspective, two commercially available rodent diets fed successfully to research colonies of *O. degus* through multiple life-stages[4] did not contain supplemental ascorbic acid. At this time, there is no evidence to support the addition of ascorbic acid to diets fed to this species.

Water

Free-ranging degus experience geographic and seasonal changes in availability of preformed water (ie, water contained in food).[18,19] They are adapted to survive during periods of limited water supply.[13]

Water influx varies seasonally: summer, 10.3 mL per day (22.8% of expected value, 45.2 mL per day); winter, 40.4 mL per day (88.8% of expected value, 45.2 mL per day).[31] As one would predict, urine osmolality also varies seasonally: summer, 3,137 mosmol per kg; winter, 1,123 mosmol per kg; mean, 4,338 mosmol per kg.[32]

One unsupported reference suggests chlorinated tap water should not be given to captive degus, because degus' "body cannot deal with" chlorine.[8] For animals in managed environments, potable water should be available at all times; however, the need to avoid chlorinated water from municipal sources requires further study.

LIFE STAGE CONSIDERATIONS
Neonates

Octodon degus are precocial, fully furred, with upper and lower teeth and eyes open at birth.[1,4,17,33] Young can support their own weight and walk in a coordinated manner at birth.[17] Mean birth weight was 14.6 plus or minus 0.4 g (males, n = 20; females, n = 15)[17] (see **Table 5**). Mean growth rate from birth (day 0) to 28 days was 2 g per day.[17]

Juveniles are weaned after 4 to 6 weeks of nursing,[7,11,34] although individuals can survive after nursing for just 2 to 3 weeks.[3,33] Free-ranging adults harvest and carry fresh grass to burrows for young to eat.[2] First solid foods may be consumed as early as day 6.5.[11] Juveniles should have access to components of the adult diet within the first week of life. No additional or modified foods are recommended at this age.

Breeding

Degus are sexually mature at 6 months (range 45 days to 20 months),[3,11] at which time breeding pairs may be formed.[4] Females have no regular estrous cycle.[1] The presence of a male to induce ovulation has been suggested.[1,9]

Table 5
Body weight of *Octodon degus* at birth and at various ages

Age	Age, d	Gender	Body Weight Mean ± SD, g	Range, g	n	Location	Source
Birth	0	B	14.6	—	35	Bronx, New York, USA	17
	0	U	14.1	—	—	—	11
Neonate (1–21 d)	7	B	22.7 ± 1.0	—	35	Bronx, New York, USA	17
	14	B	34.8 ± 2.0	—	35	Bronx, New York, USA	17
	21	B	49.4 ± 4.0	—	35	Bronx, New York, USA	17
Juvenile (22–30 d)	28	M	72.7	—	20	Bronx, New York, USA	17
	28	F	66.4	—	15	Bronx, New York, USA	17
Sub-adult (1–5 mos)	63	M	145.5 ± 3.6	—	20	Bronx, New York, USA	17
	63	F	130.3 ± 4.0	—	15	Bronx, New York, USA	17
Adult (≥ 6 mos)		B	195.0	—	52	Santiago, Chile	44
		B	177.0	—	8	Okayama, Japan	14
	—	M	—	270–273	7	Williamsburg, VA, USA	46
	—	F	113 ± 14.5	—	5	Parque Nacional Fray Jorge	21
	—	U	173.4 ± 5.2	—	5	Santiago, Chile	26
	—	U	176.8 ± 7.4	—	5	Santiago, Chile	26
	—	U	187.0 ± 8.6	—	5	Santiago, Chile	26
	—	U	192.7 ± 6.9	—	5	Santiago, Chile	26
	—	U	179.7 ± 27.1	—	10	San Carlos de Apoquindo, Chile	15
	—	M	198.3 ± 45.3	143.0–314.3	17	Santiago, Chile	5
	—	F	184.3 ± 32.3	112.4–250.5	38	Santiago, Chile	5
	—	B	186.2 ± 14.4	—	9	San Carlos de Apoquindo, Chile	31
	—	B	187.8 ± 11.8	—	6	San Carlos de Apoquindo, Chile	31
	—	B	182.2 ± 13.3	—	9	Santiago, Chile	24
	—	B	184.3 ± 15.0	—	7	Santiago, Chile	24
	—	B	181.2 ± 15.0	—	7	Santiago, Chile	24
	—	B	206.5 ± 17.8	—	5	Santiago, Chile	24
	—	M	211.3 ± 39.7	—	11	Lampa, Chile	31
	—	F	227.9 ± 5.5	—	12	Quebrada de la Plata, Chile	47
	—	F	243.3 ± 33.9	176.0–315.0	18	Washington, DC, USA	a

Abbreviations: B, both male and female; F, female; M, male; U, gender unreported.
[a] Mark S. Edwards, PhD, Smithsonian National Zoological Park, unpublished data, 2007.

In central Chile, *O. degus* has a pattern of seasonal reproduction characterized by two peaks of parturition (early and late spring) and a nonreproductive period between summer and winter.[33] Captive colonies in the northern hemisphere breed throughout the year.[1,3] Females can produce more than one annual litter.[1,3]

The diets of captive degus are higher in nutrient density and quality than those consumed by free-ranging animals. Additionally, captive diets are more consistent in nutrient and energy content. Thus, no additional or modified foods are indicated for breeding individuals.

Gestation

Gestation ranges from 90 to 93 days.[1,3,8,33] A mean litter size of 5.0 to 6.8 has been reported,[1,3,11,34] with a range of 1 to 10 young per litter.[1,3] Because of the consistent nutrient composition of captive-degu diets, no additional or modified foods are indicated for females during gestation.

Lactation

Lactation is the most energy-demanding life stage for females.[11,35] Among free-ranging degus, these higher energy demands are met through increased food intake, not through selective consumption of higher energy foods.[35] This finding suggests there is no need for supplemental or modified foods for lactating captive degus; however, the diet typically offered should not be limited during this period.

Octodon degus milk, with average total solids (DM) of 26.9 plus or minus 5.8%, is relatively dilute, with no significant variation in composition during the 35- to 40-day lactation period (see **Table 1**).[11,33] Lipids (crude fat) are the major source of milk energy (70%).[33]

Female degus possess four pairs of ventral mammae.[3] Nursing bouts average 25 minutes. While nursing, juveniles are huddled lying on their backs.[34] Offspring of multiple females may nurse a single female simultaneously (promiscuous nursing).[34] Females typically terminate nursing when they leave the nest or when the young leave them.[34]

Geriatrics

Captive *O. degus* typically live 7 to 10 years.[3,8] Diet modifications based on age alone are not appropriate; however, health and disease issues commonly associated with advanced age may necessitate diet changes (see below). Additionally, age-associated changes in dentition (eg, malocclusion, fractures, and loss) may require dietary modifications to facilitate mastication.

ASSESSMENT CRITERIA
Morphometrics

Degus are moderate-sized animals with a head and body length of 125 mm to 195 mm and a tail length of 105 mm to 165 mm.[3] Body weights range from 170 g to 300 g (see **Table 5**).[7] A target body weight for adult females (250 g) has been practically applied to the management of one population. (Mark S. Edwards, PhD, Smithsonian National Zoological Park, unpublished data, 2007).

Fecal Output

Daily fecal output has been reported at 5.04 g, 4.8 g, and 7.92 g (DMB) from degus fed 35%, 47%, and 57% NDF diets, respectively.[36] When offered *ad libitum* quantities of a pelleted, alfalfa-based diet and maintained on a photoperiod of 13 hours of light/11 hours of darkness, *O. degus* excreted 7.30 g of fecal DM, with 4.96 g excreted during the light period and 2.34 g excreted during the dark period.[16] Use of fecal output to assess food intake and gut function should take into consideration the species' coprophagic behavior.

MANAGEMENT OF CLINICAL ILLNESS RELATED TO NUTRITION
Diabetes

Spontaneous lesions, including cataracts, amyloidosis, and hyperplasia of the islets of Langerhans, most frequently associated with diabetes mellitus, have been reported in O. degus.[1,37] As with guinea pigs, degu insulin and the C-terminal region of glucagon are highly divergent from that of other mammals.[37,38] Hystricomorph rodent insulin is only 1% to 10% as biologically active as the insulin of other mammals.[38]

Despite these differences, O. degus have compensatory mechanisms, such as increased insulin receptors and potentially higher insulin concentrations, to maintain normal blood-glucose concentrations, plus physiologic responses that follow typical mammalian patterns.[38] When degus with normal circulating glucose levels (< 140 mg/dL) were compared with individuals with elevated glucose levels (> 200 mg/dL), there were no differences observed (such as unidentified pancreatic alpha-cell crystals or islet amyloidosis).[39] Glucose concentrations of O. degus documented in the laboratory and field were 4.34 mM ± 0.22 mM and 4.54 mM ± 0.58 mM (range 3.89 –5.39 mM; $n = 16$), respectively.[38]

Fibrous plants selected by free-ranging O. degus are naturally low in simple carbohydrates (eg, sugars, starch). Consumption of foods higher in nonstructural carbohydrates, combined with unique species adaptations (described above), may contribute to the increased incidence of diabetes mellitus observed in captive degus.

Cataracts and Lens Lesions

In degus, polyol compounds, converted from glucose or galactose by aldose reductase (AR), accumulate in lens fibers, resulting in swelling, rupture, and subsequent cataract formation.[40] When AR activity levels in gerbil and rat lenses are compared, degus demonstrated significantly higher AR activity.[40] Cataracts formed within 4 weeks following experimental induction of diabetes in degus.[40] Blood-glucose levels in these animals were greater than or equal to 500 mg/dL, as compared to levels of less than or equal to 120 mg/dL in clinically normal animals.[40] Elevated blood-glucose concentrations in diabetic degus, combined with an overall higher AR activity in all degus, may increase the species risk for diabetic cataract formation when compared with other rodents. The involvement of AR is further demonstrated by the prevention of cataract formation in diabetic degus receiving 0.04% sorbinil (CP 45634), a potent AR inhibitor.[40]

SOCIAL BEHAVIOR

Octodon degus is colonial, forming extended family groups of up to 100 individuals.[8,41] Neonates, juveniles, and weaned subadults maintained in isolation demonstrate behavioral and neural deficits not observed in parent-reared animals.[42] Male degus may be found with harems of up to 20 females.[8] In captivity, housing multiple males with one or more females may result in undesired aggression between males.[8]

Species communication mechanisms are tactile, visual, auditory, and olfactory. Initial contact between two O. degus may result in nose-to-nose contact, continued by sniffing and nuzzling body areas such as the perineum, rump, and neck.[34] Octodon frequently solicit allo-grooming by presenting the throat or moving the forehead under a con-specific's chin.[34] Bouts of allo-grooming may last 10 to 15 minutes.[34] Olfactory information may be exchanged when degus communicate tactiley.[34]

Octodon demonstrate a wide range of visual communication. Courting males, maintaining a submissive posture while approaching a female, will wag and vibrate their tails while trembling their forefeet or bodies.[34] Similar tail movements during agonistic encounters may be a defensive mechanism to repulse opponents.[34] A tail-up rump display may also be exhibited during agonistic encounters between males, or between a male and female.[34] A locomotor-rotational movement, or "frisky-hop," described in *Octodon*, is often associated with play.[34]

Degus make a variety of mechanical and vocal sounds.[34] Alarm calls (sharp squeaks) alert con-specifics.[34,43] Tooth chatter and hind foot thumping are warning sounds associated with agonistic behavior.[34,43] When captive degus are aroused, but not frightened, they will make a call that sounds like "chuck-wee."[43] The postcopulatory calls produced by males are very uniform and repetitive.[43]

Octodon also use chemical communication.[34] When introduced to a novel enclosure, degus often urinate and display an anogenital drag. Following contact with the scent of a strange or known con-specific, degus scent-mark the substrate.[34] During scent marking, degus deposit more urine marks over the urine of same-sexed individuals.[34] The odor of a con-specific may stimulate further scent-marking. In the wild, preferred sand bathing sites are saturated with urine and anal gland secretions, resulting in a common scent among group members.[34]

Male degus adopt a tripedal stance during enurination (ie, urine spraying on female) associated with courtship.[34] Additional behaviors reported during courtship include mutual grooming, tail wagging, and body trembling.[34]

A reproductively active but nonresponsive female may threaten or lunge at a courting male.[34] Female degus are sexually receptive for several hours.[34] Copulation involves multiple, thrusting intromissions, each 10 seconds long. Males ejaculate multiple times. Ejaculatory intromission ranges from 12 to 18 seconds.[34]

Independence from mother's milk (nutritional weaning) is not necessarily concurrent with behavioral independence from the mother (social weaning).[34] *Octodon* males do not urinate over or play with young, as seen in related species, but do spend time huddling over young.[41] Males spend less time in contact with offspring than females.[44] Pairs show contact-promoting behavior, such as grooming, at all times.[34]

ABIOTIC FACTORS
Housing, Light, Temperature, and Humidity

Degus have been successfully housed in wire-mesh or solid-bottom enclosures, although wire-mesh bottom enclosures may be associated with the development of bumble-foot.[1,8] Ground corn-cob bedding is a suitable, although indigestible, substrate.[1,4] Access one to two times a week to a container filled with a fine, clean dust commercially available for rodent bathing is recommended.[8,9]

Artificial light cycles with 12 to 14 hours of light daily have been successfully used with captive degu colonies.[1,4] The thermal neutral zone and body temperature of *O. degus* is 24°C to 32°C and 37.2°C ± 0.4°C, respectively.[45] Free-ranging animals demonstrate a cyclic, bimodal rhythm of activity, at 0830 hours and 1930 hours, retreating to underground burrows during the warmest part of the day to avoid temperatures above 32°C.[45] Recommended levels for environmental temperature and relative humidity are 24°C ± 1°C and 50%, respectively.[1]

SUMMARY

Octodon degus are herbivorous rodents that are adapted anatomically and behaviorally to utilize a fibrous diet with moderate-to-low levels of nonstructural carbohydrate.

Captive degus should consume foods containing nutrients comparable to those consumed by free-ranging animals. The species is highly social, demonstrating a broad array of communication methods that make them appealing as a companion animal species. Controlled research studies with degus have produced a wealth of information that facilitates the care of this species in captivity.

ACKNOWLEDGEMENTS

The author expresses sincere appreciation for the contributions of Smithsonian National Zoological Park (Washington, DC), Francisco Bozinovic, Laura Lickel and Cassandra Lockhart to the manuscript.

REFERENCES

1. Fine J, Quimby FW, Greenhouse DD. Annotated bibliography on uncommonly used laboratory animals: mammals. ILAR News 1986;29(4):3A–38A.
2. Fulk GW. Notes of the activity, reproduction, and social behavior of *Octodon degus*. J Mammal 1976;57:495–505.
3. Nowak RM. Mammals of the World. Sixth edition. Baltimore (MD): The Johns Hopkins University Press; 1999. p. 1681–2.
4. Lee TM. *Octodon degus*: a diurnal, social, and long-lived rodent. ILAR J 2004; 45(1):14–24.
5. Veloso C, Bozinovic F. Effect of food quality on the energetics of reproduction in a precocial rodent, *Octodon degus*. J Mamm 2000;81(4):971–8.
6. Stevens CE, Hume ID. Digesta transit and retention. In: Comparative Physiology of the Vertebrate Digestive System. Second edition. New York: Cambridge University Press; 1995. p. 118–51.
7. Woods CA, Boraker DK. Octodon degus. Mamm Species 1975;67:1–5.
8. Griffiths-Irwin D, Davis J. How To Care for Your Degu. England (UK): Kingdom Books; 2001. p. 4–34.
9. Vanderlip S. Degus: A Complete Pet Owner's Manual. New York: Barron's; 2001. p. 5–93.
10. Ebensperger L, Bozinovic F. Energetics and burrowing behaviour in the semifossorial degu *Octodon degus* (Rodentia: Octondontidae). J Zool 2000;252:179–86.
11. Langer P. The digestive tract and life history of small mammals. Mamm Rev 2002; 32(2):107–31.
12. Hackstein JHP, van Alen TA. Fecal methanogens and vertebrate evolution. Evolution 1996;50(2):559–72.
13. Gallardo P, Olea N, Sepúlveda FV. Distribution of aquaporins in the colon of *Octodon degus*, a South American desert rodent. Am J Physiol Regul Integr Comp Physiol 2002;283:R779–88.
14. Sakaguchi E, Ohmura S. Fibre digestion and digesta retention time in guinea pigs (*Cavia porcellus*), degus (*Octodon degus*) and leaf-eared mice (*Phyllotis darwini*). Comp Biochem Physiol 1992;103A(4):787–91.
15. Bozinovic F, Torres-Contreras H. Does digestion rate affect diet selection? A study in *Octodon degus*, a generalist herbivorous rodent. Acta Theriol 1998;43(2): 205–12.
16. Kenagy GJ, Veloso C, Bozinovic F. Daily rhythms of food intake and feces reingestion in the degu, an herbivorous Chilean rodent: optimizing digestion through coprophagy. Physiol Biochem Zool 1999;72:78–86.
17. Reynolds TJ, Wright JW. Early postnatal physical and behavioural development of degus (*Octodon degus*). Lab Anim 1979;13:93–9.

18. Meserve PL. Trophic relationships among small mammals in a Chilean semiarid thorn scrub community. J Mamm 1981;62(2):304–14.
19. Meserve PL, Martin RE, Rodriguez J. Feeding ecology of two Chilean caviomorphs in a central Mediterranean savnna. J Mamm 1983;64(2):322–5.
20. Simonetti JA, Montenegro G. Food preferences by *Octodon degus* (Rodentia Caviomorpha): their role in the Chilean matorral composition. Oecologia 1981; 51:189–90.
21. Gutierrez J, Bozinovic F. Diet selection in captivity by a generalist herbivorous rodent (*Octodon degus*) from the Chilean coastal desert. J Arid Environ 1998; 39(4):601–7.
22. Bozinovic F. Rate of basal metabolism of grazing rodents from different habitats. J Mamm 1992;73(2):379–84.
23. Lovegrove BG. The zoogeography of mammalian basal metabolic rate. Am Nat 2000;156(2):201–19.
24. Bozinovic F, Bacigalupe LD, Vásquez RA, et al. Cost of living in free-ranging degus (*Octodon degus*): seasonal dynamics of energy expenditure. Comp Biochem Physiol 2004;137A:597–604.
25. Robbins CE. Wildlife Feeding and Nutrition. San Diego (CA): Academic Press; 1983.
26. Bozinovic F, Novoa FF, Sabat P. Feeding and digesting fiber and tannins by an herbivorous rodent, *Octodon degus* (Rodentia Caviomorpha). Comp Biochem Physiol 1997;118A(3):625–30.
27. National Research Council. Nutrient Requirements of Laboratory Animals. Fourth revised edition. Washington, DC: National Academy Press; 1995.
28. Long CV. Degu Information. Available at: www.degutopia.co.uk. Accessed on August 28, 2008.
29. Chatterjee IB. Evolution and the biosynthesis of ascorbic acid. Science 1973; 182(4118):1271–2.
30. Jenness R, Birney EC, Ayaz KL. Variation of L-gulonolactone oxidase activity in placental mammals. Comp Biochem Physiol 1980;67B:195–204.
31. Bozinovic F, Gallardo PA, Visser GH, et al. Seasonal acclimatization in water flux rate, urine osmolality and kidney water channels in free-living degus: molecular mechanisms, physiological processes and ecological implications. J Exp Biol 2003;206:2959–66.
32. Cortes A, Rosenmann M. A field lab method to determine urine concentration in small mammals. Comp Biochem Physiol 1989;94A(2):261–2.
33. Veloso C, Kenagy GJ. Temporal dynamics of milk composition of the precocial caviomorph *Octodon degus* (Rodentia Octodontidae). Rev Chil Hist Nat 2005; 78:247–52.
34. Kleiman DG. Patterns of behaviour in Hystricomorph rodents. Symp Zool Soc Lond 1974;34:171–209.
35. Veloso C, Bozinovic F. Dietary and digestive constraints on basal energy metabolism in a small herbivorous rodent. Ecology 1993;74(7):2003–10.
36. Bozinovic F. Nutritional energetics and digestive responses of an herbivorousrodent (Octodon degus) to different levels of dietary fiber. J Mamm 1995;76(2):627–37.
37. Nishi M, Steiner DF. Cloning of complementary DNAs encoding islet amyloid polypeptide, insulin, and glucagon precursors from a New World rodent, the degu, *Octodon degus*. Molecular Endo 1990;4:1192–8.
38. Opazo JC, Soto-Gamboa M, Bozinovic F. Blood glucose concentration in caviomorph rodents. Comp Biochem Physiol 2004;137A:57–64.
39. Spear GS, Caple MV, Sutherland LR. The pancreas of the degu. Exp Mol Pathol 1984;40:295 310.

40. Datiles MB, Fukui H. Cataract prevention in diabetic *Octodon degus* with Pfizer's sorbinil. Curr Eye Res 1989;8:233–7.
41. Wilson SC, Kleiman DG. Eliciting play: a comparative study. Am Zool 1974;14: 341–70.
42. Poeggel G, Nowicki L, Braun K. Early social deprivation alters monoaminergic afferents in the orbital prefrontal cortex of *Octodon degus*. Neuroscience 2003; 116:617–20.
43. Eisenberg JF. The function and motivational basis of Hystricomorph vocalizations. Symp Zool Soc Lond 1974;34:211–47.
44. Wilson S. Cataract-promoting behaviour, social development and relationship with parents in sibling juvenile degus (*Octodon degus*). Dev Psychobiol 1982; 15(3):257–68.
45. Rosenmann M. Regulacion termica en *Octodon degus*. Medio Ambiente 1977;3: 127–31.
46. Refinetti R. Rhythms of body temperature and temperature selection are out of phase in a diurnal rodent, *Octodon degus*. Physiol Behav 1996;60(3):959–61.
47. Bozinovic F, Vasquez RA. Patch use in a diurnal rodent: handling and searching under thermoregulatory costs. Funct Ecol 1999;13:602–10.

Nutrition, Care, and Behavior of Captive Prairie Dogs

John L. Hoogland, PhD[a],*, Dianne A. James[b], Lynda Watson[c]

KEYWORDS

- Black-tailed prairie dog • Captivity • Cynomys ludovicianus
- Diet • Diseases • Housing • Injuries

Prairie dogs are burrowing mammals that inhabit the grasslands of western North America. Coloniality is perhaps the most striking feature of these plump, brown, non-hibernating, herbivorous squirrels that stand approximately 30 cm (12 in) tall, weigh approximately 700 g (1.5 lb), and forage aboveground from dawn until dusk.[1] Despite their common name, prairie dogs are not dogs. They are rodents of the squirrel family (Sciuridae), and their close taxonomic relatives include ground squirrels (Spermophilus), marmots/woodchucks (Marmota), chipmunks (Eutamias and Tamias), tree squirrels (Sciurus and Tamiasciurus), and flying squirrels (Glaucomys). Biologists currently recognize five species of prairie dogs: black-tailed (Cynomys ludovicianus), Gunnison's (C. gunnisoni), Mexican (C. mexicanus), Utah (C. parvidens), and white-tailed (C. leucurus).[2,3] We limit our discussion to the black-tailed prairie dog, the most common species and the one most likely to be found in zoos and private homes.

Approximately 150 years ago, black-tailed prairie dogs (hereafter simply referred to as "prairie dogs") inhabited 14 states/provinces (Arizona, Chihuahua, Colorado, Kansas, Montana, Nebraska, New Mexico, North Dakota, Oklahoma, Saskatchewan, Sonora, South Dakota, Texas, and Wyoming) of three countries (Canada, Mexico, and United States).[4] The overall population size probably exceeded 5 billion. Ranchers and farmers have viewed prairie dogs as pests, however, and have shot and poisoned legions of them—often with assistance from state and federal agencies.[5,6] More recently, plague has killed millions of prairie dogs,[7] and urban development has eliminated some of the best prairie dog habitat. The current overall population is less than 2% of the number that Meriwether Lewis described as "infinite" 200 years ago.[4] The prairie dog is currently under consideration for the Federal List of Endangered and Threatened Wildlife and Plants.

[a] University of Maryland Center for Environmental Science, Appalachian Laboratory, 301 Braddock Road, Frostburg, MD, USA
[b] Midwest Prairie Dog Shelter, Post Office Box 135, Arcola, IN 46704-0135, USA
[c] PMS Recycled Vermin, 7525 West 19th Street, Lubbock, TX 79407, USA
* Corresponding author.
E-mail address: hoogland@al.umces.edu (J.L. Hoogland).

Vet Clin Exot Anim 12 (2009) 255–266
doi:10.1016/j.cvex.2009.01.013
1094-9194/09/$ – see front matter © 2009 Elsevier Inc. All rights reserved.

Whether or not one likes prairie dogs, they are hard to ignore. Their colony sites sometimes contain thousands of residents and extend for kilometers in all directions. The vegetation at colony sites is unusually short, because prairie dogs systematically consume or clip grasses and other herbs that grow taller than approximately 30 cm (12 in).[8] Colony sites contain hundreds of large mounds—up to 1 m (3.3 ft) high and 2 m (6.6 ft) wide—that surround each burrow-entrance. After emerging from their burrows at dawn, prairie dogs are conspicuous as they forage, fight, chase, "kiss," vocalize, and play aboveground until they submerge for the night at dusk.[1,8]

Because it has such a profound impact on the grassland ecosystem, the prairie dog is a "keystone species."[9] Their burrows, which can be as deep as 5 m (16.4 ft) and as long as 33 m (108 ft),[1,10] affect the cycling of water and minerals. Burrows also provide shelter and homes for a diverse array of animals, including burrowing owls (*Athene cunicularia*), tiger salamanders (*Ambystoma tigrinum*), and myriad insects and arachnids.[9] Prairie dogs serve as prey not only for terrestrial predators, such as American badgers (*Taxidea taxus*), black-footed ferrets (*Mustela nigripes*), bobcats (*Lynx rufus*), and coyotes (*Canis latrans*), but also for avian predators, such as ferruginous hawks (*Buteo regalis*), golden eagles (*Aquila chrysaetos*), and prairie falcons (*Falco mexicanus*) (**Fig. 1**).[1] Prairie dogs maintain short vegetation at their colony sites, and colony sites foster the growth of certain plants that are uncommon elsewhere, such as black nightshade (*Solanum americanum*), fetid marigold (*Dyssodia papposa*, also called prairie dog weed), pigweed (*Amaranthus retroflexus*), and scarlet globemallow (*Sphaeralcea coccinea*).[8,9]

Within colonies—also called towns or villages—prairie dogs live in territorial family groups called coteries,[8] which usually contain one adult (≥ 2-year-old) male and several adult females that are genetically related to each other (eg, mothers, daughters, granddaughters, sisters, nieces). A coterie's territory is approximately one third of a hectare (1 acre), and contains approximately 70 burrow entrances.[1] Young males disperse from the natal territory, so mother-son and sister-brother matings are rare;

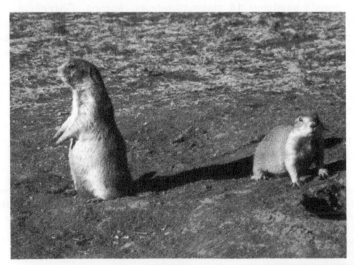

Fig. 1. Under natural conditions, prairie dogs spend about one third of their time scanning for predators, such as American badgers, coyotes, golden eagles, and prairie falcons. As seen here, scanning often occurs on a mound that surrounds a burrow entrance. (*Courtesy of* J. L. Hoogland, Frostburg, MD.)

older males do not remain in the same territory for more than 2 consecutive years, so father-daughter matings are also rare.[11] Under natural conditions, however, prairie dogs regularly mate with more distant kin, such as first and second cousins.[12]

In the wild, the mating season for prairie dogs varies with latitude but usually is in January or February. Each female is sexually receptive for only 5 to 6 hours on a single day each year, and most females mate with only the single adult male of the home territory.[1] Pregnancy lasts approximately 35 days. Neonates are blind and hairless, are approximately 1 cm long (0.4 in), and weigh approximately 15 g (0.5 oz). Nearly weaned juveniles first emerge from their nursery burrows when they are approximately 6 weeks old. Both sexes usually defer first mating until their second year. Litter size at birth can be as high as eight, but the most common litter sizes at weaning are three and four.[1]

Body mass for prairie dogs varies with season under natural conditions. In late winter and early spring, before the appearance of new vegetation, adults in South Dakota weigh approximately 700 g (1.5 lb). By late autumn, after several months of voracious feeding, adults usually weigh approximately 900 g (2 lb) and sometimes weigh as much as 1400 g (3 lb). Except when females are in late pregnancy, males are usually about 5% to 10% heavier than females.[13]

After detecting a predator and running to a burrow mound, a prairie dog sometimes gives an alarm call, which is a series of "chirk" sounds.[8,14] Approximately 50% of adults and yearlings call during an attack, and both males and females call. Prairie dogs call to warn not only offspring but also other kin, such as siblings, nieces, nephews, and first cousins.[1] After a predator has departed, a prairie dog sometimes gives a "jump-yip": while stretching the length of the body nearly vertical, the individual throws its front feet high into the air as it gives a two-syllable call (**Fig. 2**).[8,14]

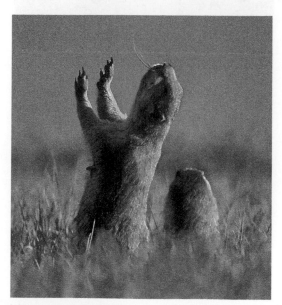

Fig. 2. Prairie dog giving a jump-yip. Prairie dogs commonly jump-yip after a predator has disappeared from view or when defending the home territory. A pet prairie dog frequently jump-yips when its owner enters the room. (*Courtesy of* R. Gehman, Waynesboro, PA.)

A single jump-yip usually initiates a chain reaction among other prairie dogs of the home and adjacent territories. The sight of 40 to 50 jump-yipping prairie dogs is amusing and remarkable.

WHY DO PRAIRIE DOGS MAKE GOOD PETS?

Prairie dogs have been popular as pets in private homes for more than 100 years.[15–18] If captured when young, a prairie dog seems to "imprint" on its human owners and is charming in many ways (**Figs. 3** and **4**). It commonly responds with a jump-yip when the owner enters the room, and, when given a blanket, it will try to mold the blanket into a "burrow mound." The pet is insatiably curious and captivates its owner with its antics and nonstop exploring. It is receptive to scratching, rubbing, and grooming by the owner, and it often tries to reciprocate. A pet prairie dog sometimes sits quietly in its owner's lap for hours and might fall asleep there. When a strange human approaches, however, a pet prairie dog might chatter its teeth and flare its tail, but it usually does not bite unless severely provoked.

One of the most fascinating and intriguing aspects of pet prairie dogs is that they, like prairie dogs under natural conditions,[1,8] have individual personalities that differ radically from each other. Some pets always wake up early each morning, for example, whereas others always sleep late into the morning, and others assume the

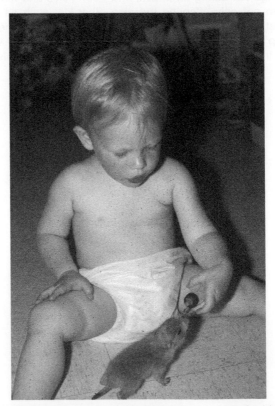

Fig. 3. Here a young child bottle-feeds evaporated milk to a 6-week-old pet prairie dog. If captured just before or shortly after weaning, prairie dogs make charming, fascinating pets. (*Courtesy of* J. L. Hoogland, Frostburg, MD.)

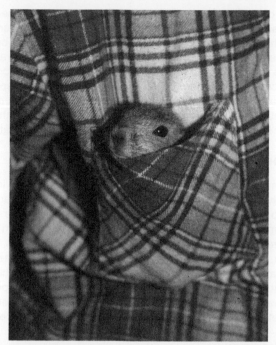

Fig. 4. Pet prairie dog in owner's pocket. (*Courtesy of* J. L. Hoogland, Frostburg, MD.)

sleeping patterns of their human owners. Some prefer to stay in the home cage, but others always appreciate time out of the cage. Some frequently jump-yip, but others rarely call. Some crave the company of other pet prairie dogs, but others prefer to be alone. The list of individual differences goes on and on.

HOUSING FOR CAPTIVE PRAIRIE DOGS

A pet prairie dog spends significant amounts of time in close contact with its owner, but a pet needs a large, safe cage when its owner is unavailable. Larger is better, but the minimal size that we recommend is a 60 cm × 60 cm × 90 cm (2 ft × 2 ft × 3 ft) two-story wire cage. (Visit http://www.bunnyrabbit.com/price/petcagecombo. htm for examples of suitable cages by Bunnyrabbit.com.) A one-story cage with the same or larger floor area also works but requires more space. These cages can house two or three adult prairie dogs. Some prairie dogs are more tolerant than others of cage mates, however, so the optimal number of prairie dogs per cage depends on individual personalities. Younger pets should be kept in a 60- to 80-L (15- to 20-gallon) aquarium until they are large enough to move into the two-story wire cage.[19]

Several features of a pet prairie dog's housing are especially important. (1) The wire mesh of the cage should be 1.25 cm × 1.25 cm (0.5 in × 0.5 in). Prairie dogs get their feet caught in larger or smaller squares. (2) The cage should contain cotton clothing that the prairie dog can use for bedding. The clothing should be immune to unraveling so that thread does not become entangled in the pet's toes. T-shirts in good condition work well, and they should be washed every week or so. (3) We recommend connecting the first and second levels of a two-story cage with polyvinyl chloride (PVC) tubing so that the prairie dog can move easily between levels of the cage. (4) Door latches should be secure or the prairie dog will learn how to escape. (5) The cage should be placed out of direct sunlight (because prairie dogs can easily overheat) and away from drafts and heating/air conditioning vents. (6) Toys should be added to the cage to encourage exercise and keep the pet busy. Good options available at most pet stores include toys for domestic dogs and parrots. Other options include cardboard boxes and cardboard tubing. (7) Finally, we recommend newspaper, pine shavings, or aspen shavings to catch urine and feces that fall below a pet prairie dog's cage. Owners should avoid cedar chips or "kitty litter" underneath the cage because ingestion of either by the pet can lead to sickness and possible death.

WHICH SEX AND WHAT AGE FOR PETS?

Both male and female prairie dogs make excellent, engaging pets. In general, males are more aggressive than females to human strangers. On the other hand, a male is also more likely to sit quietly on its owner's lap. Females are more restless and are more likely to damage furniture by chewing and scratching. When getting two pet prairie dogs, we recommend two of the same sex. For three pets, we recommend all of the same sex, or one male and two females. The best age for a new pet is approximately 10 weeks after birth, when it is fully weaned. A young pet at this age "imprints" with and accepts its owner more easily and more quickly than older pets, and is easier to handle. With patience from the owner, prairie dogs first received as adults also make excellent pets, even if the prairie dog has been abused by previous owners.

URINATION AND DEFECATION

Under natural conditions, prairie dogs usually urinate and defecate aboveground and do not have specific sites where they concentrate their urine and feces.[1] Urination is infrequent, and fecal pellets are hard and dry. Most pet prairie dogs can learn to restrict urination and defecation to their cages. Training involves taking the new pet out of its cage for short periods only (10–15 minutes). After a month or so of training, the pet will consistently return to the cage to urinate or defecate if the cage door is open and easily accessible.

DIET FOR CAPTIVE PRAIRIE DOGS

Prairie dogs under natural conditions are herbivorous, and what they eat depends on plants that are available in the home territory.[8,20–22] Choices throughout the year commonly include buffalo grass (*Buchloe dactyloides*), grama (*Bouteloua* spp), prickly pear cactus (*Opuntia* spp.), rabbitbrush (*Chrysothamnus* spp.), scarlet globemallow, thistle (*Cirsium* spp.), and wheatgrass (*Agropyron* spp). Plants that prairie dogs usually avoid include horseweed (*Conyza ramosissima*), fetid marigold, sage (*Artemisia* spp), and threeawn (*Aristida* spp). Wild prairie dogs commonly go for months without access to puddles of water, and evidently they can obtain all the water they need from moisture on the surface of, and within, plants.

Prairie dogs under natural conditions show three deviations from herbivory.[1] First, individuals sometimes consume fresh or old scats of American bison (*Bison bison*). Second, when they find them and can catch them, prairie dogs sometimes eat insects such as cutworms (Noctuidae), ground beetles (Carabidae), and short-horned grasshoppers (Acrididae). Third, individuals sometimes cannibalize other prairie dogs that die of natural causes. In addition, adults of both sexes commonly kill and cannibalize unweaned prairie dogs that have not yet emerged from the nursery burrow. This combination of infanticide and cannibalism accounts for the partial or total demise of 39% of litters and has a major impact on the demography and social behavior of prairie dogs.[1,23] Killers remove future competitors and obtain important sustenance via the cannibalism.

Owners of pets almost never have access to the plants that prairie dogs eat under natural conditions. **Box 1** lists plants that are nutritious, acceptable, and easily available for captive adult prairie dogs or fully weaned juveniles. Box 1 also lists foods that are not acceptable for prairie dogs. In addition to the foods listed in **Box 1**, captive prairie dogs should have access to gravity-fed water bottles.

Box 1 shows foods for captive adult prairie dogs or juveniles that are fully weaned. Unweaned prairie dog juveniles require syringe-feeding with an unusual formula that includes one part goat's (*Capra hircus*) milk, one part pureed sweet potato (*Ipomoea batatas*), and two parts water or Pedialyte (Abbot Nutrition Consumer Relations, Columbus, OH).[19]

Healthy adult prairie dogs usually weigh 700 to 900 g (1.5–2 lb) under natural conditions. Healthy pets should weigh about the same or perhaps as much as 200 to 300 g more. At one extreme, failure to follow the recommendations in **Box 1** can lead to starvation; at the other extreme, failure can lead to obesity, which is probably the most common dietary problem for pets. As for humans, obesity for prairie dogs leads to numerous physiologic problems and ultimately to a shorter lifespan. If an owner is uncertain about whether a pet is seriously overweight, then he or she should take the prairie dog to a veterinarian.

DISEASES OF PRAIRIE DOGS

Under natural conditions, prairie dogs are susceptible to several diseases, including tularemia and plague. Also known as rabbit fever, tularemia is caused by a bacterium (*Francisella tularensis*), usually spreads via ticks, and can be lethal for prairie dogs. Tularemia has been documented in only two wild colonies of prairie dogs,[24] and to

---

Box 1
Recommended foods for pet prairie dogs

Nutritious foods that can be offered in unlimited quantities (free choice)

Bermuda-grass hay, brome, fescue, grass, and timothy-hay; if timothy-hay is unavailable, acceptable substitutes are either American Pet Diner's Timbo Cubes (Healthy Hay Products Company, Eureka, NV) or Brisky's Prairie Dog Pellets (Brisky Pet Products, Franklinville, NY)

Nutritious foods that can be offered on limited basis (approximately 0.125 cup every other day per prairie dog)

American Pet Diner's Timmy Pellets, Prairie Dog Delight (Oxbow Animal Health, Murdock, NE), Bunny Basic/T (Oxbow Animal Health, Murdock, NE)

Nutritious foods that can be offered as occasional treats (small amounts every other day or so)

Carrots, Basic T Pellets (Oxbow Animal Health, Murdock, NE), Cheerios (General Foods, Minneapolis, MN), plain shredded mini-wheat cereal (General Foods, Minneapolis, MN), sweet potatoes, whole oats, and whole wheat toast

Foods that should never be fed to captive prairie dogs

Alfalfa, bird-food, candy, cheese, coffee, corn, gerbil food, hamster food, ice cream, lettuce, liquids other than plain water, nuts/peanuts, pizza, potato chips, rodent/lab block, tobacco

our knowledge, only one case of tularemia has been reported among captive prairie dogs.[25] Because it responds to antibiotics, tularemia is rarely fatal for humans.

Plague is an introduced disease to which prairie dogs have been exposed for only approximately 60 years. In this short time, prairie dogs have been unable to evolve a good defense; consequently, they are highly susceptible. Plague—also called bubonic plague, wild rodent plague, or sylvatic plague—is caused by a bacterium (*Yersinia pestis*) that most commonly spreads via fleas. When plague infects a prairie dog colony, it spreads quickly and mortality usually approaches 100%.[7] Humans usually first suspect plague among prairie dogs by the sudden disappearance of most or all residents within a colony. Most victims show no aboveground symptoms and perish underground. The time between initial exposure to plague and mortality varies among prairie dogs but usually is less than 14 days. *Y pestis* is the same bacterium that killed approximately 40% of the human population in Europe during the "Black Death" from 1347 to 1352.[26] Plague among humans responds to antibiotics, but because its early symptoms are similar to those of influenza, plague often advances to a dangerous stage before a physician recognizes the problem. Because captive prairie dogs are routinely quarantined for a minimum of 14 days before sale, plague among pet prairie dogs ready for sale, or transfer of plague from pet to owner, has not been reported.

In spring 2003, a viral disease known as monkeypox was introduced into the United States from Africa via other rodents; the most likely culprits were Gambian giant rats (*Cricetomys gambianus*) imported from Ghana. In a pet store in Illinois, monkeypox evidently then spread from caged Gambian giant rats to prairie dogs in adjacent cages.[27] From their pet prairie dogs, several people contracted monkeypox, which can be fatal for prairie dogs and humans.[28] Mainly because of monkeypox, the sale and transport of captive prairie dogs was illegal from June 2003 through September 2008.[27,29]

Some people worry about rabies among prairie dogs. Rabies has never been reported among wild or captive prairie dogs, however, so the risk of contracting this disease from a pet prairie dog is small.

ODONTOMA

Odontoma occurs when a tumor develops at the base of one of the prairie dog's upper incisors. The tumor invades the nasal cavity, interferes with normal breathing, and eventually can be fatal.[19] Some pet owners have lost several prairie dogs to odontoma, but an accurate estimate of the frequency of odontoma among pets is unavailable. Odontoma has not been reported among prairie dogs living under natural conditions. Some evidence indicates that odontoma results after trauma to one of the incisors (eg, after a fall or after continual chewing on hard surfaces). Other evidence indicates that poor nutrition might be the cause. No cure is currently available for this puzzling malady among pet prairie dogs.

EXTERNAL AND INTERNAL PARASITES

Under natural conditions, prairie dogs harbor fleas, lice, ticks, and mites.[1,3,8,30] Fleas are especially common and can transmit plague. External parasites that occur naturally on prairie dogs are usually absent from pets, because reputable dealers always remove the parasites before sale and pets usually have no later exposure to wild prairie dogs and their natural parasites. Pets can temporarily harbor fleas and other parasites that are normally found on domestic dogs, domestic cats, and other kinds of pets, however. These parasites are easy to remove with commercial insecticides for domestic cats/kittens. Under natural conditions, prairie dogs also harbor numerous internal parasites, including protozoans, roundworms, spiny-headed worms, and tapeworms.[31,32] We know little about the prevalence of internal parasites among pet prairie dogs, but probably they pose little threat to the pets or their owners.

INJURIES

Pet prairie dogs easily climb upward, but have difficulty climbing downward. Pets also have little fear of heights. Consequently, the most common serious injuries for pet prairie dogs result from falls. To reduce the probability of falls, a pet needs constant supervision when out of its cage.

WHERE TO OBTAIN A PET PRAIRIE DOG

Until 2003, pet prairie dogs were available from hundreds of vendors in the United States and many other countries. Then came the outbreak in 2003 of monkeypox (see previous discussion), which affected a minimum of 37 people, most of whom had pet prairie dogs. To deter the spread of monkeypox among captive and wild prairie dogs, the United States Department of Health and Human Services issued a ruling in June 2003 that prohibited the capture of wild prairie dogs and the sale/trade of prairie dogs.[27] This ruling, which many regarded as unfair to persons who wanted to obtain a pet prairie dog, was revoked in September 2008.[29] Prairie dogs will soon be available in pet stores again, or people can obtain one by contacting Dianne James (Midwest Prairie Dog Shelter, Post Office Box 135, Arcola, IN, 46704-0135; phone: 260-704-7364; "Dianne James" midwestpd@hotmail.com) or Lynda Watson (PMS Recycled Vermin, 7525 West 19th Street, Lubbock, TX, 79407; phone: 806-799-5806; "Robert Parrish" vs-41@suddenlink.net).

Some persons argue that having pet prairie dogs is unethical. We disagree for three reasons. First, most pets come from wild colonies that are destined to be devastated by shooting, poisoning, bulldozing, or some other destruction. Taking prairie dogs from these colonies is better than allowing them to simply die (ie, it's making the best of a bad situation). Using offspring from captive prairie dogs as pets is also acceptable in our opinion. We emphasize, however, that we strongly oppose the capture of prairie dogs as pets from natural, healthy populations that are in no imminent danger of elimination. Such action, if ubiquitous, could threaten the long-term persistence of prairie dogs under natural conditions.[33] Second, pet prairie dogs bring years of satisfaction and enjoyment to their owners. Finally, pets profoundly and positively affect the thinking of people regarding the conservation of prairie dogs. Many people first experience prairie dogs as their own or others' pets. Thousands of people cherish prairie dogs because they have had or seen them as pets, and these owners speak favorably about prairie dogs to their friends, coworkers, neighbors, and politicians. Such positive commentary promotes the long-term survival of prairie dogs.

LONGEVITY OF PRAIRIE DOGS

Juvenile mortality rate of wild prairie dogs is high. In a typical year, only approximately 50% of offspring born survive to weaning[1,23]; of those that survive to weaning, only approximately 50% survive until the next spring.[1,34] The mortality rate is also high among older prairie dogs.[1,34] Males that survive the first year do not live longer than 5 years in the wild; some females, however, live as long as 8 years. In captivity, male pet prairie dogs can live as long as 14 years, and females can live as long as 12 years.

NEUTERING OF PET PRAIRIE DOGS (CASTRATION AND SPAYING)

We recommend neutering of male and female pet prairie dogs by a qualified veterinarian. Neutered prairie dogs are more amicable to humans and other prairie dogs, and they live longer. The best time to neuter is autumn of the prairie dog's first year,[19] when it is approximately 6 months old. Neutered prairie dogs cannot reproduce, of course, but prairie dogs do not usually mate and rear offspring in captivity anyway.

RETURN TO THE WILD?

Ownership of a pet prairie dog is a lifelong commitment. An owner never should consider returning a pet to the wild, where it will be quickly and viciously attacked by other prairie dogs and will be highly vulnerable to predators. An owner who can no longer care for a pet prairie dog should contact Dianne James or Lynda Watson (see contact information given previously).

VETERINARY CHECK-UPS

In general, captive prairie dogs remain healthy if owners follow the guidelines in this article and other resources.[19] Obtaining a pet prairie dog from a reliable vendor and providing safe housing with the proper diet promotes long-term vitality. If a pet incurs a serious injury or suffers from a disease or other condition, however, the owner should promptly seek veterinary care. Finding top-notch care can be difficult, because most veterinarians have never seen captive prairie dogs and are not familiar with their common ailments. For assistance in finding veterinary care for pet prairie dogs in a particular geographic area, please contact Dianne James or Lynda Watson (see previous contact information).

FINAL THOUGHTS ABOUT PRAIRIE DOGS AS PETS

We cannot figure out if a pet prairie dog thinks that it is a member of its owner's human family or if the pet regards its owner as a member of its prairie dog coterie. In any event, if the owner follows the recommendations in this article, a pet prairie dog will provide many years of delightful, devoted, and entertaining companionship.

ACKNOWLEDGMENTS

For financial assistance for John Hoogland's research with prairie dogs living under natural conditions, we thank The Denver Zoological Foundation, The National Geographic Society, The National Science Foundation, and The University of Maryland.

REFERENCES

1. Hoogland JL. The black-tailed prairie dog: social life of a burrowing mammal. Chicago (IL): University of Chicago Press; 1995.
2. Hollister N. A systematic account of the prairie dogs. North American Fauna 1916; 40:1–37.
3. Pizzimenti JJ. Evolution of the prairie dog genus *Cynomys*. Occasional Papers of Museum of Natural History, University of Kansas 1975;39:1–73.

4. Proctor J, Haskins B, Forrest SC. Focal areas for conservation of prairie dogs and the grassland ecosystem. In: Hoogland JL, editor. Conservation of the black-tailed prairie dog. Washington, DC: Island Press; 2006. p. 232–47.

5. Forrest SC, Luchsinger JC. Past and current chemical control of prairie dogs. In: Hoogland JL, editor. Conservation of the black-tailed prairie dog. Washington, DC: Island Press; 2006. p. 115–28.

6. Reeve AF, Vosburgh TC. Recreational shooting of prairie dogs. In: Hoogland JL, editor. Conservation of the black-tailed prairie dog. Washington, DC: Island Press; 2006. p. 139–56.

7. Cully JF, Biggins DE, Seery DB. Conservation of prairie dogs in areas with plague. In: Hoogland JL, editor. Conservation of the black-tailed prairie dog. Washington, DC: Island Press; 2006. p. 157–68.

8. King JA. Social behavior, social organization, and population dynamics in a black-tailed prairie dog town in the Black Hills of South Dakota. Contributions of Laboratory of Vertebrate Biology, University of Michigan 1955;67:1–123.

9. Kotliar NB, Miller BJ, Reading RP, et al. The prairie dog as a keystone species. In: Hoogland JL, editor. Conservation of the black-tailed prairie dog. Washington, DC: Island Press; 2006. p. 53–64.

10. Sheets RG, Linder RL, Dahlgren RB. Burrow systems of prairie dogs in South Dakota. J Mammal 1971;52:451–3.

11. Hoogland JL. Prairie dogs avoid extreme inbreeding. Science 1982;215:1639–41.

12. Hoogland JL. Levels of inbreeding among prairie dogs. Am Nat 1992;139:591–602.

13. Hoogland JL. Sexual dimorphism in five species of prairie dogs. J Mammal 2003;84:1254–66.

14. Waring GH. Sound communications for black-tailed, white-tailed, and Gunnison's prairie dogs. Am Midl Nat 1970;83:167–85.

15. Jilson BC. Habits of the prairie dog. Am Nat 1871;5:24–9.

16. Squire L. Cutie, a prairie pet. Nature 1925;6:135–9.

17. Dale HF. Prairie dogs as pets. Outdoor Nebraska 1947;24:22.

18. Ferrara J. Prairie home companions. Nat Widl 1985;23:48–53.

19. Stoica K, Callis B, Watson L. Bringing a prairie dog pup into your home. Canton (OH): Karen Stoica; 2001.

20. Koford CB. Prairie dogs, whitefaces, and blue grama. Wildlife Monographs 1958;3:1–78.

21. Summers CA, Linder RL. Food habits of the black-tailed prairie dog in western South Dakota. Journal of Range Management 1978;31:134–6.

22. Rogers-Wydeven P, Dahlgren RB. A comparison of prairie dog stomach contents and feces using a microhistological technique. J Wildl Manage 1982;46:1104–8.

23. Hoogland JL. Infanticide in prairie dogs: lactating females kill offspring of close kin. Science 1985;230:1037–40.

24. Long D, Bly-Honness K, Truett JC, et al. Establishment of new prairie dog colonies by translocation. In: Hoogland JL, editor. Conservation of the black-tailed prairie dog. Washington, DC: Island Press; 2006. p. 188–209.

25. Avashia SB, Petersen JM, Lindley CM, et al. First report of prairie dog-to-human tularemia transmission: Texas, 2002. Emerg Infect Dis 2004;10:542–3.

26. Orent W. Plague: the mysterious past and terrifying future of the world's most dangerous disease. New York: Free Press; 2004.

27. Gerberding JL, McClellan MB. Joint order of the Centers for Disease Control and Prevention and the Food and Drug Administration, Department of Health and Human Services. Rockville (MD): Food and Drug Administration; 2003.

28. CDC (Center for Disease Control). Questions and answers about monkeypox. Available at: http://www.cdc.gov.ncidod/monkeypox/qa.htm. Accessed June 2008.
29. Shuren J. Control of communicable diseases: restrictions on African rodents, prairie dogs, and certain other animals. Fed Regist 2008;73:51912–9.
30. Hoogland JL. Aggression, ectoparasitism, and other possible costs of prairie dog (Sciuridae: *Cynomys* spp) coloniality. Behaviour 1979;69:1–35.
31. Vetterling JM. Endoparasites of the black-tailed prairie dog of northern Colorado [master's thesis]. Fort Collins (CO): Colorado State University; 1962.
32. Buscher HN, Tyler JD. Parasites of vertebrates inhabiting prairie dog towns in Oklahoma. II. Helminths. Proceedings of the Oklahoma Academy of Science 1975;55:108–11.
33. Miller BJ, Reading RP. A proposal for more effective conservation of prairie dogs. In: Hoogland JL, editor. Conservation of the black-tailed prairie dog. Washington, DC: Island Press; 2006. p. 248–60.
34. Hoogland JL. Black-tailed, Gunnison's, and Utah prairie dogs all reproduce slowly. J Mammal 2001;82:917–27.

Behavior, Nutrition, and Veterinary Care of Patagonian Cavies (*Dolichotis patagonum*)

David S. Kessler, BA[a],*, Katharine Hope, DVM[b], Michael Maslanka, MS[c]

KEYWORDS

• Patagonian cavy • Mara • *Dolichotis patagonum*
• Nutrition • Behavior • Captive management

DESCRIPTION

Patagonian cavies (*Dolichotis patagonum*), also known as maras, are long-legged, large rodents of the family Caviidae, which also includes capybaras, guinea pigs, and other cavies. Though they are rodents, their body confirmation is similar to that of hoofed stock, with long legs adapted for cursorial life. Their hind legs are slightly larger and more muscular than their forelimbs.[1] They have a grayish-brown dorsal and facial coat, a white ventrum, and a white patch on the rump separated from the dorsal fur by a black stripe.[2] They are generally 610-mm to 810-mm long and weigh 7 kg to 9 kg.[2,3] They have a short tail (40 mm–50 mm) that is almost hairless[4] (**Fig. 1**). They can live up to 14 years in captivity. Captive Patagonian cavies breed well and are available on the commercial exotic animal market, though the authors strongly discourage keeping Patagonian cavies as pets.

Native only to Argentina, they are found in lowland arid grass and brush lands of the Pampas between 28°S and 50°S.[5] Fossil remains of *Dolichotis* species dating from the Late Pleistocene have been discovered in Argentina.[6] The International Union for Conservation of Nature Red List classifies Patagonian cavies as "Low Risk/Near

[a] Small Mammal Unit, Smithsonian's National Zoological Park, PO Box 37012 MRC 5507, Washington, DC 20013-7012, USA
[b] Department of Animal Health, Smithsonian's National Zoological Park, PO Box 37012 MRC 5502, Washington, DC 20013-7012, USA
[c] Department of Nutrition, Smithsonian's National Zoological Park, PO Box 37012 MRC 5503, Washington, DC 20013-7012, USA
* Corresponding author.
E-mail address: kesslerd@si.edu (D.S. Kessler).

Vet Clin Exot Anim 12 (2009) 267–278
doi:10.1016/j.cvex.2009.01.009
1094-9194/09/$ – see front matter. Published by Elsevier Inc.

vetexotic.theclinics.com

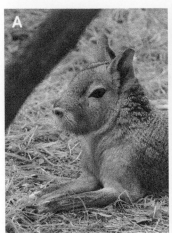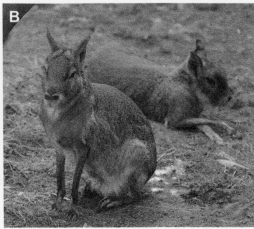

Fig. 1. (*A* and *B*) Patagonian cavies. (*Courtesy of* Ann Batdorf, Smithsonian's National Zoologic Park, Washington, DC.)

Threatened" because of human-induced habitat loss and degradation and to competitive invasive of alien species.[7]

BEHAVIOR IN THE WILD

Patagonian cavies are diurnal. They are herbivorous, eating mostly grasses and leaves and spending at least 36% of the day grazing over ranges of approximately 200 ha.[3,8,9] Their long hind limbs are well suited for running and they can reach speeds of over 60 km per hour when alarmed.[9] In an interesting case of convergent evolution, Patagonian cavies exhibit "stotting" as part of their predator response repertoire.[10] Stotting consists of an animal jumping in the air from all four legs when in the presence of a predator, and is considered to be either an alarm call for con-specifics or a demonstration of fitness to potential predators.

The mating and social structure of Patagonian cavies is unusual and well researched. Unlike most mammals, Patagonian cavies are monogamous, forming strong, life-long pair-bonds[3,10–12] in which the breeding male and female stay in close proximity. The female initiates most activities, including resting, walking, grazing, and moving toward communal burrows. Although there is very little physical contact between mates other than breeding, pairs communicate with each other through vocalizations when they are within a few meters of each other. They do not allogroom. If a male approaches his mate, attempting contact during a nonbreeding encounter, she will occasionally spray urine toward his face. The male responds by marking the ground with his anal glands and feces, dragging his rump across areas previously occupied by the female, and moving in figure-eight patterns around her.[12,13]

Monogamously pair-bonded, Patagonian cavies may rear their young in isolated dens or they may live in groups of up to 70 individuals, maintaining communal burrows each housing as many as 33 pups.[14] Home ranges tend to be flexible, with animals occupying and defending territories until resources are depleted, after which time the Patagonian cavies drift to more promising areas.[3] The pairing of communal dens with monogamy is a behavior unique to Patagonian cavies. Large settlements may offer protection from predators and better access to limited resources. Dens are for the exclusive use of young and nursing females, though adult females and sometimes males will re-excavate burrows about 2 weeks before females give birth.[14]

Gestation is between 91 and 111 days, and the young are precocial, born fully furred with their eyes open.[13,15] Seventy percent of births are twins, 25% are singletons, and 5% are triplets. Estrus lasts for as little as half an hour and occurs a few hours after a female gives birth.[12] Most breeding occurs from mid-August to November or December.[14,16] Mortality of pups is high because of predation by felids, grisons, foxes, and birds of prey. Communal denning offers increased protection for both pups and adults.[14]

Pups nurse once a day in their dens for their first 6 weeks of life. The mother stays in the den for approximately 65 minutes, typically nursing one to two (up to four) pups at a time. Nursing occurs only during daylight. Once the pups are 6 weeks old, they emerge from the dens to nurse in the scrub and to forage with their parents. They are weaned at 11 weeks. Females can identify their own pups via smell and vocalizations and carefully sniff rumps and flanks of pups before allowing them to nurse. Unrelated pups will try to steal milk from unrelated females. Nursing females will attack interloping pups by chasing, lunging, and even biting or shaking. Pups attempting to nurse from a female other than their mother will occasionally be sprayed with urine, possibly to communicate the female's identity to the pups. Despite the nursing female's vigilance, interloping pups are often able to "steal" 2 to 6 minutes worth of milk per adult female's visit to the warren, a communal breeding area.[14]

Adult aggression occurs when the male of one pair attempts to sniff or mount the female of another pair. Agonistic interactions can last up to an hour. Females do not leave their mates during these encounters.[14] A male will perform urine and scent marking displays directed toward his mate if another adult male approaches within 10 m of the female, again using urine for identification purposes.[12,14] Direct contact is negligible; pairs generally remain separated from other pairs by at least 20 m.[10] The complex social system of Patagonian cavies presents challenges to maintaining them successfully in captivity.

CAPTIVE MANAGEMENT

Patagonian cavies have been displayed at zoos in many different social groupings: pairs, families, single-sex groups, and singletons. Ideally, they should be exhibited in large groups with several breeding pairs, though most institutions do not have the space available to maintain a large breeding group. Aggression often occurs in single-sex groups, which can sometimes be mitigated by castration, though even castrated males may be too aggressive to be housed together. Females may or may not be compatible with one another. Compatibility of single-sex groups may depend on enclosure space and environmental complexity (eg, multiple dens, hiding spaces, natural topography), though it may simply be a matter of individual differences among animals.

Patagonian cavies are fairly hardy animals that can be housed outdoors in temperate climates. They require dirt and grass substrate and burrows, which can be constructed of concrete, polyvinyl chloride, or other materials. Each burrow should have at least two tunnel entrances, each at least 1.5-m long. If the temperature goes below 5°C, heat should be supplied to the burrow. Patagonian cavies gnaw, so electrical cables and connections should be well-shielded. Patagonian cavies tolerate heat well, but they should be offered shade and a variety of resting places. Because of their shyness, they should be provided with several hiding areas in each enclosure. They are excellent diggers and will dig under and out of most fences. Patagonian cavies will eat just about anything planted in an exhibit, so toxic plants should be avoided and enclosures should be periodically re-planted to ensure a constant source of material for chewing.

Patagonian cavies can be trained to hand-feed, step on scales, and go into crates. Though shy by nature, they can be trained with simple operant conditioning. Animals housed alone should be given extra enrichment and training to compensate for lack of con-specific social stimulation. Enrichment items include sturdy polyethylene plastic balls, wooden logs, sticks, cardboard tubes for shredding, cat litter pans for digging, timothy hay for bedding, and spices and oils for olfactory stimulation. Though they are beautiful, gentle, and fascinating creatures, Patagonian cavies are not suitable as private pets.

NUTRITIONAL CARE

Patagonian cavies are herbivorous caviomorphs (South American rodents that include cavies and guinea pigs). Little work has been performed specifically on the nutritional ecology and physiology of maras. Zoo diets tend to be relatively straightforward, taking into consideration their natural foraging strategy, gastrointestinal tract morphology, and target dietary-nutrient values.

Natural Foraging Ecology

In the wild, Patagonian cavies consume green vegetation and fruits.[1] In the Monte Desert region, they have large dietary overlap with plains vizcachas (Lagostomus maximus), livestock, and European hares (Lepus europaeus). In the central Monte Desert, they consume leaves of monocot species (70%) and dicot species (30%).[1] In this area, monocot preferences include Chloris, Pappophorum, and Trichloris, and the perennial dicots, Atriplex lampa, Lycium, and Prospis. Patagonian cavies also are opportunistic browsers on new herb growth and fruits (eg, Prosopis flexuosa) and distribute fruit seeds via their feces. In the southernmost part of the Monte Desert, Patagonian cavies mostly browse on shrubs, with seasonal shifts to annual and perennial grasses and forbs.[17] Some studies show Patagonian cavies prefer grasses over shrubs and forbs, regardless of precipitation regime.[18]

Gastrointestinal Tract Morphology

Patagonian cavies have a simple, large, single cavity, glandular stomach.[19] The majority of the small intestine resides on the left side of the abdominal cavity, caudal to the stomach. The cecum is large in relation to rest of the gastrointestinal tract, typical of a hindgut fermenter. Cecal contents of a similar hindgut fermenting caviomorph rodent, the guinea pig, are reported as 5% to 10% of total gastrointestinal tract volume.[19] The voluminous cecum and ascending colon lie on the right side of the abdominal cavity, caudal to the liver. The descending colon is coiled and lies on the left side of the body.[20]

Fiber digestibility in Patagonian cavies is believed to be similar to that of guinea pigs; however digestibilities of crude protein and ash are reported to be lower in Patagonian cavies than in guinea pigs.[21] Even though they are closely related to coprophagous guinea pigs, it is unclear whether Patagonian cavies are coprophagous.

Mean retention time of fluid and particles in the gastrointestinal tract of Patagonian cavies is reported to be 27 hours.[21] In a study with dwarf cavies (Microcavia australis; small caviomorph rodent, 250 g), spatial and seasonal plasticity in gastrointestinal morphology was observed.[22] When low-quality, high-fiber diets were consumed during the dry season, cecum weights were significantly larger than when high-nitrogen diets were consumed during the wet season.

Target Nutrient Values

For Patagonian cavies, as with many other nondomestic species, studies to determine specific nutrient toxicities and deficiencies are not possible. Thus, target nutrient values are derived from a variety of sources that include: applied research with the species in question; applied and basic research performed on nearly-related domestic animal models; well-studied species within the same genus or family; other species with similar foraging strategies; or gastrointestinal morphology. The closest, well-studied species to the Patagonian cavy is the guinea pig (*Cavia porcellus*); however, extensive studies with rats (*Rattus* spp.) and hamsters (*Cricetus cricetus*) also provide valuable target nutrient information. Based on guinea pigs' specific dietary requirement for ascorbic acid[23] (vitamin C), this nutrient is also recommended for Patagonian cavies. As a hindgut fermenter, Patagonian cavies also have a recommended dietary fiber level. The target dietary nutrient values for Patagonian cavies (**Table 1**) are based on this information.

Diets for Animals Maintained in Zoo Settings

A variety of diets have been used to maintain Patagonian cavies in zoo settings. Most commercially produced rodent or primate diets will provide adequate nutrients to maintain Patagonian cavies. In addition to these nutritionally complete food items, greens, vegetables, and fruits also are recommended. Because of their herbivorous nature, Patagonian cavies likely should be fed leafy greens as the largest proportion

Table 1
Target nutrient values for Patagonian cavy (*Dolichotis patagonium*); dry matter basis

Nutrient	Target Nutrient Value
Crude protein, %	5.0–18.0
Fat, %	4.0–5.0
Fiber, %	15.0
Vitamin A, IU/g	2.3–3.6
Vitamin C, mg/kg	200.0
Vitamin D, IU/g	1.0
Vitamin E, mg/kg	18.0–27.0
Choline, mg/kg	1,800.0
Folic acid, mg/kg	3.0–6.0
Niacin, mg/kg	10.0
Pantothenic acid, mg/kg	20.0
Pyridoxine, mg/kg	2.0–3.0
Riboflavin, mg/kg	3.0
Thiamin, mg/kg	2.0
Calcium, %	0.5–0.8
Phosphorus, %	0.3–0.4
Magnesium, %	0.05–0.1
Iron, mg/kg	35.0–70.0
Manganese, mg/kg	10.0–40.0

of their diet on a wet-weight basis (Table 2). Target body-weight ranges and regular body-condition observations, paired with routine intake measurements, are recommended to better monitor the success of the diet offered.

Hand-Rearing Considerations

Patagonian cavies have been successfully hand-reared,[24,25] although mother-reared animals are always preferable, as mother-reared offspring tend to integrate better with con-specifics and are more successful in rearing their own young upon reaching maturity. Caviidae rodents are born with their second set of teeth.[26] As with hoofed mammals, the number of young is low and offspring are highly developed at birth.

As a group, rodent milks are variable in dry matter (18%–29%) and energy (1.0 kcal –2.5 kcal gross energy per gram).[27] Rodent milks are higher in fat, lower in carbohydrate, and more concentrated than human or bovine milks. Information specific to Patagonian cavy milk is lacking, so hand-rearing formula recommendations are made for rodents in general.[27]

Esbilac (Pet Ag, Hampshire, Illinois), KMR (Pet Ag), and Milk Matrix (Pet Ag) have been used, either alone or in combination, to hand-rear rodents. A Patagonian cavy was successfully hand-reared using SMA Gold infant-milk powder formula (Berks, UK) with an added multivitamin.[25] This Patagonian cavy was weaned at 49 days of age, but began to consume solid foods as early as 20 days, suggesting that weaning from the bottle formula could have occurred sooner, if needed.

VETERINARY CARE

The Patagonian cavy is a unique animal in terms of veterinary care in that, although a rodent and closely related to the guinea pig, the Patagonian cavy has longer legs and is more flighty and difficult to restrain that its caviidae relatives. This section will cover common diseases and health concerns of captive Patagonian cavies, as well as clinical techniques for diagnosing and treating illnesses in these animals.

Anatomy

The gastrointestinal tract of the Patagonian cavy is similar to that of other Caviidae, as described above. The Patagonian cavy's dental formula is I 1/1, c 0/0, p 1/1, m 3/3, and the teeth are hypsodont, continuously growing throughout life in response to constant wear on the grinding surfaces.[1] The Patagonian cavy's unique musculoskeletal anatomy sometimes causes it to be confused with a hare, rather than a rodent. Patagonian cavies have relatively longer legs than other rodents, with the

---

Table 2
Sample daily diet for one (one female) Patagonian cavy (as-fed basis, Smithsonian Institution's National Zoologic Park, Washington, DC)[a]

Items	Amount, Grass	Percent of Diet
Leaf-eating primate biscuit	150	14.8
Apple	240	23.6
Sweet potato	125	12.3
Green beans	130	12.8
Kale	370	36.5
Total	1050	100

[a] Produce rotations within food groups are recommended and used.

antebrachium significantly longer than the humerus and the hind legs slightly longer than the front legs. Patagonian cavies have three digits on their hind feet, four digits on their front feet, and are digitigrade, standing and walking on their toes.[1]

Clinical Techniques

Handling and anesthesia

Patagonian cavies are relatively large, fast, and flighty animals; therefore, when a Patagonian cavy is handled and restrained for examination, it is imperative to minimize stress. Additionally, they are difficult to safely restrain for examination while awake. Hyperthermia can result from a stressful or prolonged capture, and although hyperthermia is often transient and correctable by cooling the body with water once Patagonian cavies are anesthetized, hyperthermia can kill these animals.[28]

Sedation or anesthesia is recommended to perform a full veterinary examination. Patagonian cavies do not need to be fasted before anesthesia, as they are rodents and cannot vomit. Anesthetic agents that have been successfully used in the Patagonian cavy and other cavies include dissociative agents, benzodiazepines, and inhalant anesthestics (**Table 3**). Once anesthetized, Patagonian cavies can be intubated if a prolonged anesthesia is expected. However, they can be very difficult to intubate. A stylet can be passed through the eye at the end of the endotracheal tube and then passed just through the glottis to help guide the tube into the trachea. If a short procedure is planned, it is possible to maintain sedation through inhalation of gas anesthesia via a face mask.

Venipuncture and clinical pathology

The jugular vein in the Patagonian cavy is fairly prominent, and it is an easy site from which to obtain diagnostic blood samples. The cephalic and medial and lateral saphenous veins can also provide adequate sites for blood sampling or intravenous catheter placement. When placing an intravenous catheter, however, one must be careful to ensure that the catheter is adequately secured, so that the animal will not be able to remove it once it is awake. Reference ranges for hematologic and chemistry values for Patagonian cavies are reported in **Table 4**.[33]

Reported Diseases and Health Concerns

Malocclusion

As with other members of the rodent family, Patagonian cavies can develop cheek teeth malocclusion. Although malocclusion is often traumatic in origin, it can be related to nutritional or congenital problems, as well.[34] Clinical signs include ptyalism, "slobbers," weight loss, dropping food, or difficulty swallowing. Diagnosis can be made with a thorough oral examination. Teeth can be trimmed with a dremmel tool

Table 3 Sedatives and anesthestic agents used in Caviidae	
Drug	**Dose**
Acepromazine	0.5 mg/kg–1.0 mg/kg intramuscularly (IM)[29]
Diazepam	0.5 mg/kg–3.0 mg/kg IM[30]
Isoflurane	2%–5% induction; 0.25–4.0% maintenance[31]
Ketamine	22 mg/kg–44 mg/kg IM[32]

Combinations are frequently used at varying dosages.

Table 4
Reference ranges for hematologic and chemistry values of Patagonian cavies

CBC	Mean ± SD	Chemistry	Mean ± SD
WBC (× 10^3/ul)	7.151 ± 4.233	Calcium (mg/dl)	10.7 ± 1.5
RBC (× 10^6/ul)	7.43 ± 1.14	Phosphorus (mg/dl)	5.2 ± 2.5
Hb (g/dL)	17.7 ± 2.5	Sodium (mEq/L)	149 ±5
HCT (%)	50.5 ± 6.2	Potassium (mEq/L)	4.1 ± 0.6
MCV (fL)	69.2 ± 10.9	Chloride (mEq/L)	109 ±6
MCH (pg/cell)	24.1 ± 3.0	CO_2 (mEq/L)	20.8 ± 13.4
MCHC (g/dL)	35.5 ± 4.3	Iron (ug/dl)	296 ± 49
Platelets (× 10^3/ul)	597 ± 262	Blood urea nitrogen	23 ±10
nRBC (/100 WBC)	2± 1	Creatinine (mg/dl)	1.5±0.5
Reticulocytes (%)	1.4 ± 0	Total bilirubin (mg/dl)	0.5 ± 0.2
Neutrophils (×10^3/ul)	4.831 ± 3.343	Glucose (mg/dl)	213±52
Lymphocytes (×10^3/ul)	1.882 ± 1.482	Creatine phosphokinase (IU/L)	1,179 ±1,789
Monocytes (×10^3/ul)	0.255 ± 0.231	Lactate dehydrogenase (IU/L)	421 ± 317
Eosinophils (×10^3/ul)	0.144 ± 0.152	Alkaline phosphatase (IU/L)	60 ± 40
Basophils (× 10^3/ul)	0.164 ± 0.414	Alanine aminotransferase (IU/L)	34 ± 22
Bands (× 10^3/ul)	0.476 ± 0.836	Aspartate aminotransferase (IU/L)	60 ± 33
		Total protein (g/dl)	5.7 ± 0.7
		Globulin (g/dl)	2.0 ± 0.6
		Albumin (g/dl)	3.8 ± 0.7

Abbreviations: CBC, Complete blood cell; HCT, Hematocrit; MCH, Mean cell hemoglobin; MCHC, Mean cell hemoglobin concentration; MCV, Mean cell volume; RBC, Red blood cell; WBC, White blood cell.

Data from International Species Information System. Reference ranges for physiological values in captive wildlife. Eagan, MN: ISIS, 2002.

or nail clippers, and frequent trimming may be necessary to maintain proper occlusion. Proper diet is also important in helping to maintain normal occlusion.

Gastrointestinal diseases

The majority of reported gastrointestinal diseases in Patagonian cavies are caused by gastrointestinal parasites. Nematodes reported in Patagonian cavies include *Wellcomia dolichotis*, *Trichostrongylus retortaeformis*, and *Graphidioides affinis*.[1] Captive Patagonian cavies in North America should be screened routinely and treated for endoparasitic infections. **Table 5** lists antiparasitic drugs that may be used safely in Patagonian cavies.

Other reported gastrointestinal diseases include *Yersinia pseudotuberculosis* infections, bacterial enteritis, and gastric mucosal erosions.[28] As Patagonian cavies are closely related to guinea pigs, they may be sensitive to antibiotic-induced dysbiosis and enterotoxemia. Oral administration of beta-lactam drugs, lincosamides, macrolides, bacitracin, and vancomycin should be avoided, if possible, as they can lead to clostridial enterotoxemia.[36] Antibiotics that have been safely used in caviidae are listed in **Table 6**.

There have been a few reports of histoplasmosis in Patagonian cavies. This species has a unique, primarily gastrointestinal presentation of the disease.[38] *Histoplasma capsulatum var capsulatum* is a fungal infection contracted via inhalation of spores from the environment. Patagonian cavies with histoplasmosis had primary clinical signs of weakness and anorexia, progressing to death quickly. On necropsy, they

Table 5
Selected antiparasitic drugs used in Caviidae

Drug	Dose
Fenbendazole	20 mg/kg q 24 hr for 5 days[32]
Ivermectin	0.2 mg/kg–0.4 mg/kg subcutaneously SC or PO q 10 d–14 d[32]
Metronidazole	25 mg/kg PO q12 h[32]
Praziquantel	6 mg/kg–10 mg/kg PO,[29] SC repeat in 10 d[32]
Pyrethrin powder	0.1% topically q 7 d for three treatments[30]
Sulfadimethoxine	25 mg/kg–50 mg/kg PO q24 hr for 10 d[32]
Thiabendazole	100 mg/kg PO q 24 hr for 5 d[35]

had depleted fat stores, ascites, enlarged sternal and gastrohepatic lymph nodes, splenomegaly, and hepatomegaly. Additionally, the liver, lymph nodes, and adrenals had epithelial cells and macrophages containing cytoplasmic, yeast-like organisms, 2 to 4 microns in diameter, surrounded by a clear halo. While granulomatous pneumonia is the most common lesion with disseminated histoplasmosis in most mammals, Patagonian cavies with histoplasmosis had yeast in some alveolar walls, but they did not develop characteristic pneumonia. Histoplasmosis in Patagonian cavies appears to be primarily an intestinal disease. A partial list of antifungal therapies that have been used safely in Caviidae is described in **Table 7**.

Cardiopulmonary diseases
A large percentage of Patagonian cavies appear to have hypertrophic cardiomyopathy, often associated with pulmonic arteriosclerosis.[28] This pathology is rarely associated with morbidity but is the cause of death in some cases. Additionally, endocarditis of the right atrioventricular valve has been reported in some Patagonian cavies.[28]

In one large, captive Patagonian cavy colony in Mexico, several animals had significant pulmonary lesions secondary to *Besnoitia* infections.[40] *Besnoitia* is a coccidia that infects carnivores as definitive hosts and many other mammals, including rodents, as intermediate hosts. This parasite encysts in lungs and other tissues, including myocardium, pancreas, and esophagus, and may cause pneumonia in cavies.[40]

Musculoskeletal and integumentary diseases
Because of their long-legged anatomy and flighty nature, Patagonian cavies are commonly susceptible to traumatic fractures. Successful repair in a Patagonian

Table 6
Selected antibiotics used in Caviidae

Drug	Dose
Cephalexin	50 mg/kg PO or IM, divided q 12 h–24 h[31]
Chloramphenicol	50 mg/kg PO q 8 h–12 h[32]
Ciprofloxacin	5 mg/kg–15 mg/kg PO q12 h–24 h[32]
Doxycycline	2.5 mg/kg PO q12 h[35]
Enrofloxacin	5 mg/kg–10 mg/kg PO, IM q 12 h[29]
Metronidazole	20 mg/kg PO q 12 h[31]
Neomycin	8 mg/kg–15 mg/kg PO q 12 h[32,37]
Trimethoprim-sulfa	15 mg/kg–30 mg/kg PO, SC q12 h[32]

Table 7 Selected antifungal agents used in Caviidae	
Drug	**Dose**
Griseofulvin	15 mg/kg–25 mg/kg PO q 24 h for 14 d–28 d[39]
Itraconazole	5 mg/kg PO q 24 h[36]
Ketoconazole	10 mg/kg–40 mg/kg PO q 24 h for 14 d[36]

cavy of a comminuted tibia/fibula fracture using external skeletal fixation has been reported.[41] Pododermatitis associated with tendon sheath infections from *Staphylococcus*, *Streptococcus*, or *Pseudomonas* also has been reported.[28]

Patagonian cavies are susceptible to infestation by fleas, mites, and flies. Flea or mite infestation may cause dorsal hypotrichosis, alopecia, and skin crusting or ulceration. Mites can be treated with ivermectin (0.2 mg/kg–0.4 mg/kg subcutaneously every 10–14 days), and fleas and flies can be treated with topical pyrethrin-based powders. **Table 5** lists antiparasitic drugs that have been used safely in caviidae.

Cowpoxvirus has been reported in Patagonian cavies at an animal park in the Netherlands.[41] Clinical signs of cowpoxvirus include conjunctivitis, anorexia, multifocal ulcers on the nose, tongue, buccal mucosa, hard palate, and genital skin and mucosa. In one case, all affected animals died or were euthanized. On necropsy, multifocal, intracytoplasmic, eosinophilic inclusion bodies were found in the skin and mucosa epithelium. Additionally, pericardial effusion, pulmonary edema, and focal acute necrosis of the liver and kidneys were seen on necropsy. It is likely that cowpoxvirus was transmitted to the Patagonian cavies via rat carriers.[42] Because of the potential for zoonotic transmission of this poxvirus, gloves should be worn when captive Patagonian cavies or infected animals are handled.

SUMMARY

Patagonian cavies, with their unique combination of monogamy, communal denning, and atypical rodent morphology, are excellent subjects for field studies and exhibition at zoologic parks. These attributes make them poor candidates for private ownership as pets. They are difficult to maintain in proper social groups in private settings. Veterinary care of Patagonian cavies is challenging, because they are thin-limbed, flighty, and easily stressed.

REFERENCES

1. Campos C, Tognelli F, Ojeda R. Dolichotis patagonum. Mammalian Species 2001; 652:1–5.
2. Redford KH, Eisenberg JF. Mammals of the Neotropics. The southern cone University of Chicago Press, (IL); 1992;2:1–403
3. Macdonald DW, Herrera EA, Taber AB, et al. Social organization and resource use in capybaras and maras. In: Wolff JO, Sherman PW, editors. Rodent Societies: an ecological and evolutionary perspective. Chicago/London: University of Chicago Press; 2007. p. 393–402.
4. Cabrera A. Los roedores argentinos de la familia Caviidae. Publicaciones de la Escuela Veterinaria, Universidad de Buenos Aires 1953;6:1–93 [in Spanish].
5. Honacki JH, Kinman KE, Koeppl JW, editors. Mammal species of the World: a taxonomic and geographic reference. Lawrence (KS): Allen Press and the Association of Systematics Collections; 1982.

6. Verzi DH, Quintana CA. The caviomorph rodents from the San Andrés formation, east-central Argentina, and global Late Pliocene climate change. Palaeogeogr Palaeoclimatol Palaeoecol 2005;219:303–20.
7. Available at: http://www.iucnredlist.org. Accessed June 3, 2008.
8. Campos C, Ojeda R, Monge S, et al. Utilization of food resources by small and medium-sized mammals in the Monte Desert biome, Argentina. Austral Ecology 2001;26:142–9.
9. Erize F. Patagonian "Hares". Animals 1971;13:548–9.
10. Taber AB, Macdonald DW. Spatial organization and monogamy in the mara Dolichotis patagonum. J Zool (Lond) 1992;227:417–38.
11. Ganslosser U, Wehnelt S. Juvenile development as part of the extraordinary social system of the mara Dolichotis patagonum (Rodentia: Caviidae). Mammalia 1997;61(1):3–15.
12. Genest H, Dubost G. Pair-living in the mara (Dolichotis patagonum). Mammalia 1974;38(2):155–62.
13. Kleiman D. Patterns of behaviour in hystricomorph rodents. In: Rowlands IW, Weir BJ, editors. The biology of hystricomorph rodents. London: Academic Press. Symposia of the Zoological Society of London 1974;34:171–209
14. Taber AB, Macdonald DW. Communal breeding in the mara, Dolichotis patagonum. J Zool 1992;227:439–52.
15. Dubost G, Genest H. Le comportment social d'une colonie de maras, Dolichotis patagonum z. dans le Parc de Branfere. Z Tierpsychol 1974;35:225–302 [in French].
16. Baldi R. Breeding success of the endemic mara Dolichotis patagonum in relation to habitat selection: conservation implications. Journal of Arid Environments 2007;68:9–19.
17. Bonino N, Sbriller A, Manacorda M, et al. Food partitioning between mara (Dolichotis patagonum) and the introduced hare (Lepus europaeus) in the Monte Desert, Argentina. Studies on Neotropical Fauna and Environment 1997;32:129–134.
18. Sombra MS, Mangione AM. Obsessed with grasses? The case of mara Dolichotis patagonum (Caviidae: Rodentia). Rev Chil Hist Nat 2005;78:401–8.
19. Stevens CE, Hume ID. Comparative physiology of the vertebrate digestive system. Cambridge (UK): Cambridge University Press; 1995. p. 67–70.
20. Weissengruber GE. Anatomisch-topographische Darstellung des Magens, des Dunndarmes, des Dickdarmes sowie deren arterielle GefaBversorgung beim GroBen mara (Dolichotis patagonum Desmarest 1820). Anat Histol Embryol 2000;29:87–95 [in German].
21. Sakaguchi E, Nippashi K, Endoh G. Digesta retention and fibre digestion in maras (Dolichotis patagonium) and guinea pigs. Comp Biochem Physiol 1992;101(4):867–70.
22. Sassi PL, Borghi CE, Bozinovic F. Spatial and seasonal plasticity in digestive morphology of cavies (Microcavia australis) inhabiting habitats with different plant qualities. J Mammal 2007;88(1):165–72.
23. National Research Council (NRC). Nutrient requirements of laboratory animals. Subcommittee on Lab Animal Nutrition, National Research Council. Washington, DC: National Academy Press; 1995. p. 104.
24. Rosenthal MA. Hand-rearing Patagonian cavies or maras (Dolichotis patagonum). International Zoo Yearbook 1974;14:214–5.
25. Prior N. The hand-rearing of an 8-day-old mara (Dolichotis patagonum) and its subsequent reintroduction into the group at Suffolk Wildlife Park. Ratel 2000;27(6):204–8.

26. Stahnke A, Hendrichs H. Cavy rodents. In: Parker SP, editor. Grzimek's encyclopedia of mammals. New York: McGraw-Hill; 1990. p. 325–36.
27. Edwards ME. Handrearing members of rodentia. AZA Animal Health Committee. In: Amand WB, editor. AZA Infant Diet Notebook. Wheeling (WV): American Association of Zoological Parks and Aquariums; 1994. p. 91–937.
28. Rosas-Rosas AG, Juan-Salles C, Garner MM. Pathological findings in a captive colony of maras (Dolichotis patagonum). Vet Rec 2006;158:727–31.
29. Harkness JE, Wagner JE. The Biology and medicine of rabbits and rodents. 4 edition. Philadelphia: Williams and Wilkins; 1995. p. 76–80.
30. Andersen NL. Basic husbandry and medicine of pocket pets. In: Birchard SJ, Sherding RG, editors. Saunders manual of small animal practice. Philadelphia: WB Saunders; 1994. p. 1363–89.
31. Ness RD. Rodents. In: Carpenter JW, editor. Exotic Animal Formulary. St. Louis (MO): Elsevier; 2005. p. 377–408.
32. Morrisey JK, Carpenter JW. Formulary. In: Quesenberry KE, Carpenter JW, editors. Ferrets, rabbits, and rodents: clinical medicine and surgery. 2nd edition. St Louis (MO): WB Saunders; 2004. p. 436–44.
33. Physiological reference values for the Patagonian cavy. International Species Information System, Apple Valley, Minn. March 2002.
34. Sainsbury AW. Rodentia (Rodents). In: Fowler ME, Miller RE, editors. Zoo and wild animal medicine. St. Louis (MO): Elsevier Science; 2003. p. 420–42.
35. Allen DG, Pringle JK, Smith DA, editors. Handbook of veterinary drugs. Philadelphia: JB Lippincott; 1998. p. 612–22.
36. Adamcak A, Otten B. Rodent therapeutics. In: Fronefield S.A, editor. Vet Clin North Am: Exotic animal practice: therapeutics. Philadelphia: WB Saunders; 2000. p. 221–37.
37. Collins BR. Antimicrobial drug use in rabbits, rodents and other small mammals. In: Antimicrobial therapy in caged birds and exotic pets. International Symposium North Am Vet Conf, Orlando (FL): Veterinary Learning Systems; 1995. p. 3–10.
38. Rosas-Rosas A, Juan-Salles C, Rodriguez-Arellanes G, et al. Disseminated Histoplasma capsulatum var capsulatum infection in a captive mara (Dolichotis patagonum). Vet Rec 2004;155:426–8.
39. Quesenberry KE. Guinea pigs. Vet Clin North Am Small Anim Pract 1994;24:67–87.
40. Juan-Salles C, Rico-Hernandez G, Garner MM, et al. Pulmonary besnoitiasis in captive Patagonian cavys (Dolichotis patagonum) associated with interstitial pneumonia. Vet Pathol 2004;41:408–11.
41. Joyner PH, Rochat MC, Hoover JP. Use of a hybrid external skeletal fixator for repair of a periarticular tibial fracture in a Patagonian cavy. JAVMA 2004; 224(8):1298–301.
42. Kik MJL, Liu PL, van Asten JAM. Cowpoxvirus infection in the Patagonian cavy (Dolichotis patagonum): emerging diseases in an educational animal park: the first reported case. Vet Q 2006;28(2):42–4.

Determinants for the Diet of Captive Agoutis (*Dasyprocta* spp.)

Deborah A. McWilliams, MSc[a,b,*]

KEYWORDS

- Dasyprocta • Diet • Rodentia • Agouti • Captive
- Nutrition • Frugivore • Omnivore

Sparse attention in the literature has been given to the considerations for an appropriate, practical diet for captive animals of the genus *Dasyprocta* (order Rodentia, family Dasyproctidae, common name agouti). *Dasyprocta* includes 11 extant species distributed throughout Central America, South America, and some associated islands (Coiba Island Panama, Roatan Island Honduras, and the Lesser Antilles). The species name, common name and average weights of the species in this genus are listed in **Table 1.**[1,2] These species are terrestrial rodents that prefer neotropical savannas and evergreen forests.[3,4] All species of *Dasyprocta* are diurnal[5] and are classified as scatter-hoarding frugivores.[6–9] Current species holdings in zoos that participate in the International Species Information System (ISIS) include *Dasyprocta azarae, D cristata, D fuliginosa, D leporine* (and subspecies), *D mexicana, D prymnolopha,* and *D punctata* (and subspecies).[10]

Species in the genus *Dasyprocta* resemble pacas but they are larger and more slender.[11] *Dasyprocta* are not burrowers,[8,11,12] although they use crevices or existing burrows for birthing and raising pups.[11–13]

DIET CLASSIFICATION

There is much evidence supporting classification of *Dasyprocta* species as a frugivore.[6–9] For example, *D leporine* is reported to have a wild diet that is 87% fruit, 6% animal matter, 4% fibrous foods, and 2% leaves.[8,9] There is an equal—if not overwhelming—amount of evidence that species of *Dasyprocta* are omnivores, however.

Dasyprocta, as members of the order Rodentia, have the generalist feeder, rodent dentition to support an omnivorous adaptation.[14] Similar to most caviomorphs, the

---

[a] American Association of Zoos and Aquariums Rodent, Insectivore and Lagomorph Taxon Advisory Group (AZA RIL-TAG), USA

[b] Canadian Association of Zoos and Aquariums Nutrition Advisory Group (CAZA-NARG), 807-40 Vanier Drive, Guelph, ON, N1G 2X7 Canada

* Canadian Association of Zoos and Aquariums Nutrition Advisory Group (CAZA-NARG), 807-40 Vanier Drive, Guelph, ON, N1G 2X7 Canada.

E-mail address: monogastricnutrition@yahoo.ca

Vet Clin Exot Anim 12 (2009) 279–286
doi:10.1016/j.cvex.2009.01.001
1094-9194/09/$ – see front matter © 2009 Elsevier Inc. All rights reserved.

METABOLIC RATE

The metabolic rate of *Dasyprocta* species varies according to territorial conditions or the housing conditions of captives.[16] For example, males bonded to a female are more active and have higher respiration rates and body temperatures (use more energy) than animals housed alone, male/male or all-male groups, or male and female non-bonded pairs. The activity of bonded males seems to be related to territoriality, and behaviors include digging, scrape-marking, and scenting.[26] Adult males defend their territory against any male at any time but adult females only defend their territory when food is scarce.[11]

An equation for estimating basal metabolic rate for *Dasyprocta* species from 2.7 to 3.3 kg is 8.78 × weight (kg).[27] In general, females weigh more than males.[9]

APPARENT DIETARY REQUIREMENTS

Studies on the captive diets of *Dasyprocta* are nonexistent. Captive *Dasyprocta* are reported to eat carrots, potatoes, cassava, and cooked ground beef.[23] In general, they eat meat only if cooked but this does not mean they will not eat uncooked flesh. For example, a group of captive *Dasyprocta* killed and ate an adult male *Liomys pictus* (painted spiny pocket mouse).[23]

The high proportion of seeds and nuts in the diets of wild *Dasyprocta* along with the selection of foods higher in energy and lower in water content in captive animals[7] suggest a preference for foods that offer sufficient protein and fats. Protein and fats are minimally available in most fruit pulp.[3] For example, avocado is a preferred food of captive *Dasyprocta* and this fruit is high in protein and fat.[7]

Dietary fiber levels for wild *Dasyprocta* seem to be consistent year-round, because of the availability of fruit when in season and the consumption of roots and plant matter during the off-season.[9] A suggested level of dietary crude fiber for a 2.7 kg animal is 157 g crude fiber/kg dry matter feed (DM).[28] Calculation of dietary fiber levels must be based on fruit without peels, because of the penchant of *Dasyprocta* to peel fruit before ingestion.[23]

Captive *Dasyprocta* seem to prefer foods high in ascorbic acid.[7] Again, whether the preference is for the ascorbic acid or the palatable fruit (mango, papaya, melon, oranges, pineapple, and tomato) remains to be determined.

Dasyprocta prefer eating either on elevated surfaces or under and within vegetation. They eat by sitting on their haunches and holding food with their forepaws. Food is often examined and tasted before ingestion, and spherical food or objects from 1.5 cm to 15 cm in diameter seem to be the most appealing.[23] The practice of handling and tasting food before ingestion is probably a form of examination and determination for suitability as a food. For example, wild *Dasyprocta* do not eat seeds containing quinolizidine alkaloids (QA) although they do cache these seeds.[29] QAs can disrupt neural function and they are also a teratogen.[21]

LIFE STAGE NUTRITION: REPRODUCTION

Sexual maturity in *Dasyprocta* can occur as early as 6 months of age.[8] Gestation is approximately 120 days and the precocial pups (one to two) are born furred with their eyes open.[11,23,30] Neonates weigh about 22.7 g, and the young are tolerated within a territory even after weaning.[23,31] The mating season of wild *D punctata* is February to April,[23] but in captivity *D punctata* often has two litters per year with about 4 months between litters.[8,11]

In the wild, pregnant *Dasyprocta* increase the amount of seeds (protein, fat, and energy) in their diets.[3] In captive guinea pigs (*C procellus*), another precocial rodent, the average daily energy intake during gestation was 16% greater than normal intake and energy intake while lactating was 92% greater than normal intake.[12] Female agoutis were observed to continue nursing pups as long as 7 weeks post partum.[29] As with many species, lactating females should be fed ad lib to guarantee provision of sufficient energy.

Despite the precociality of the pups, they will nurse even while eating solid food.[12] In the wild, at 1 day old, pups nurse, groom, and search leaf litter.[29] The lactating female does not provide the pups with solid food, but the pups do follow her and eat from her foods. Learning is probably a dominant factor in food choice, although pups eventually explore and eat foods not introduced by the dam.[29]

DIABETES

Rodent species have been used for decades as models for human diabetes.[31] In addition, wild caviomorph rodents (not including *Dasyprocta* species) have a low physiologic activity of insulin (1%–10% of the activity of most mammals),[32] and in serum glucose tests, caviomorph species produced more insulin than most mammals.[31] The current hypothesis states that the higher insulin response in these species is a compensatory mechanism for the lower physiologic activity of their insulin.[31] This compensatory response may also predispose them to developing diabetes, however.[33]

Field studies support the hypothesis that a higher insulin response in caviomorph species may predispose them to diabetes. Three wild caviomorph individuals, two *Abrocoma bennetti* (chinchilla rat) and one *Microcavia niata* (Andean Mountain cavy), had abnormal serum glucose concentration values and cataracts, and all three animals were obese. These are typical symptoms of diabetes.[33] A captive agouti diagnosed with diabetes was also obese and had cataracts.[31]

Extrapolating these findings to *Dasyprocta* species suggests that captives are at extremely high risk for developing diabetes, especially when fed as frugivores. Diabetes in general has become nearly epidemic in captive wild animals. For example, diabetes was once only believed to be a risk factor for sedentary, obese nonhuman primates.[34,35] Diabetes is increasingly identified in captive animals of other species, however.[36]

DENTAL CARIES AND PATHOLOGY

Studies of wild *Dasyprocta* suggest that captives are at high risk for developing dental caries and dental pathology. Dental caries were found in wild populations of caviomorphs, and this seems related to dietary carbohydrates (mainly those containing fructose, glucose, and sucrose)[37,38] that promote plaque and bacteria.[39] Dental caries have been induced in laboratory animals by feeding a soft diet high in carbohydrates.[40] In wild populations of caviomorphs, frugivores had the highest incidence of dental caries (10.5%–19.8%) in comparison with grazers (1.1%–8.7%).[38] Moderate fresh fruit consumption actually decreases the incidence of dental caries in humans.[41]

SUMMARY

Although there is no existing research on the dietary physiology and nutrition of captive *Dasyprocta* species, there are several recommendations that can be made for feeding captives. These include:

Feed as omnivores: There is overwhelming evidence that these species are omnivorous despite a preference for fruit when given food choices. Captive diets should have a high percentage (40% as fed) of foods providing protein and fats (avocado, seeds, nuts, legumes) supplemented with plant matter (40% as fed). Other foods, such as corn, oats, rice, rye, wheat, roots (carrots, parsnips), grasses, leaves, hibiscus flowers, and grains should be fed at about a 10% as-fed level. An estimated dietary crude fiber for a 2.7 kg animal is approximately 157 g crude fiber/kg DM.[27] Fruit and insects should be provided as environmental enrichment at approximately 10% of foods (as fed).

Provide opportunities for caching: Scatter-hoarding seems to be an innate behavior of *Dasyprocta* species. In captivity, caching of food would provide activity at the time of burial and later when food is retrieved. Most exhibits could accommodate an area of dirt of sufficient depth for this activity.

Prevent obesity: Caviomorph species are prone to obesity. Vigilant body condition scoring and weighing is the only way to reliably monitor weight gain or loss. In addition, provision for activity, such as caching opportunities, mazes, elevations, burrows, and puzzle boxes with novel items, encourages activity and energy use.

Gestation and lactation: The dietary percentage of foods providing protein and fats (seeds, nuts, and so forth) should be increased for gestating females, and the energy content should be increased by at least 16%.[12] Food should be provided ad lib for lactating females.

Prevent the development of diabetes: Current evidence suggests that wild and captive caviomorphs are at risk for diabetes. To date, it seems that caviomorphs produce more insulin than most mammals to compensate for the lower physiologic activity of their insulin.[31] This atypical physiologic factor may predispose *Dasyprocta* to developing diabetes. Feeding captive *Dasyprocta* as omnivores and feeding a diet low in fermentable carbohydrates seems to be preventative.[33]

Prevent dental caries: Individuals in wild populations of frugivorous caviomorphs had a 10.5%–19.8% incidence of dental caries.[38] This information seems to support that if fed as frugivores, captive *Dasyprocta* are also at high risk for developing dental caries. Feeding captive *Dasyprocta* as omnivores and feeding a diet low in fermentable carbohydrates seems to be a preventative.

REFERENCES

1. Redford KH, Eisenberg JF. Mammals of the neotropics, The Southern Cone: Chile, Argentina, Uruguay. Chicago: University of Chicago Press; 1992.
2. McNab MK. The influence of food habits on the energetics of eutherian mammals. Ecological Monographs 1986;56:1–20.
3. Henry O. Frugivory and the importance of seeds in the diet of the orange-rumped agouti (*Dasyprocta leporine*) in French Guiana. J Trop Ecol 1999;15:291–300.
4. Guimarães PR, Lopes PFM, Lyra ML, et al. Fleshy pulp enhances the location of *Syagrus romanzoffiana* (Arecaceae) fruits by seed-dispersing rodents in an Atlantic forest in southeastern Brazil. J Trop Ecol 2005;21:109–22.
5. Emmons LH, Feer F. Neotropical rainforest mammals: a field guide. 2nd edition. Chicago: University Press; 1997.
6. Arends A, McNab BK. The comparative energetics of caviomorph rodents. Comp Biochem Physiol A Mol Integr Physiol 2001;130:105–22.
7. Laska M, Baltazar JML, Luna ER. Food preferences and nutrient composition in captive pacas, Agouti paca (Rodentia, Dasyproctidae). Mamm Biol 2003;68: 31–41.

8. Dubost G, Henry O, Comizzoli P. Seasonality of reproduction in the three largest terrestrial rodents. Mamm Biol 2005;70(2):93–109.
9. Dubost G, Henry O. Comparison of diets of the acouchy, agouti and paca, the three largest terrestrial rodents of French Guianan forests. J Trop Ecol 2006;22: 641–51.
10. ISIS. International Species Information System. Available at: www.ISIS.org. Accessed December 2008.
11. Eisenberg JF, Redford KH. Mammals of the neotropics: the central neotropics, vol. 3. Chicago: The University of Chicago Press; 1999.
12. Kunkele J. Energetics of gestation relative to lactation in a precocial rodent, the guinea pig (*Cavia procellus*). J Zool (Lond) 2000;250:533–9.
13. Dubost G. Ecology and social life of the red acouchy, *Myoprocta exilis*; comparison with the orange-rumped agouti, *Dasyprocta leporina*. J Zool 1988;214: 107–23.
14. Landry SO Jr. The Rodentia as omnivores. Q Rev Biol 1970;45(4):351–72.
15. Townsend KEB, Croft DA. Enamel microwear in caviomorph rodents. J Mammal 2008;89(3):730–43.
16. Lee TE Jr, Hartline HB, Barnes BM. Dasyprocta ruatanica. Mammalian Species 2006;800:1–3.
17. Hoch GA, Adler GH. Removal of black palm (*Astrocaryum standleyanum*) seeds by spiny rats (*Proechimys semispinosus*). J Trop Ecol 1997;13:51–8.
18. Peres CA, Schiesari LC, Diasleme CL. Vertebrate predation of Brazil-nuts (*Bertholletia excelsa, Lecythidaceae*), an agouti-dispersed Amazonian seed crop: a test of the escape hypothesis. J Trop Ecol 1997;13:69–79.
19. Silva MG, Tabarelli M. Seed dispersal, plant recruitment and spatial distribution of Bactris acanthocarpa Martius (Arecaceae) in a remnant of Atlantic forest in northeast Brazil. Acta Oecol 2001;22:259–68.
20. Guimarães PR Jr, Gomes BZ, Ahn YJ, et al. Cache pilferage in red-rumped agoutis (*Dasyprocta leporina*) (Rodentia). Mammalia 2005;69(3–4): 431–4.
21. Panter KE, Keeler RF. Quinolizidine and piperidine alkaloid teratogens from poisonous plants and their mechanism of action in animals. Vet Clin North Am Food Anim Pract 1993;9(1):33–40.
22. Silvius KM. Spatio-temporal patterns of palm endocarp use by three Amazonian forest mammals: granivory or "grubivory"? J Trop Ecol 2002;18:707–23.
23. Smythe N. The natural history of the Central American agouti (*Dasyprocta punctata*). Smithsonian Contrib Zool 1978;257:1–52.
24. Yess NJ, Hegsted DM. Biosynthesis of ascorbic acid in the acouchi and agouti. J Nutr 1967;92(3):331–3.
25. Guimarães PR Jr, Kubota U, Zacarias B, et al. Testing the quick meal hypothesis: the effect of pulp on hoarding and seed predation of Hymenaea courbaril by red-rumped agoutis (*Dasyprocta leporine*). Austral Ecol 2006;31:95–8.
26. Korz V, Hendrichs H. Spontaneous behavior and body temperature in male Central American agoutis (*Dasyprocta punctata*) under different social conditions. Physiol Behav 1995;58(4):761–8.
27. Huesner AA. Size and power in mammals. J Exp Biol 1991;160:25–54.
28. Langer P. The digestive tract and life history of small mammals. Mamm Rev 2002; 32(2):107–31.
29. Guimarães PR Jr, Jose J, Galetti M, et al. Quinolizidine alkaloids in Ormosia arborea seeds inhibit predation but not hoarding by agoutis (*Dasyprocta leporina*). J Chem Ecol 2003;29(5):1065–72.

30. Galef BG, Clark MM. Non-nurturent functions of mother-young interaction in the agouti (*Dasyprocta punctata*). Behav Biol 1976;17:255–62.
31. Montiani-Ferreira F, Pachaly JR, Lange RR, et al. Cataract and diabetes in an agouti. In: Anais 15th Congresso Panamericano de Caencias Veterinarias. Campo Grande: Pan American Association of Veterinary Sciences; 1996. p. 71.
32. Opazo JC, Soto-Gamboa M, Bozinovic F. Blood glucose concentration in caviomorph rodents. Comp Biochem Physiol A Mol Integr Physiol 2004;137:57–64.
33. Garca-Rubi E, Calles-Escandon J. Insulin resistance and type 2 diabetes mellitus—evidence for a role of insulin. Arch Med Res 1999;30(6):459–64.
34. Diamond J. The double puzzle of diabetes. Nature 2003;423:599–602.
35. Sandrick K. Zoo nutrition: a walk on the wild side. J Am Diet Assoc 2001;101(8):868–9.
36. Sanchez C, Bronson E, Deem S, et al. Diabetes mellitus in a cheetah: attempting to treat the untreatable? In: Proceedings of the American Association of Zoo Veterinarians/American Association of Wildlife Veterinarians. 2005. p. 101–3.
37. Pollard MA. Potential cariogenicity of starches and fruits as assessed by the plaque-sampling method and an intraoral cariogenicity test. Caries Res 1995;29:68–74.
38. Sonea K, Koyasuc K, Tanakab S, et al. Effects of diet on the incidence of dental pathology in free living caviomorph rodents. Arch Oral Biol 2005;50:323–31.
39. Navia JM. Experimental periodontal disease. Animal models in dental research. Alabama: University of Alabama Press; 1977. p. 312–37.
40. Miles AEW, Grigson C. Variations and diseases of the teeth of animals. Cambridge (UK): Cambridge University Press; 1990.
41. Edgar WM. Extrinsic and intrinsic sugars: a review of recent UK recommendations on diet and caries. Caries Res 1993;27(Suppl):64–7.

Nutrition of Tree-dwelling Squirrels

Kerrin Grant, MS

KEYWORDS

- Tree squirrels • Flying squirrels • Nutrition
- Hand-rearing • Milk formulas

North American squirrels are categorized into one of three main groups based on physical characteristics, ecologic niche (including diet and food-hoarding strategies), and social structures. Animals designated as "tree squirrels" are divided into one of two genera. *Sciurus* (which means "shade tail") includes the larger tree squirrels with large, bushy tails, such as the eastern gray (*Sciurus carolinensis*), western gray (*Sciurus griseus*), Abert's (*Sciurus aberti*), fox (*Sciurus niger*), and Arizona gray squirrel (*Sciurus arizonensis*). The genus *Tamiasciurus* includes two smaller tree squirrels, the Douglas (*Tamiasciurus douglasii*), which is native to areas west of the Rockies, and the eastern US analog red squirrel (*Tamiasciurus hudsonicus*). These small squirrels are commonly called "chickarees," referring to the chattering call they emit. Another group of tree-dwelling squirrels is the flying squirrels (*Glaucomys sabrinus* and *Glaucomys volans*). The third main group is the ground-dwelling squirrels, which includes members of the genus *Spermophilus* (eg, California ground squirrel), chipmunks (*Eutamias* spp), prairie dogs (*Cynomys* spp), and marmots (*Marmota* spp), which are mentioned only briefly in this article.

WILD DIETS OF SQUIRRELS
Tree Squirrels

Tree squirrels are primarily native to forest environments, with the larger species found in deciduous and mixed forests and the chickarees found in coniferous forests. The eastern gray and fox squirrels are more utopian and have evolved to exploit other habitats, including parks and suburban neighborhoods.[1] The diet of tree squirrels is predominantly seeds (including nuts), fruit, buds, leaves, bark, and fungi growing on trees, although they also consume invertebrates such as beetles, caterpillars, and larvae of various insects (**Table 1**). They also have been known to gnaw on bones and eat soil (geophagy), presumably to consume minerals such as sodium, calcium, and magnesium, which are somewhat deficient in seeds and nuts.[2]

Eastern gray and fox squirrels are the most recognizable squirrel species in suburban and urban communities because they raid bird feeders and harvest food

Intensive Care Unit (ICU), The Wildlife Center, PO Box 246, Espanola, NM 87532, USA
E-mail address: zoonutrition@msn.com

Vet Clin Exot Anim 12 (2009) 287–297
doi:10.1016/j.cvex.2009.01.015
1094-9194/09/$ – see front matter © 2009 Elsevier Inc. All rights reserved.

Table 1
Natural food items of various species of squirrels

Douglas Squirrel	Red Squirrel	Eastern Gray Squirrel	Fox Squirrel	Townsend's Chipmunk	Flying Squirrel
Seeds from: pine, ash, mountain ash, Pacific silver fir, Douglas fir, spruce, Western hemlock, salal, filberts, caterpillars, beetles, larvae	Hazelnuts (filberts), beech nuts, spruce cones, pine cones	Acorns, pine, hickory, dogwood, beech, mushrooms, spruce, blackberry, cherry, caterpillars, beetles, larvae	Walnut, maple, serviceberry, elm, chokecherry, ash, cherry, corn, blackberry, acorns, hickory, huckleberry, beech, blueberry, grape, mulberry, willow, raspberry, beetles, butterflies, caterpillars	Common snowberry, black hawthorn (berries), Himalayan blackberries, purple peavine (flowers, peapods), springbank clover (flowers), Queen Anne's lace (flowers), dandelion (flowers), smooth hawksbeard (flowers), pumpkin seeds, wheat grass (seeds), mushrooms, bent grass (seeds), serviceberry, canary grass (seeds), perennial fescue, sumac, gooseberry, Brome grass (seeds)	Truffles, mushrooms, lichen, vegetation, invertebrates, tree sap, birds' eggs

from nut-producing trees. Burying acorns in the autumn months is a common sight in much of the country. In addition to providing an important energy source for squirrels in cold winter months, acorns contain secondary plant compounds known as tannins. Tannins are a plant defense for warding off predator attack by animals and have some deleterious effects on animals that consume them.[3] The bitter taste associated with tannins acts as a deterrent as the concentration of the compound increases. Tannins are also known to bind with dietary protein and iron, reducing the bioavailability of those nutrients to the animals.[3] Many species, such as deer, have adaptations for neutralizing tannins (eg, tannin-binding salivary proteins) and reducing the adverse effects of the plant compounds.[3] It is unclear whether squirrels have physiologic adaptations to bind tannins, but they have demonstrated adaptations in foraging behavior to minimize the negative effects of these secondary plant compounds. Studies indicate that fox squirrels preferentially collect and eat acorns from white oak trees early in the autumn rather than bury them.[2] This is because the tannin content of white oak acorns is relatively low (> 2%) and these acorns provide a good energy source as squirrels begin to store additional body fat. Any white oak acorns that are buried are first "modified" by the squirrels as they bite off the endocarp to prevent germination, which allows the seeds to be harvested at a later date by the squirrels. Acorns of the black oak group are also harvested by squirrels but contain higher concentrations of tannins (≥ 6% by weight), which affects the taste and has a greater effect on binding important nutrients.[4] Acorns from black oaks are harvested and buried by fox squirrels for later use; once buried, the tannins leach out, and these foods are retrieved and eaten later, after the tannins have leached out of the nut.

Red squirrels prefer hazelnuts/filberts (*Corylus* spp) over other seeds, followed by beech nuts *(Fagus spp),* spruce cones (*Picea* spp), and pine cones (*Pinus* spp).[2] Douglas squirrels prefer the cones from Pacific silver fir (*Abies amabilis*), followed by Douglas fir (*Pseudotsuga menziesii*), then spruce and Western hemlock (*Tsuga heterophylla*)[2] and hypogeous fungi.[5] Abert's squirrels feed on the inner bark of Ponderosa pine (*Pinus ponderosa*) twigs during winter.[6]

Flying Squirrels

Flying squirrels preferentially consume hypogeous mycorrhizal fungi (truffles) over other food items.[7,8] These fungi have moderate nutritional value compared to seeds.[9,10] They also readily consume all mast-crop nuts, tree sap, insects, carrion, bird eggs, and nestlings, buds, and flowers.[11]

Ground Squirrels

The natural diet of ground squirrels varies depending on subgroup but is typically more herbivorous than that of tree squirrels. Grasses, forbs, flowers, and buds form the bulk of the diet, with nuts, seeds, and invertebrates taken more opportunistically.[1]

CAPTIVE DIET

Captive squirrels must be fed a diet that provides adequate protein and supplies all the essential amino acids. Because squirrels commonly raid bird feeders, it is a common but inaccurate assumption that sunflower seeds are a normal part of their diet. Sunflower seeds are the equivalent of "junk food" and are deficient in the essential amino acid lysine. Lysine interferes with calcium absorption.[12] Sunflower seeds contain 8.5 times more phosphorus than calcium.[13] When squirrels fill up on these seeds, they are unable to obtain the proper ratio of calcium to phosphorus (1:1 to 2:1) needed to maintain proper bone growth, which increases the likelihood of metabolic bone disease in young squirrels. Peanuts are another inappropriate food for squirrels and are deficient in methionine. In the wild, squirrels have access to flowers, buds, stems, and other nuts and are able to balance their diet as needed. Unfortunately, when captive squirrels consume a high proportion of sunflower seeds and peanuts, they can develop health problems such as obesity, alopecia, and other maladies related to poor nutrition.[12] The recommended captive squirrel diet consists of 60% rodent lab chow or primate chow (do not offer rabbit or guinea pig chow, hamster or rat/mouse seed mixture), 30% fruit and vegetables, and 10% nuts and seeds. Examples of appropriate food items are provided in **Table 2**. Sunflower seeds and peanuts should be restricted to occasional treats and training vehicles only.

Weight ranges for adult tree squirrels are eastern gray: 410–710 g; fox: 504–1062 g; western gray: 340–964 g; chickarees: 140-300 g.[1]

Table 2
Appropriate captive diet items for tree squirrels and chipmunks

| | | Nuts and Seeds | |
Fruit	Vegetables	*Sciurus* spp	*Tamiasciurus* spp
Apples	Yam, raw	Pumpkin seeds	Beech nuts
Grapes	Carrots + leafy tops	Acorns	Scotch pine cones
Watermelon + seeds	Celery tops	Hazelnuts/ filberts	Norway spruce
Berries	Corn	English walnuts	Lodgepole pine cones
—	Peas	—	Western hemlock
—	Greens (collards, dandelion, mustard greens)	—	Douglas fir cones
—	Broccoli	—	—
—	Mushrooms	—	—

HAND-REARING INFANT SQUIRRELS

Often people find themselves with an orphaned squirrel pup. This scenario typically occurs when the nest is destroyed during storms and subsequent destruction of the habitat or when cats or dogs attack. It is preferable that concerned citizens contact an appropriate wildlife rehabilitation center and release the infant to them for proper care. Rehabilitators are more likely to have other squirrel pups, which allows squirrels to be raised with their own kind. This reduces the incidence of imprinting onto human caregivers and provides better preparation (through socialization) to squirrel life once they are released. Although cute and enjoyable when young, imprinted squirrels kept as pets tend to be destructive and aggressive when they reach puberty and generally do not adapt well to long-term captivity.

In the event that an appropriate rehabilitation facility is not available and hand-rearing is required, the following diet information should be incorporated into the hand-rearing protocol. **Table 3** contains information regarding the preferred substitute milk formula and recipe. It is imperative that squirrels (and most other wild animals) not be fed cow's milk, even on an emergency, short-term basis. The nutritional composition of cow's milk only provides approximately 35% of the protein and 27% of the fat requirement for squirrels and contains approximately 1.5 times more lactose than squirrel milk.[13] Protein is the limiting nutrient for growth, so giving a protein-deficient milk formula results in retarded growth during the phase when organ and muscle development is still occurring. Lactose is another limiting nutrient. Excess amounts of lactose cause an overgrowth of pathogenic intestinal bacteria, which results in chronic diarrhea and potentially death from enteritis. Finally, cow's milk contains twice as much water as squirrel milk and so does not provide adequate energy from an equivalent volume fed.

Condensed or evaporated milk also should be avoided because these products are cow's milk in a different form (ie, water removed and sugar added). Sweetened condensed milk contains 18 times more sugar than squirrel milk.[13] Homemade recipes for infant mammals that contain sugar in any form (eg, refined sugar, honey, corn syrup) never should be fed to squirrels because they increase the already excessive levels of sugar in the diet and result in enteritis and death of the infants.

Table 3
Comparison of gray squirrel maternal milk composition and appropriate substitute milk formulas (as-fed basis)

	Dry Matter (%)	Crude Protein (%)	Fat (%)	Milk Sugar (%)	kcal/mL
Maternal Milk[18]	25.4	9.0	12.1	3.0	1.57
Recommended substitute formula for squirrels	26.68	9.40	13.38	2.58	1.67
Esbilac liquid	18.1	6.2	7.9	2.5	0.98
Substitute milk formula recipe for squirrels					
1 part Esbilac or Milk Matrix 33/40					
1 part Multi-Milk or Milk Matrix 30/55					
2 parts water					

In order to reduce the carbohydrate content of milk formulas made with cow or goat milk, they would have to be diluted significantly to provide a lactose level appropriate for squirrels. By diluting the lactose component, however, fat and protein content are also diluted to levels that are insufficient for proper growth and development, resulting in death from chronic starvation. A milk formula must be constructed using commercial products that provide appropriate percentages and absolute values of fat and protein while limiting the amount of lactose.

The Pet Ag (261 Keyes Ave., Hampshire, IL 60140) formula for canine pups (Esbilac powder) is used as the base formula for replacement squirrel milk. Esbilac alone is insufficient in protein and fat and is inadequate for long-term nutrition, although it may be used initially until the preferred diet components are obtained. The author has successfully used the recommended milk formula listed in **Table 3** for tree squirrels (eastern gray, western gray, fox), ground squirrels (California, Washington, and Belding's), Northern flying squirrels, and Townsend's chipmunk. Douglas squirrels have been reared successfully on a slightly modified version of this diet, which is addressed in **Table 3**.

Before 1993, Pet Ag used coconut oil as the fat source in their KMR, Esbilac, and Multi-Milk recipes. In 1993, the ingredients were changed, with coconut oil being replaced by butterfat. The change was the result of research indicating that butterfat was more digestible in domestic dogs and cats. Wildlife rehabilitators and zoo facilities, which hand-raised infants, noticed that various species were developing digestive problems, however. Coconut oil has a high concentration of medium-chain fatty acids, which are generally more digestible than the long-chain fatty acids present in butterfat.[3] Pet Ag responded to the situation by marketing the Zoologic Milk Matrix line of milk formulas. It is essentially the pre-1993 version of their milk formulas and contains coconut oil instead of butterfat as the fat source. The Milk Matrix line uses formula numbers, which refer to the concentration of protein and fat, as the product names. Multi-milk = Milk Matrix 30/55; Esbilac = Milk Matrix 33/40. The Milk-Matrix version of Esbilac and Multi-Milk are the preferred products to use in rodent hand-rearing formulas.

The Milk Matrix line is easy to mix when the powder is added to cold water in equal parts and stirred in a "whisking" fashion. Then the additional water is added to the slurry and mixed completely. There are usually a lot of air bubbles right after mixing, but they dissipate within a few hours. The consistency is much thicker when the

full-strength stock milk formula is advisable; then it should be given every 2 to 3 days after that until the pup is consuming solid food. All of the probiotics may be discontinued during the weaning process but given as needed if loose stool/diarrhea occurs. *Acidophilus* comes in tablet form and may be crushed and added to the milk formula. The author has given small mammals (rodents and rabbits) *acidophilus* at the rate of 0.5 to 1 tablet in a batch of formula, which lasts 2 to 3 days, and has observed no ill effects from that dose. As a general guideline, one-half tablet per pup per day may be adequate. Yogurt contains *acidophilus* in much lower doses and may be used initially or on an emergency basis until a more concentrated form is obtained. Dannon's (White Plains, NY) Activia (plain or vanilla flavor, no sugar added) is the preferred brand.

WEANING DIET

Addition of solid foods to the squirrel diet may begin after 4 weeks of age. Solid foods are initially comprised of pureed items, such as vegetable baby foods, oatmeal. Continue offering normal milk formula volumes as solid food items are introduced to pups. As they consume solids on a regular basis, greens (dandelion, kale, mustard greens, parsley) also may be provided. Start decreasing milk formula feedings, one per day, each week as you increase the amount of solid foods. At 6 weeks of age, pieces of nuts (walnuts, pine nuts, filberts) may be offered as treats. Weaning from milk formula may be completed by 8 to12 weeks of age. Solid foods offered at that time are the same as for adults and are based on species (see **Tables 1** and **2**).

HEALTH PROBLEMS COMMONLY ASSOCIATED WITH SQUIRRELS

Diarrhea is commonly seen in infant squirrels and is caused by any combination of the following:

- Improper feeding technique—feeding too much (overextending the stomach) or too fast. Limit milk intake to 5% of the squirrel's body weight (when calculated in grams) per feeding and 20% to 25% body weight per day.
- Feeding a diet that lacks the proper percentage of dry matter (total solids) and carbohydrates. It is essential that the milk formula closely mimic the natural milk composition and not exceed the percent of carbohydrates or be deficient in protein and fat.
- Bacterial or parasitic infections, such as enteritis, can occur within 5 to 7 days of consuming an improper milk formula diet. White diarrhea accompanied by hypothermia, dehydration ($\geq$10%) and emaciation has a poor prognosis. Animals in good to fair condition may be given subcutaneous fluids (Normosol-R or NaCl + 2.5% dextrose) and antibiotics. Oral antibiotics should be limited to enrofloxacin (Baytril) and sulfonamides (Bactrim).

    Coccidiosis (*Eimeria* spp) can occur in squirrels $\geq$ 8 days of age. Most squirrels harbor *Eimeria* oocysts, but disease is self-limiting in healthy adults and does not require treatment if asymptomatic.[14,15] In young squirrels and injured adults that exhibit diarrhea and heavy loads of oocysts, sulfadimethoxine (Albon) is the treatment of choice and is given at the dose for coccidiosis for companion animals.

    Ascariasis from *Baylisascaris procyonis*: Rodents are the intermediate host for the raccoon roundworm. Infestation typically presents with neurologic signs as the larvae migrate to the brain and central nervous system.[16] Torticollis, nyotagmus, and incoordination are typical. The differential diagnosis is head trauma. It can also mimic signs of rabies and tetanus.[17] Because the larvae migrate to the central nervous system, ova are not expelled in the feces. The only way to definitively diagnose this parasite is to necropsy and take brain tissue for analysis. The likelihood of this condition is regional and is more typical in animals from wooded areas inhabited by large populations of raccoons, because contact with raccoon feces is the mode of transmission.

- Side effects of antibiotic therapy, With the exception of enrofloxacin (Baytril) and sulfonamides (Bactrim, Albon), oral antibiotics are not recommended. As they pass through the gastrointestinal tract, beneficial bacteria required to break down plant material are also killed by the drugs. The following modifications to antibiotic treatment protocols should include:

  Add probiotics to the diet (on a daily basis) while on oral antibiotics to provide an influx of beneficial bacteria while the gastrointestinal tract is stressed by bactericidal medications.

  Limit antibiotic therapy to 2 to 3 days. With the exception of severe bacterial infections, this time frame is typically adequate. Squirrels have a strong constitution and recover quickly from wounds and bacterial infection, so 7 to 10 days of antibiotic therapy is generally not warranted and tends to have deleterious effects.

  Enrofloxacin is a good first-line choice for wound management. A suspension may be formulated and flavored with fruit baby food to use it as an oral medication. Penicillin-G and analogs (eg, amoxicillin) should never be used in rodents.

OTHER HEALTH ISSUES
Mange

Mange can be caused by *Sarcoptes scabiei* or *Notoedres cati* mites. Sarcoptic mange most commonly occurs in the extremities, groin, and face, whereas *Notoedres* more typically localizes in the head and neck region, although other areas may be affected from grooming. Diagnosis is by microscopic identification of the mites. *Notoedres* resembles *Sarcoptes*, but the slit-like anus is subterminal on the dorsal abdomen rather than terminal, as it is in *Sarcoptes* (R. Haveman, DVM, personal communication, 1988). Treatment is similar for both species of mange. Ivermectin (Ivomec 0.27% injectible) is the treatment of choice. Administer 2.7mg/kg bodyweight subcutaneously and repeat dose in 2 weeks.

Abscesses

Puncture wounds from tree branches and cat bites result in localized abscesses. Treatment includes antibiotic therapy, with enrofloxacin being the treatment of choice.

Seizures

Tremors and seizures can result from several physiologic abnormalities, including nutritional imbalances and head trauma. Diets deficient in absolute amounts of calcium or ones that have a skewed calcium to phosphorus ratio (Ca:P) can result in seizure-like activity, especially in young, growing squirrels. The proper Ca:P in growing squirrels is 2:1; in adults it is 1:1. Nuts and seeds are highly skewed toward phosphorus and may have deleterious effects in maintaining a proper Ca:P ratio unless balanced with other foods, such as rodent chow and greens. In the wild, squirrels are able to access bones and soil that contain high levels of minerals that are deficient in their seasonal diet. In captivity, they are at the mercy of the diet they are offered and are generally unable to access other nutrients they need to maintain proper health.

Head and Spinal Trauma

Seizure activity not associated with nutritional imbalances or parasitism is an indication of brain trauma. Spinal trauma commonly occurs in squirrels that have been hit by cars. Dragging the hind limbs, with or without deep pain reflex, indicates spinal trauma. Supportive care and administration of antibiotics (eg, enrofloxacin) and steroid therapy have limited success, and these cases typically have a poor prognosis.

SUMMARY

The diet of tree squirrels is predominantly seeds, nuts, fruit, buds, leaves, bark, and fungi growing on trees, although they also consume invertebrates such as beetles, caterpillars, and larvae of various insects. Flying squirrels preferentially consume hypogeous mycorrhizal fungi (truffles) over other food items but also consume mast-crop nuts, tree sap, insects, carrion, bird eggs, and nestlings, buds, and flowers. The recommended captive squirrel diet consists of 60% rodent lab chow or primate chow, 30% fruit and vegetables, and 10% nuts and seeds. The appropriate hand-rearing formula for infant squirrels consists of one part Esbilac or Milk Matrix 33/40, one part Multi-Milk or Milk Matrix 30/55, and two parts water.

REFERENCES

1. Whitaker JO Jr. Squirrels. In: Audubon Society Field Guide to North American Mammals. New York: Alfred A. Knopf; 1985. p. 370–424.
2. Gurnell J. Natural history of squirrels. New York: Christopher Helm Publ. Ltd; 1987.
3. Robbins CT. Wildlife feeding and nutrition. 2nd edition. San Diego (CA): Academic Press; 1993.
4. Thorington RW, Ferrell K. Food and feeding. In: Squirrels: the animal answer guide. Baltimore (MD): Johns Hopkins Univ Press; 2006. p. 102–13.
5. Pyare S, Longland WS. Patterns of ectomycorrhizal fungi consumption by small mammals in remnant old-growth forests of the Sierra Nevada. J Mammal 2001; 82:681–9.
6. Snyder MA. Abert's squirrel in ponderosa pine: the relationship between selective herbivory and plant host fitness. Am Nat 1993;141:866–79.
7. Hall DS. Diet of the northern flying squirrel at Sagehen Creek, California. J Mammal 1991;72:615–7.
8. Maser Z, Maser C, Trappe JM. Food habits of the northern flying squirrel in Oregon. Can J Zool 1985;63:1084–8.
9. Claridge A, Trappe JM, Cork SJ, et al. Mycophagy by small mammals in the coniferous forests of North America: nutritional value of sporocarps of Rhizopogon vinicolor, a common hypogeous fungus. J Comp Physiol [B] 1999;169:172–8.
10. Cork SJ, Kenagy GJ. Rates of gut passage and retention of hypogeous fungal spores in two forest dwelling rodents. J Mammal 1989;70:512–9.
11. Mitchell D. Spring and fall diet of the endangered West Virginia northern flying squirrel (Glaucomys sabrinus fuscus). Am Midl Nat 2001;146:439–43.
12. Sheldon WG. Alopecia of flying squirrels. J Wildl Dis 1971;7:111–4.
13. USDA. National Nutrient Database SR17. Available at: www.nal.usda.gov/fnic/foodcomp. Accessed July 15, 2008.

14. McAllister CT, Upton SJ. *Eimeria lancasterensis* (Apicompexa: Eimeriidae) from the eastern fox squirrel, *Sciurus niger* (Rodentia:Sciuridae), in North-Central Texas. J Parasitol 1989;75(4):642-4.
15. Schmidt GD, Roberts LS. Foundations of parasitology. 4th edition. St Louis (MO): Times Mirror/Mosby Publ; 1989. p. 116–22.
16. Nance D. *Baylisascaris procyonis* and the wildlife rehabilitator. Wildl J 1986;9(3): 12–5.
17. Kasacos KR. Raccoon ascarids as a cause of larval migrans. Parasitol Today 1986;2(9):253–5.
18. Nixon CM, Harper WJ. Composition of gray squirrel milk. Ohio J Sci 1972;72(1): 3–6.

Nutrition and Behavior of Fennec Foxes (*Vulpes zerda*)

Janet L. Dempsey, MS[a], Sherilyn J. Hanna[b], Cheryl S. Asa, PhD[c], Karen L. Bauman, BS[c],*

KEYWORDS

- Fennec fox • *Vulpes zerda* • Nutrition • Behavior
- Hand-rearing

The fennec fox (*Vulpes zerda*) is the smallest canid. Native to the arid desert regions of northern Africa and the Sinai Peninsula,[1] these tiny foxes are well adapted for desert life. Fennec foxes have sand- or cream-colored fur with black-tipped tails and extremely large ears that are believed to aid in cooling and in locating prey. The soles of the paws are furred to protect against the hot sand. Fennec foxes are nocturnal, although a few reports suggest that they may be crepuscular.[2,3]

Fennec foxes make popular pets because of their small size, minimal odor, and highly social behaviors. They are kept in zoos for conservation and educational programs. The number of individuals remaining in the wild is unknown.[1,4] It is likely that a sustainable wild population exists, because the fennec fox is commonly trapped and sold for the pet and fur trades.[1,4] The uncertain political climate within their native range makes it difficult to obtain current population data; thus, these foxes are listed by the International Union for Conservation of Nature (IUCN) Red List of Threatened Animals as "data deficient"[5] and by Convention on International Trade of Endangered Species as Appendix II. In 2007, the IUCN Canid Specialist Group listed the fennec fox as one of its priority species to emphasize the vital need for more information.

Fennec foxes have few unique nutritional or behavioral problems and are fairly easy to maintain in captivity. They can be nervous, especially if not hand-raised, and are sensitive to disturbances, making breeding challenging. An understanding of the natural behaviors is essential. For example, fennec foxes dig in the wild to create dens and locate food; with these animals in homes, this can lead to unwanted digging in furniture or to individuals escaping. The exotic animal practitioner is most likely to be presented with overweight fennec foxes on inappropriate diets or receiving too much food. As with domestic dogs and cats, obese fennec foxes may suffer from health

[a] Technical Services, Nestlé Purina PetCare Company, Checkerboard Square, Saint Louis, MO 63164, USA
[b] Exotic Endeavors, Camarillo, CA, USA
[c] Research Department, Saint Louis Zoo, 1 Government Drive, Saint Louis, MO 63110, USA
* Corresponding author.
E-mail address: kbauman@stlzoo.org (K.L. Bauman).

Vet Clin Exot Anim 12 (2009) 299–312
doi:10.1016/j.cvex.2009.01.004
1094-9194/09/$ – see front matter © 2009 Elsevier Inc. All rights reserved.

vetexotic.theclinics.com

vertebrate and invertebrate, which are commercially raised and fed to captive carnivores (**Table 1**). Analysis of entire vertebrate carcasses shows less variability in nutrient composition across species than invertebrate carcasses. These data, although limited, are still important to consider when developing diets for captive fennec foxes. The nutrient content of commercially raised prey is likely to be different from wild prey. The finding that commercially raised prey items are high in energy and fat should be taken into account when formulating captive diets.

Nutrient Requirements

There are currently no published nutrient requirement data for fennec foxes. The most appropriate animal models for developing diets for fennec foxes are the domestic dog and cat. The National Research Council's[25] estimated nutrient requirements for dogs and cats provide a basis for comparison to nutrient content of diets developed for captive fennec foxes. In addition, the Association of American Feed Control Officials publishes minimum nutrient levels for foods manufactured for dogs and cats.[26] These data also provide valuable guidelines for evaluating captive fennec fox diets. Whenever possible, the total diet provided should be chemically analyzed by a professional nutrition laboratory to determine nutrient concentrations, and the results should be compared with data in **Table 2**. At a minimum, diets should be analyzed for moisture, crude protein, crude fat, crude fiber, and ash. These values enable calculation of estimated metabolizable energy using the modified Atwater method.[26] Software programs are also available to calculate dietary nutrient content.

Food Availability and Practical Captive Diets

When formulating diets for captive fennec foxes, caretakers must identify the foods available and appropriate for meeting probable nutrient needs. Commercially manufactured diets for domestic dogs and cats (dry, canned, or raw/frozen) can provide the basis for captive fennec fox diets. These commercial products can supply most essential vitamins and minerals if they are included in the diet in the appropriate amounts. Observations of fennec foxes at zoos and private breeding facilities that

Table 1
Nutrient composition of selected vertebrate and invertebrate prey on a dry matter basis

Species	Body Mass (g)	Dry Matter (%)	Crude Protein (%)	Fat (%)	Ash (%)	Calcium (%)	Phosphorus (%)
Rat, adult	280.0	34.0	59.7	23.6	15.7	4.0	1.8
Rat, pup	5.9	14.0	77.1	7.1	15.7	—	—
Mouse, adult	27.6	31.5	58.3	23.9	11.0	3.4	1.8
Mouse, pup	1.6	16.7	74.9	12.6	12.6	—	—
Mouse, pup	5.9	25.8	59.2	23.6	9.8	2.3	1.9
Chick, domestic	34.3	33.0	67.9	16.8	8.2	1.7	0.9
House cricket	—	29.9	66.1	17.3	6.1	0.18	0.86
Mealworm larvae	—	36.1	48.4	41.7	4.6	0.07	0.60
Waxmoth larvae	—	43.9	30.8	61.5	1.8	0.03	0.39

Data from Allen ME, Oftedal OT, Baer DJ, et al. The feeding and nutrition of carnivores. In: Kleinman DG, editor. Wild mammals in captivity: principles and techniques. Chicago: University of Chicago Press; 1996. p.139–47.

successfully raise these animals have shown that captive fennec foxes readily accept these types of products. **Table 2** compares five diets with recommended minimum dietary nutrient levels. Nutrient recommendations have been extrapolated from information for domestic dogs and cats. Dogs do not require fat and protein levels as high as those required by cats, however, likely because cats are carnivores and canids are omnivores. It is therefore not necessary to feed solely meat-based products to captive canids, such as fennec foxes. Dry foods or a mixture of canned or raw/frozen meat-based products with dry food are more appropriate for fennec foxes. The recommended percentage of commercial foods within the total diet by weight, as fed, is 30% to 50%, with at least one half of the diet as dry dog or cat food. Additional nutritional supplements are not necessary if nutritionally complete foods make up most of the diet.

Fresh produce may be included in the diet to mimic the plants wild fennec foxes consume. Produce includes fruits, vegetables, and leafy green vegetables that provide additional sources of certain nutrients and fiber. Produce should be restricted to 10% to 20% of the diet, by weight, as fed, to prevent dilution of essential nutrients.

Prey items, including vertebrates and invertebrates, also may be fed regularly. In general, vertebrate prey, such as rats, mice, and chicks (domestic chicken or quail), are substantially more expensive than commercial diets, and their nutrient content is highly variable. It is therefore recommended that these items be used only as enrichment one to three times per week. Invertebrate prey consists of commonly available insects, such as crickets and mealworms. Insects tend to be low in calcium and if fed in large amounts may lead to inadequate intake of dietary calcium. Vertebrate prey should not make up more than 5% to 15%, by weight, as fed, and invertebrate prey should be limited to no more than 5% to 10% of the diet. Clean water should be available at all times to captive fennec foxes, even though wild fennec foxes subsist for extended periods without access to free water.

Fennec foxes should be fed at least once daily, although a recent survey of feeding practices in zoos and private breeding facilities indicates that most institutions feed two times daily. The total amount of food offered per day depends not only on the animal's activity and physiologic state but also on the diet's energy and nutrient density. A common assumption is that animals consume enough food to meet their energy needs and self-regulate intake. The prevalence of obesity in captive exotic animals illustrates that relying on the animal to regulate its intake of an "unnatural" diet is problematic. Institutions keeping adult fennec foxes (weighing an average of 1–2 kg each) generally feed a total daily quantity of diet (as fed) equal to 5% to 10% of body weight. This formula can serve as a rule of thumb for determining the daily amount of diet to offer. The body condition of individual foxes should be assessed regularly. Guidelines for assessing body condition in domestic dogs and cats can be applied to captive foxes.[27–30] Animal nutritionists, veterinarians, biologists, and animal managers all may be helpful in developing successful nutritional husbandry programs for captive exotic species, such as fennec foxes.

HAND-REARING

Maternal care is the best for the newborn. Hand-rearing may be undertaken, however, when the dam is unable to produce an adequate supply or quality of milk, with maternal rejection or aggression, or when the pups are unable to nurse properly because of weakness or competition. Hand-rearing may also be elected for behavioral reasons to promote the human–animal bond and to produce pups that are easily handled and are calmer in captivity. Hand-rearing for behavioral reasons is a common

Table 2
Composition and nutrient content of sample diets fed to captive fennec foxes (*Vulpes zerda*) compared with minimum nutrient recommendations

Food Category	Diets (% of the Diet as Fed)				
	Diet 1	Diet 2	Diet 3	Diet 4	Diet 5
Nutritionally complete dry canine diet	20.8	6.1	19.3	—	43.5
Nutritionally complete dry feline diet	—	—	—	30.1	—
Nutritionally complete canned canine diet	—	—	18.6	—	—
Nutritionally complete canned feline diet	52.2	18.2	—	—	28.4
Nutritionally complete raw meat–based diet	—	26.3	—	—	—
Fresh produce (fruits and/or vegetables)	22.7	39.3	57.7	31.7	3.2
Whole prey	3.9	7.7	2.6	2.7	3.0
Insects	0.3	1.2	1.8	15.2	5.5
Nutritional supplements	0.1	1.2	—	1.5	—
Miscellaneous	—	—	—	18.8[a]	16.4[b]
Total	100.0	100.0	100.0	100.0	100.0

Nutrients	Units	Minimum Recommended Dietary Nutrient Range for Fennec Foxes[c]	Diets (Calculated Nutrient Levels on a Dry Matter Basis)				
			Diet 1	Diet 2	Diet 3	Diet 4	Diet 5
Crude protein[d]	%	22.0–30.0	22.4	35.2	25.7	30.5	41.6
Crude Fat	%	5.0–9.0	9.4	23.4	10.1	13.3	21.3
Linoleic acid	%	1.0–2.0	NA[e]	1.2	1.2	4.0	NA
Arachidonic	%	0.02–0.1	0.03	NA	NA	NA	NA
Vitamins and other							
Vitamin A	IU/g	5.0–50.0	38.4	45.4	169.2	6.6	34.3
Vitamin D	IU/g	0.5–3.0	2.1	0.9	1.1	1.0	2.0
Vitamin E	IU/g	0.05–0.75	0.21	0.12	NA	0.07	0.14

Vitamin K	mg/kg	0.1	NA	NA	NA	NA	NA
Thiamine	mg/kg	5.0	24.8	9.1	5.6	NA	8.5
Riboflavin	mg/kg	4.0	5.0	9.1	3.8	4.2	9.8
Pantothenic acid	mg/kg	10.0	12.2	24.5	13.4	21.2	20.5
Niacin	mg/kg	60.0	NA	59.4	NA	NA	76.4
Pyridoxine	mg/kg	4.0	4.3	6.8	7.4	4.5	11.2
Folic acid	mg/kg	0.8–1.0	1.2	1.0	1.0	NA	1.9
Biotin	mg/kg	0.07	0.14	NA	0.08	0.1	0.2
Vitamin B_{12}	mg/kg	0.02–0.05	0.02	0.06	0.02	0.02	0.17
Choline	mg/kg	1200	NA	NA	NA	NA	2913
Minerals							
Calcium	%	0.6–1.0	0.6	1.2	1.1	0.87	1.7
Phosphorus	%	0.5–0.8	0.5	0.8	0.7	0.78	1.4
Potassium	%	0.6	NA	0.8	1.0	0.6	0.7
Sodium	%	0.2	NA	0.3	NA	NA	NA
Chloride	%	0.3	NA	NA	NA	NA	NA
Magnesium	%	0.08	NA	0.31	0.13	0.16	0.13
Iron	mg/kg	80	NA	156	136	138	238
Copper	mg/kg	10.0	NA	24.9	10.3	10.2	17.5
Manganese	mg/kg	7.5	9.3	30.3	39.5	44.4	28.9
Zinc	mg/kg	100–1000	NA	158	NA	NA	146
Iodine	mg/kg	1.5	NA	1.1	1.4	NA	3.0
Selenium	mg/kg	0.11	0.16	NA	NA	NA	0.20

[a] Miscellaneous items consisted of a nutritionally complete primate biscuit, which contributed significantly to the overall nutrient content.
[b] Miscellaneous items consisted of cooked chicken egg whites, which contributed significantly to the overall dietary crude protein content.
[c] Recommended values from this article based on National Research Council 2006 and Association of American Feed Control Officials 2008 data.
[d] Values for individual amino acids were not calculated because of lack of these data for most of the diet ingredients used.
[e] NA, not available (indicates values for this nutrient were not available in database for one or more of the nutritionally complete feeds and therefore were not calculated).

practice in the private sector where fennec foxes are bred and raised as pets. The decision to hand-rear should be made early, and a consistent plan should be followed to be successful.

Maintaining body temperature of hand-reared pups is vital. Normal body temperature for pups is the same as that for domestic dogs. Body temperature at birth is 35.5° to 36°C (96°–97°F) increasing incrementally to 37.8°C (100°F) by 4 weeks old. Keeping pups in a small crate with a heating pad (Sunbeam, Boca Raton, FL; king size) under one end of the crate may be more successful than an incubator. Unlike in an incubator, where temperature is constant, an under-crate heating pad allows pups to regulate their body temperatures by moving toward or away from the heat source (S. J. Hanna, unpublished observation, 1998). This crate method uses a small (17 × 12 × 8) under-seat airline carrier with an open metal frame top (Petmate, Arlington, TX), with a hand towel and a stuffed animal toy placed inside the crate for snuggling to substitute for the dam. The heating pad is set on low-medium setting, depending on the ambient temperature, and can be adjusted according to the pups' behavior. Pups sleep huddled together if they are cold or far apart and away from the heating pad if they are too warm. If necessary, pups removed for hand-rearing should be warmed to normal body temperature before feeding to help ensure proper digestive function.

Even fennec fox pups that are to be hand-raised should be allowed to nurse from the dam shortly after birth if possible, to obtain colostrum, or first milk, produced by the dam. Colostrum contains immunoglobulins and other immune factors that are absorbed across the intestinal mucosa and provide passive immunity to the pups. The neonatal intestine can absorb these intact proteins for approximately the first 48 hours of life.[27,31] Pups hand-reared for behavioral reasons are generally not removed from the dam until 10 days of age to allow them adequate colostrum intake; this practice has been successful in private breeding collections (S.J. Hanna, unpublished observations, 1998).

MILK COMPOSITION

The major components of milk are water, protein, fat, sugar, and mineral matter (ash). The proportion of these components in milk and milk output vary not only with species but also with stage of lactation.[31,32] A comprehensive review of milk composition in domestic and nondomestic mammalian species categorized data based on general trends in nutrient composition. Only those species with a minimum of three milk samples taken during midlactation were included. This review showed that canid milk tends to be high in dry matter and protein, moderately high in fat, and low in sugar. Additional data have been published on the milk composition of certain fox species and the domestic dog.[33–37]

FORMULA SELECTION

The nutrient composition of formula should mimic dam's milk as closely as possible. The use of inappropriate formulas to hand-rear can lead to complications, such as diarrhea, dehydration, growth failure and, ultimately, death. **Table 3** shows milk composition data available for other fox species and the domestic dog. **Table 3** also lists the nutrient composition of the commercially available puppy milk replacer, Esbilac (Pet Ag Inc., Hampshire, IL), the most commonly and successfully used formula among zoos and private breeders. Esbilac is available in two forms: powder, which is more economical and easier to store, and liquid, which is more convenient to use and requires less preparation time. The nutrient composition of both forms falls within the recommended range for canid species and also adequately meets the

Table 3
Comparison of nutrient composition of milk for selected species of domestic and nondomestic Canidae with commercial milk replacer formulas

Species	N	Nutrient Composition (As-Fed Basis)					Reference
		Dry Matter (%)	Gross Energy (kcal/mL)	Fat (%)	Protein (%)	Sugar (%)	
Domestic dog (Canis familiaris)	25	22.7	—	9.5	7.5	3.8	Offedal 1980[31]
Domestic dog (C familiaris)	5+	—	0.80	4.5–5.2	4.0–6.0	4.0–5.0	Lonnerdal et al 1981[36]
Red Fox (Vulpes vulpes)	3	18.1	—	5.8	6.7	4.6	Young and Grant 1931[37]
Arctic Fox (Alopex lagopus)	100+	28.6	—	13.5	11.1	3.0	Dubrovskaya 1967[35]
Commercial milk replacer formulas							
Esbilac powder diluted 1:2[a]	—	18.5	0.90	8.2	6.5	2.9	PetAg Inc., 2006
Esbilac powder half-strength formula[b]	—	9.3	0.45	4.1	3.3	1.4	PetAg Inc., 2006
Esbilac liquid[c]	—	15.1	0.82	6.4	5.1	2.9[d]	PetAg Inc., 2006
Esbilac liquid half-strength formula[e]	—	7.6	0.55	3.2	2.5	1.4	PetAg Inc., 2006

[a] Calculated from manufacturer's information, one part Esbilac powder to two parts water, where one part Esbilac = 1 cup = 106 g dry Esbilac and 1 cup water = 226.8 g, on an as-fed basis.
[b] Esbilac formula prepared as in previous footnote and then further diluted 1:1 (50%:50% by weight) with water or Pedialyte.
[c] Manufacturer's information.
[d] Calculated from manufacturer's information.
[e] Esbilac liquid diluted 1:1 (50%:50% by weight) with water or Pedialyte.

needs of fox species. Esbilac is formulated to be nutritionally complete and to provide adequate energy and essential vitamins and minerals to meet the requirements of growing domestic dogs.

FEEDING REGIMEN: FORMULA PREPARATION, FEEDING FREQUENCY AND AMOUNT

The correct preparation of formula is important. Formula that is too dilute does not support growth and may encourage overeating. Formula that is too concentrated may cause gastrointestinal upset, diarrhea, and dehydration, eventually resulting in failure to grow. When young are first removed from the dam for hand-rearing, it may be necessary to rehydrate the pups by giving an oral electrolyte solution, such as Pedialyte (Abbott Nutrition, Columbus, OH) for the first feeding. It is not uncommon for the pups to initially refuse Pedialyte; apple-flavored Pedialyte seems to help in the transition (S.J. Hanna, unpublished observations, 1998).

Esbilac powder, prepared according to package directions using boiled or bottled water, or liquid, ready-to-feed Esbilac can be used for feeding. The first feeding should consist of 100% Pedialyte to rehydrate the pup; all subsequent feedings for the first 24 hours should consist of prepared formula diluted with Pedialyte. The concentration of formula should be increased by 25% and the concentration of Pedialyte decreased by 25% with each successive feeding. The last feeding before moving to full-strength formula should consist of 75% formula with 25% boiled or bottled water replacing the Pedialyte to ease the transition off electrolytes. The temperature of the formula should be as close to the pup's normal body temperature as possible. If signs of gastrointestinal upset occur at any point, return to the previous dilution for a few feedings until symptoms cease. Pups may take up to 24 hours to accept formula, so a small drop in body weight is expected. If there is no rebound in body weight within 1 to 2 days, the pup should be examined to rule out other problems.

Some pups accept and do well on full-strength formula after the first 24 hours if the feeding frequency and amount are strictly controlled. Alternately, some pups respond better when fed dilute formula (two parts formula to one part water) and allowed to feed ad lib throughout hand-rearing, until solid food is introduced at weaning. Any symptoms of gastrointestinal distress, especially diarrhea or failure to gain weight over a 2-day period, are a clear sign to provide more dilute formula or to decrease the amount fed at each feeding until symptoms cease. If problems persist, or the pups continue to lose weight, a veterinarian should be consulted immediately.

The feeding frequency is also adjusted throughout hand-rearing based on the pup's age and the formula dilution. Pups pulled from birth to 10 days of age should be fed more frequently, approximately every 2 to 2.5 hours per 24 hours. From approximately 11 to 26 days of age, pups can be fed every 3 to 3.5 hours per 24 hours. Some facilities adopt an 18-hour feeding period when pups are 11 days old, and feed every 2 to 3 hours with success. Once pups reach 26 to 28 days old, small amounts of solid food in the form of baby rice cereal (Gerber, Fremont, MI; single grain rice) can be introduced into formula at a concentration of two parts Esbilac to one part water to one part cereal. At this time, the interval between feedings can be extended to every 4 to 4.5 hours, with no feedings for 6 to 7 hours overnight. Weaning can begin when the pups are 28 to 30 days of age.

The amount of formula fed is just as important as the nutrient composition, formula preparation, and feeding frequency. The daily quantity of formula should provide adequate nutrition to maintain health and to support normal weight increases while avoiding gastrointestinal upset. Most mammalian young consume a quantity of formula equivalent to 10% to 25% of body weight per day at peak lactation.[31] General recommendations for hand-reared carnivores are to feed a volume equivalent to 10% to 15% of body weight per day from birth through 3 weeks of age, gradually increasing to 20% to 25% of body weight per day by 4 weeks of age.[27,31,38] Milk replacer formulas tend to be highly palatable, which can promote overfeeding and lead to gastrointestinal upset. A volume not greater than 5% to 7% of body weight should therefore be fed at each feeding.[39] Pups should be weighed daily, preferably in the morning before the first feeding; the total daily amount to be fed and the number of feedings should be calculated from this body weight. Because the concentration of prepared milk replacer is close to 1 g/mL, 1 g of formula (calculated as a percent of body weight) is equivalent to 1 mL. The percentage of body weight used to determine the daily feeding volume should be adjusted as necessary to promote daily weight gain and to avoid gastrointestinal upset.

Experienced breeders who are able to devote extensive time to hand-rearing pups for behavioral reasons often use an observational approach to determine feeding quantities. This method's success hinges on using dilute formula throughout hand-rearing, usually two parts prepared formula to one part water, with a 24-hour feeding schedule, until pups are 26 days of age. Pups are allowed to consume as much formula as they will take at each feeding until the stomach is full but not tight, and they are not restricted to a specified volume unless they have gastrointestinal distress. Pups on this system must be observed carefully to avoid under- or overfeeding. This method may also involve more frequent changes in formula dilution based on individual variation among pups. Accurate and detailed records are essential to success.

When hand-rearing pups, the first few feedings should be given with either a 2-oz bottle, such as the Nurser (Pet Ag, Hampshire, IL), or with a 1-mL syringe. A syringe should only be used by an experienced feeder, because pups can easily aspirate formula into the lungs when they feed eagerly. Syringe feeding works well, because the exact amount of formula consumed is known, formula flow is easily regulated, and less air may be ingested. Pups that show distress after feeding not attributed to aspiration of formula may need to be burped by holding them upright for a few minutes. After each feeding, the pups must be stimulated to urinate and/or defecate by rubbing the anal region with a warm, damp towel, the same as domestic puppies.

A quantity of formula equal to what will be needed per 24-hour period should be prepared and refrigerated. Immediately before feeding, a portion of formula should be poured into a 4-oz human baby bottle (Advent, Andover, MA) and heated using an electric bottle warmer. At the end of the day, unused heated formula should be discarded, along with unused refrigerated formula, to prevent spoilage. Pups should be weighed at the same time each day, preferably before the first morning feeding. Information, such as daily weights, feeding time, feeding amounts, urination, feces, and any other observations (eg, eager feeder, slow response, lethargy, medications given) should be recorded for each pup. The back of each pup's ear should be marked for quick identification with a small dot from a different colored marker. Identification of each pup facilitates tracking an individual pup's progress and early identification of potential problems (**Fig. 1**).

WEANING

Weaning begins when the pups reach 28 to 30 days of age. By this time, pups can be removed from supplemental heat sources and provided with more space. Solid food may be introduced slowly, while formula is still being fed. Nutritionally complete foods should be introduced first, followed by produce. Nutritionally complete foods should be offered early to increase their acceptance and to provide a concentrated source

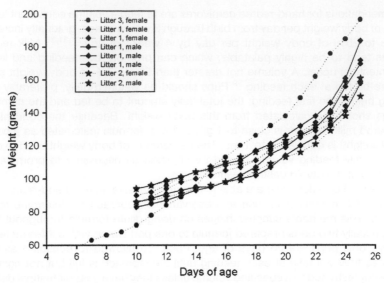

Fig. 1. Examples of body weights of hand-reared fennec fox pups. (*Data courtesy of* S. J. Hanna, Camarillo, CA.)

of essential nutrients to help pups through the stressful weaning period. Neither vertebrate nor invertebrate prey items should be introduced until pups are fully weaned and ideally not until they are at least 6 months old.

Acceptance of dry, nutritionally complete feed can be increased by soaking food in water or formula until it is soft. Pups may take a day or more to realize the kibble is food. Be careful to avoid giving too much too soon. Most pups thrive on gradual introduction of solid food while still receiving formula. After they have readily accepted dry food soaked in formula for 3 to 4 days, pups may be offered canned nutritionally complete food if it is typically fed as a part of the adult diet. Begin with small portions (approximately 2 g) of canned food. After 3 or more days of the dry food/formula/canned food mixture, pups may be offered quarter-inch cubes (approximately 2 g each) of vegetables, but should not be given vegetables high in starch, such as lima beans and corn. Formula should be continued by syringe and on top of the food in the dish. Water should be introduced into the diet at the same time as solid food, beginning with 1 to 2 mL twice a day by syringe, progressing to 1 mL per feeding, once the pups are consuming vegetables. When pups are readily consuming solid food out of a dish, water should also be offered in a dish ad lib. The proportion of solid food should gradually increase as weaning proceeds. When pups are approximately 6 to 6.5 weeks old, they should be fed a total amount equivalent to 25% of the total adult daily diet (by weight, as fed) divided into three daily feedings, with fresh water offered ad lib in a small dish. The amount of formula offered should be decreased and eliminated completely by the time the pups are about 6 to 7 weeks old, provided they are consistently eating from a dish. When the pups are 8 weeks old, the number of feedings should be reduced to two per day. The amount of solid food offered per feeding should be increased when the pups are consistently consuming all foods offered. The amount of solid food offered may be increased every 2 to 3 days in increments of 10% of the total adult daily diet if pups consume all food offered at each feeding, with no decrease in frequency or quality of feces.

Weaning is a stressful time. New foods should be offered slowly, and changes in fecal quality should be monitored. If an individual has difficulty accepting a new food, discontinue the new food, continue with formula, and try the new item again in another day or so. Weaning requires patience and flexibility, because each pup has its own timing and needs.

REFERENCES

1. Asa CS, Valdespino C, Cuzin F. Fennec fox. In: Sillero-Zubiri C, Hoffmann M, Macdonald DW, editors. Canids: foxes, wolves, jackals and dogs: status survey and conservation action plan. Gland (Switzerland): International Union for Conservation and Nature, IUCN/SSC Canid Specialist Group; 2004. p. 205-9.
2. Ortolani A, Caro TM. The adaptive significance of color patterns in carnivores: phylogenetic tests of classic hypotheses. In: Gittleman JL, editor. Carnivore behavior, ecology and evolution. vol. 2. Ithaca (NY): Cornell University Press; 1996. p. 132-88.
3. Gauthier-Pilters H. The fennec Fennecus zerda. African Wildlife 1967;21:117-25.
4. Ginsberg J, McDonald D. Fennec fox (Fennecus zerda). In: Ginsberg J, McDonald DW, editors. Foxes, wolves, jackals and dogs: an action plan for the conservation of canids. Gland (Switzerland): International Union for Conservation and Nature, IUCN/SSC Canid Specialist Group; 1990. p. 48-9.
5. International Union for Conservation and Nature. Red Data List. Switzerland: International Union for Conservation and Nature; 2008.
6. Bekoff M, Diamond J, Mitton J. Life-history patterns and sociality in canids: body size, reproduction, and behavior. Oecologia (Berl) 1981;50:386-90.
7. Bauman KL. Fennec fox (Vulpes zerda) North American Regional Studbook. 4th edition. Saint Louis (MO): Saint Louis Zoo; 2006.
8. Koenig VL. Zur Fortpflanzung und Jungendentwicklung des wustenfuchses. Zeitschrift fur Tierpsychologie 1970;27:205-46.
9. Valdespino C, Asa CS, Bauman JE. Estrous cycles, copulation, and pregnancy in the fennec fox (Vulpes zerda). J Mammal 2002;83:99-109.
10. Valdespino C. The reproductive system of the fennec fox (Vulpes zerda) [dissertation]. Saint Louis (MO): University of Missouri; 2000. p. 123.
11. Asa CS, Valdespino C. Canid reproductive biology: integration of proximate mechanisms and ultimate causes. Amer Zool 1998;38:251-9.
12. Petter F. La reproduction du fennec. Mammalia 1957;21:307-9 [in French].
13. Volf J. A propos de la reproduction du Fennec. Mammalia 1957;21:454-5 [in French].
14. Saint Girons MC. Notes sur les dates de reproduction en captivité du fennec, Fennecus zerda (Zimmerman, 1780). Z Säugetierk 1962;27:181-4 [in French].
15. Gangloff L. Breeding fennec foxes Fennecus zerda at Strasbourg zoo. Int Zoo Yearbk 1972;12:115-6.
16. Dragesco-Joffe A. La Vie Sauvage au Sahara. Lausanne, Delachaux et Niestle; 1993 [in French].
17. Bueler LE. Fennec. In: Wild dogs of the world. New York: Stein and Day Publishers; 1973. p. 182-5.
18. Cuzin F. Repartition actuelle et statut des grands mammiferes sauvages du Maroc (Primates, Carnivores, Artiodactyles). Mammalia 1996;60:101-24.
19. Sowards RK. Observations on breeding and rearing the fennec fox (Fennecus zerda) in captivity. Animal Keepers' Forum 1981;8:175-7.

20. Allen ME, Oftedal OT, Baer DJ. The feeding and nutrition of carnivores. In: Kleinman DG, editor. Wild mammals in captivity: principles and techniques. Chicago: University of Chicago Press; 1996. p. 139–47.

21. Gauthier-Pilters H. Beobachtungen an Feneks (*Fennecus zerda* Zimm). Z Tierpsychol 1962;19:441–64 [in German].

22. Nolls-Banholzer U. Body temperature, oxygen consumption, evaporative water loss and heart rate in the fennec. Comp Biochem Physiol 1979;62:585–92.

23. Stevens CE, Hume ID. The mammalian gastrointestinal tract. In: Comparative physiology of the vertebrate digestive system. New York: Cambridge University Press; 1995. p. 57–60.

24. Nolls-Banholzer U. Water balance and kidney structure in the fennec. Comp Biochem Physiol 1979;62:593–7.

25. National Research Council. Nutritient requirements of dogs and cats. Washington, DC: National Academies Press; 2006. p. 354–70.

26. Association of American Feed Control Officials. Dog and cat food nutrition profiles. Oxford (IN): Association of American Feed Control Officials Inc; 2008. p.130–41.

27. Case LP, Carey DP, Hirakawa DA. Nutritional care of neonatal puppies and kittens. In: Case LP, Carey DP, Hirakawa DA, Daristole L, editors. Canine and feline nutrition: a resource for companion animal professionals. 2nd edition. Saint Louis (MO): Mosby; 2000. p. 233–43.

28. Iams Company. How to visually assess cat and dog body condition. Iams Food for Thought Technical Bulletin 1996;77R:1–3.

29. LaFlamme D. Development and validation of a body condition score system for cats: a clinical tool. Fel Pract 1997;25:13–8.

30. LaFlamme D. Development and validation of a body condition score system for dogs. Canine Pract 1997;22:10–5.

31. Oftedal OT. Milk composition and formula selection for hand-rearing young mammals. In: Maschgan ER, Allen ME, Fisher LE. First Annual Dr. Scholl conference on nutrition of captive wild mammals. Chicago: Lincoln Park Zoological Gardens; 1980. p. 67–83.

32. Oftedal OT. Milk composition, milk yield and energy output at peak lactation: a comparative review. Symp Zool Soc Lond 1984;51:33–85.

33. Oftedal OT. Lactation in the dog: milk composition and intake by puppies. J Nutr 1984;114:803–12.

34. Adkins Y, Lepine AJ, Lonnerdal B. Changes in protein and nutrient composition of milk throughout lactation in dogs. Am J Vet Res 2001;62(8):1266–72.

35. Dubrovskaya RM. Characteristics of milk of arctic foxes. Dairy Science Abstracts 1967;29:115.

36. Lonnerdal B, Keen CL, Hurley LS, et al. Developmental changes in the composition of beagle dog milk. Am J Vet Res 1981;42:662–6.

37. Young EG, Grant GA. The composition of vixen milk. J Biol Chem 1931;93: 805–10.

38. Greenwall MG. Hand-rearing canids. In: American zoo and aquarium association infant diet notebook. Bethesda (MD): American Zoo and Aquarium Association; 1991. p. 10.1–10.13.

39. Evans RH. Rearing orphan wild mammals. Vet Clin North Am Small Anim Pract 1987;17(3):755–83.

Nutrition and Behavior of Striped Skunks

Jerry W. Dragoo, PhD

KEYWORDS

- Health • Mephitidae • *Mephitis mephitis*
- Natural history • Striped skunk

THE STRIPED SKUNK (*MEPHITIS MEPHITIS*)

When people think of skunks, two things usually come to mind: bad odor and rabies. Skunks are one of the most recognized mammals in North America, and just about everyone has a skunk story to share. Sometimes these stories are positive; other times they are not so positive. The purpose of this article is to provide a better understanding of these maligned and often misunderstood mephitids.

Historically, skunks have been classified with ferrets, weasels, otters, and badgers in the family Mustelidae.[1] This relationship was based on skunks' enlarged anal scent glands and a handful of primitive traits associated with the skull and dentition.[2–5] Genetic evidence has been used since the late 1960s to suggest that skunks are different from mustelids. Early chromosomal research indicated that the skunk karyotype was remarkably different from that of the weasel family.[6] In fact, new chromosomal data involving fluorescence *in-situ* hybridization has supported this earlier chromosomal research.[7]

Recent phylogenetic data have been used to better understand carnivore relationships. Results based on DNA hybridization suggested that Procyonidae (raccoons and allies) and pinnipeds (three families of marine carnivores: seals, sea lions, and walruses) are more closely related to mustelids than are skunks.[8] Studies that included comprehensive taxonomic sampling of zorillas (African striped weasels) and oriental stink badgers and DNA sequence analyses from both mitochondrial DNA and nuclear genes showed that New World skunks and stink badgers represent a distinct family, the Mephitidae.[9–11]

Striped skunks are one of 12 species in the family Mephitidae in the order Carnivora.[12] Other skunk species include the hooded skunk (*Mephitis macroura*), four species of spotted skunks (*Spilogale*), four species of hog-nosed skunks (*Conepatus*), and two species of stink badgers (*Mydaus*).[9,12] Stink badgers occur in Borneo, Sumatra, and a few other Philippine islands. The other three genera of skunks are

Museum of Southwestern Biology, Department of Biology, MSC03 2020, 1 University of New Mexico, Albuquerque, NM 87131, USA
E-mail address: jdragoo@unm.edu

Vet Clin Exot Anim 12 (2009) 313–326
doi:10.1016/j.cvex.2009.01.012
1094-9194/09/$ – see front matter © 2009 Elsevier Inc. All rights reserved.
vetexotic.theclinics.com

distributed over most of the New World, from southern Canada to the Strait of Magellan in South America.[3] The focus of this article is the striped skunk.

DESCRIPTION AND NATURAL HISTORY

Striped skunks (**Fig. 1**) are approximately the size of small housecats, and they have small, triangular-shaped heads. The nose pad is relatively small, as are the ears, which are rounded. The tail is long and, from the base to the last vertebrae, is less than half the total body length. The tail can appear longer depending on the length of long flowing hairs.[13] The basic pelage color of skunks is black and white, but other colors, such as brown and red, occur in the wild. As a result of domestic breeding of striped skunks for the fur and pet trade, colors such as brown, gray, cream, apricot, completely white (non-albino), and albino have been genetically selected. The typical stripe pattern in striped skunks is the white "V" down the back and a white bar running between the eyes from the forehead to the middle of the rostrum. Color pattern in striped skunks is highly variable and ranges from completely black to completely white. Skunks are born with stripes on the skin before they have hair.[3]

Striped skunks have short, stocky legs with five toes on each foot. They walk on the soles (plantigrade) of their feet. Occasionally, the heels of the hind feet are lifted off the ground when they walk or run. The claws on the front feet are longer than those of the back feet.[3] Striped skunks have six upper and six lower incisors (three upper and lower on each side of the jaw), two upper and lower canines, six upper and lower premolars, and one upper and two lower molars, for a total of 34 teeth. The dental formula is I 3/3, C 1/1, P 3/3, M 1/2 = 34.[13]

Mephitis mephitis can be found from southern Canada, throughout most of the United States (excluding hot deserts of the southwest), down to central Mexico.[13] Recently, they have been reported north of the Arctic Circle in the community of Kuujjuaraapik, Nunavik.[14] Striped skunks use a variety of habitats and tend to be more numerous where good cover and abundant food are available. This habitat can be in open grassy areas to mixed woodlands. Striped skunks also occur around agricultural areas in cultivated areas and pastures. They are often found in urban environments, usually denning under man-made structures and around parks, golf courses, buildings, and dumps.[13,15-20] Skunks den in open areas by burrowing into banks or

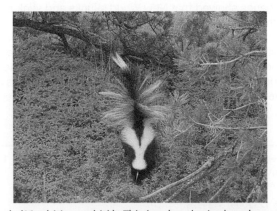

Fig. 1. Striped skunk (*Mephitis mephitis*). This is a hand-raised orphaned female that was released back to the wild. (*Courtesy of* J. W. Dragoo, PhD, Albuquerque, NM.)

will den above ground. Skunks sometimes use multiple den sites and a variety of den types (eg, above ground, holes, buildings). Usually, they are solitary when denning, except during late spring and summer, when females still are with their litters. In more northern, colder climates, striped skunks den in small groups (usually females) in the winter to conserve body heat.[16,21–23] Striped skunks are crepuscular or nocturnal.[3] In the northern part of their range, although they are not true hibernators, they may go into a torpor during cold spells or when snow is particularly deep.[24,25] In the southern parts of their range, however, they may be active during milder winters.[26]

In general, striped skunks do not defend their territories, but they do have home ranges. Aggressive encounters can occur when two skunks (especially males) with overlapping home ranges come in contact. Home ranges can be variable (0.5 km^2 to > 12 km^2), depending on availability of resources and time of year. Striped skunks become more sedentary and cover less area in colder winter months in the northern part of their ranges, whereas in warmer climates, their home ranges stay about the same size.[17,26–28]

Striped skunks usually breed from February through March, and young are born starting in April until early June. These skunks usually only go into estrus once a year. If a litter is lost early, however, a second litter may be produced.[23] Striped skunks breed in their first year, and young males exhibit breeding behavior in mid- to late summer of their first year, although they are not yet in reproductive condition (**Fig. 2**).[20] Given the opportunity, males breed with many females.[23] Females are usually in estrus for about a week and a half, and most become pregnant by the end of the breeding season. Gestation in striped skunks usually lasts from 59 to 77 days. Females that breed early in the season may undergo a short period of delayed implantation.[23,29] Young usually are born from late April through June. Striped skunks can have as many as 12 offspring per litter but average 5 to 7. Females usually have 12 mammae, but they can range from 10 to 15.[23] Young skunks are born blind, deaf, and naked. Within a couple of days after birth, black and white hairs cover their pink and white skin. They are born with their scent glands intact and are capable of scenting within the first week of birth. Their scent is more gas-like than liquid at this age.[3] Their eyes and ears open after approximately 28 days (sometimes earlier). After 6 to 8 weeks, the young are weaned. They begin to forage and explore with their mothers at this time. By the end of summer or early fall, the young begin to disperse.[3]

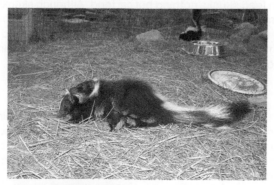

Fig. 2. Young skunks (approximately 3 months old) exhibiting breeding behavior. (*Courtesy of* J. W. Dragoo, PhD, Albuquerque, NM.)

FEEDING

With the exception of lima beans, skunks eat almost anything. Although they eat other legumes, many captive skunk caretakers report that skunks do not eat lima beans. Striped skunks are opportunistic omnivores. They feast primarily on insects, such as beetles, grasshoppers, crickets, moths, cutworms, caterpillars, bees, and wasps. They also eat earthworms, snails, clams, crayfish, fish, frogs, snakes, mice, moles, rats, squirrels, wild fruits, grains, corn, nuts, bird's eggs, carrion, and garbage. Striped skunks use their long foreclaws to dig for insects and grubs. They search in rotten or fallen logs for mice and insects. Around gardens, they forage for ripe fruits and vegetables, but they primarily look for insects that potentially damage garden crops. They also consume pet food left outside.[3]

Wild skunks cannot afford to be picky. They tend to be more active than captive skunks and as a result, they burn more calories. Wild skunks rarely die from a poor diet but can starve from a lack of food. Wild skunks are more likely be killed by predators, hit by cars, or infected by diseases or parasites than killed by an improper diet. Underweight skunks in wildlife rescue operations may be fed a higher caloric diet to help them regain weight before their release back into the wild. With captive skunks, however, which are more sedentary and are not threatened by the same risks as their wild counterparts, diet becomes a more limiting factor to their survival. Many captive skunks are overweight. They eat nutritious food but take in too many calories.

For captive skunks, a healthier diet rather than a "natural" one may be better in the long run. Many diets have been described for captive skunks and can be found on the Internet. Without controlled dietary studies, it is hard to know which diet is best for skunks. One diet may be chosen not because it is better but because caretakers have more experience with that diet. Some diets include raw meat, whereas others suggest cooked meat. Although raw meat may be higher in some nutrients than cooked meat, feeding raw meat is not recommended, because it may contain some potentially zoonotic disease organisms, such as *Salmonella* or *Campylobacter*. Vitamins (eg, vitamin D) and other nutrients (ie, taurine and L-carnitine) can be added after cooked meat has cooled. Meat products also can be added to grains and cereals, such as wheat, oats, barley, and rice, and included in the diet.

Skunks also consume fruits and vegetables. They eat broccoli, cauliflower, corn, peas, green beans, spinach, collard greens, carrots, melons, apples, bananas, raisins, grapes, and nuts. They should not be fed all of these items every day to avoid obesity. The trick is not to overfeed captive skunks and to provide variety in the diet from day to day to ensure proper long-term nutritional needs.

Caretakers often feed skunks nothing but cat food. Although skunks are classified in the order Carnivora, they are omnivorous. Cat food is too high in protein for skunks and can lead to severe diarrhea in the short-term and kidney and liver damage in the long-term. Similar symptoms occur when dogs are fed nothing but cat food. Ideally, skunks should not be fed cat food.

PROBLEM SKUNKS

Skunks are not the problem; they are a symptom of a problem. Residential areas can be inviting to skunks. Homes with large backyards or brushy vegetation are prime skunk habitat. Many such homes have a variety of resources for skunks, including bird baths, bird feeders, gardens, and pet food. Striped skunks den under homes and under backyard storage sheds. They often are removed from cluttered garages where a lot of cover is available for denning. Den sites are usually near areas where readily available foods sources abound.

Proactive measures can be taken to prevent skunks from entering buildings. Skunk-proof fences can be used to seal off entry holes under porches, buildings, and foundations. Wire mesh fencing 1 m high can be used to exclude skunks from gardens. To prevent skunks from digging beneath the fence, the bottom of the fencing should be buried 22.9 to 30.5 cm deep. The buried portion can be bent outward into an "L" shape. Skunks dig at the corner until the realize they cannot get under.[20]

Securing garbage and storing garbage cans in an enclosed space with tight-fitting lids helps discourage skunks from moving in to residential areas. Garbage cans stored outside should be attached to secure objects so that they are not tipped over by skunks (or other wildlife). Heavier trash containers are not as easily tipped over by skunks. Trash should not be left out overnight but instead set out the morning of scheduled pick-up. Compost piles also attract skunks and should be kept in sealed containers. Skunks are also readily attracted to dog and cat food left out at night. Pet food should be placed in areas inaccessible to skunks. Cat food, for example, can be placed on a bench or table above ground level.

Flour or finely sifted sand that shows paw prints when animals walk through it can be sprinkled at the entrance to the den to determine if a skunk has entered or exited the building, depending on the track direction. If it still is unclear whether all skunks have exited, a one-way hardware cloth door, folded into an "L" shape, can be placed over the exit hole. This allows skunks to push their way out but prevents them from re-entering. When the skunks have left for the evening, the hole can be sealed permanently. Ensure all skunks, young and adult, have been removed before sealing the hole. Young skunks may be left in the den unattended during May and June. It is best to avoid sealing buildings or foundations during this time to ensure that they do not starve.

One solution that homeowners have used for nuisance animals is relocation of the skunk. Homeowners do not want the animal in their environment, but they do not want them killed, either. Various state, county, and city ordinances regulate how wildlife species are to be dealt with, depending on political boundaries. The same is true for injured and orphaned skunks. Certain states do not allow rehabilitation of some wildlife species (primarily rabies vectors). Homeowners should check with local officials before trapping and relocating skunks, because not all agencies support skunk relocation or release.[30]

Striped skunks run away at the first sign of a potential threat. If running away does not work, they spray a noxious chemical from their anal scent glands.[31] Before spraying, however, skunks display a series of threat behaviors. They stomp the ground with both front feet. Sometimes they raise their tails, charge forward a few paces, and then stomp or edge backwards while dragging their front feet. Each scent gland has a nipple associated with it, and skunks can aim and direct the spray with highly coordinated muscle control (**Fig. 3**).[3]

Occasionally, the scent from a skunk can be difficult to eliminate. The anal secretions of striped skunks are composed of several major volatile components, including (E)-2-butene-1-thiol, 3-methyl-1-butanethiol, S-(E)-2-butenyl thioacetate, S-3-methylbutanyl thioacetate, 2-methylquinoline, 2-quinolinemethanethiol, and S-2-quinolinemethyl thioacetate.[31] To neutralize the odor, sulphur compounds need to be oxidized. Odor problems in the house can be eliminated or reduced by closing all windows and doors and then boiling apple cider vinegar. After boiling begins, the vinegar can be left to simmer for approximately 20 to 30 minutes. Windows then can be opened to ventilate the house. This approach may leave a lingering vinegar smell for a short time. Household bleach or vinegar can be added to a wash or rinse cycle to remove odor from clothes. The musk sprayed on decks and walls can be removed with a little household bleach.

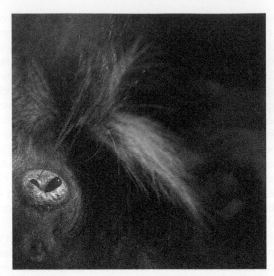

Fig. 3. Adult female skunk spraying the author in the face. Note the nipples extruding from the anal sphincter. These nipples, associated with the scent glands, allow the skunk to direct the spray. (*Courtesy of* the Nature series, WNET.ORG, New York, NY. Copyright © 2000 WNET.ORG; used with permission.)

Pets, especially dogs, return home with strong odors after encounters with skunks. Paul Krebaum provided a recipe for a solution to oxidize odor-producing thiol compounds in skunk spray. In the event that a person or pet gets sprayed, this remedy usually works: add one-fourth cup baking soda to 1 quart of 3% hydrogen peroxide and 1 tsp of liquid (pet) shampoo. Mix these ingredients immediately before and apply while foaming. The oxygen released by foaming neutralizes the thiols, and the detergent removes the oily part that holds the odor in animal's fur.[32] After approximately 5 minutes, rinse with tap water. Avoid getting this solution in the pet's eyes, because it may cause corneal ulcerations. This is an oxidation reaction, so it may cause fading of fur color. If all else fails, the odor will fade over time.

HEALTH AND DISEASES

Rabies has been recognized as a disease of mammals for more than 4000 years.[33] In addition to bats, many terrestrial mammals, especially carnivores, maintain and transmit rabies. Domestic, privately owned, community owned, and feral dogs are the primary reservoirs of the rabies virus worldwide.[34] In the United States, however, because of an aggressive program to vaccinate pets, wildlife species are the predominant reservoirs and vectors of rabies. Rabies has been reported in skunks for at least 175 years,[35] and before 1990, striped skunks were the primary species represented in reported cases of rabid animals in the United States. In 1990, raccoons became the most common species associated with rabies reported in wildlife, followed by skunks.[36–38] During 2006, 21.5% of all rabid animals reported to the Centers for Disease Control and Prevention were skunks.[38]

Skunks also are mistakenly described as being rabies carriers that transmit, but do not succumb, to the virus. Skunks, like other mammals, die from rabies once symptoms occur. Once the virus begins shedding in saliva, skunks may go as long as 6 days (usually fewer) before exhibiting any clinical symptoms of disease. Clinical signs of rabies in skunks have lasted from 1 to 18 days before the animal died.[39] Skunks can be infected and incubate the virus for up to 18 months (usually not longer than 2–6 weeks), but they cannot transmit the virus by biting before the virus reaches the salivary glands. There is no evidence of a true carrier state.[39] Skunks can neither excrete virus in saliva and remain clinically free of symptoms for long periods of time nor recover from clinical signs and continue to excrete virus. If an animal is merely incubating the virus and bites someone, it does not transmit the virus. Unfortunately, currently there is no way to detect this latent form in a living animal. Animals can be exposed to and contract the virus at any time. The amount of virus and the body part exposed may affect the duration of incubation. For an animal to contract rabies, it has to be exposed to another animal shedding the virus, usually through a bite.[39]

Currently, there are at least three recognized skunk strains of rabies virus in the United States. The northern skunk strain found in the north central midwestern plains and eastern states is similar to the fox and dog strains of Texas and Arizona. The southern skunk strain occurs in the south central states. This strain is more similar to the raccoon strain found on the east coast. A third strain occurs in California and is similar to the gray fox strain in Texas.[36] Recently, new strains of skunk rabies were found in Mexico.[40,41] Skunks do succumb to rabies in the eastern states, but the strain in that area is associated with raccoons. Skunks are not yet known to maintain that strain in their populations. The potential for spillover of this raccoon strain into skunks in this area and establishment of this raccoon strain in eastern skunks is worrisome, however, because current oral vaccines that targeting raccoons do not effectively immunize skunks.[42] Oral vaccines and delivery methods currently are being developed for skunks.[43,44] Rabies vaccines (injectable or oral) have not yet been developed for skunks. However, a trap-vaccinate-release program was successfully conducted in Ontario, Canada to reduce the incidence of rabies in skunks.[45]

Skunks are susceptible to various strains of rabies found in terrestrial mammals and bats. Massachusetts and Rhode Island, where only the raccoon strain occurs, had more rabid skunks than raccoons reported in 1999,[46] which suggests that the raccoon strain potentially could become enzootic in skunk populations. This trend has not been sustained, however, but skunks still are susceptible to the raccoon strain.[38] In 2001, several skunks were diagnosed with a bat strain (big brown bat, *Eptesicus fuscus*) of the rabies virus in Flagstaff, Arizona.[47] A similar method of trap-vaccinate-release was used during this outbreak; Imrab3 (Merial Ltd., Athens, GA) was the vaccine used off-label to manage that outbreak.[48]

Transfer of rabies virus from skunks to humans is a well-recognized health threat in urban areas. Striped skunks are often attracted to housing areas because of the presence of pet food, water, garbage, and high populations of invertebrates in urban landscaping. Consequently, they are more likely to encounter humans and their pets. Striped skunks are believed to account for a substantial number of animal-to-human rabies exposures (not infections) each year.[36] Most information on prevalence and molecular biology of rabies virus in terrestrial wildlife comes from animals submitted for testing after potential human exposure. Little is known about the prevalence of rabies in natural populations and how enzootic or epizootic levels of the disease interact with the ecology of various species.[27,36,49,50] Data are needed on the population dynamics and genetics, space use, and mortality patterns of skunks in urban and remote areas to enhance our knowledge of the ecology and disease status of these species. For example, Greenwood and others[27] noted that 36 of 40 cases of reported skunk rabies in North Dakota during 1992 would have gone unnoticed if not for their study.

Much of the data regarding skunk ecology and rabies have been collected in Canada and the northern United States.[27,45,51–54] Rabies occurrences may be seasonal.[52] In the winter, female skunks den together in communal dens, which makes rabies transmission easier. In addition to increased contact, the stress involved with communal denning may contribute to the onset of rabies.[23,51,55] During breeding season, skunks interact with each other more frequently, and the fierce breeding behavior is ideal for rabies transmission. Rabies in skunks occurs more frequently during breeding season, and females may be more likely to become rabid.[49,51] During the summer, males are more solitary, and females can be found with their young but do not interact much with other con-specifics. The occurrence of rabies at this time of year is less detectable. Fall is when young skunks disperse. They tend to be solitary but do encounter other dispersing skunks. Other ecologic factors may influence the spread of rabies, including such variables as population density, age structure, reproductive rate, survival rate, home range size, dispersal distances, and population genetics.

People often forget that not all skunks have rabies. A skunk that is aggressive and attacks someone should be tested not only for rabies but also for other diseases, such as distemper virus. A skunk that is digging for grubs in the backyard and runs away when approached is acting normally. We are constantly learning more about rabies. Rabies is virtually 100% preventable if the postexposure prophylaxis is given before the onset of rabies symptoms. Most people are aware when they have contacted a skunk, so death from skunk rabies is preventable. It is more likely that an unvaccinated pet will contract the skunk strain of rabies and pass it on to a human than it is for a human to contract the skunk strain directly from a skunk.

Skunks are prone to other diseases and infections (**Table 1**). These diseases are caused by bacteria, fungi, and viruses carried by internal and external parasites.

Table 1
Some additional disease organisms reported in striped skunks

Disease	Organism
Bacteria	
Leptospirosis[56,57]	Various genera
Rocky Mountain spotted fever[56]	*Rickettsia*
Tularemia[58,59]	*Francisella*
Suppurative arthritis[60]	*Mycoplasma*
Fungus	
Pulmonary adiaspiromycosis[61]	*Emmonsia*
Histoplasmosis[62]	*Histoplasma*
Helminths (Acanthocephalans, Cestodes, Nematodes, Trematodes)	
Lung flukes[56]	*Paragonimus*
Filarial Dermatitis[63]	*Filaria*
Parasites[64]	Various species
Protozoans / Protists	
American trypanosomiasis[65]	*Trypanosoma*
Toxoplasmosis[56,66]	*Toxoplasma*
Sarcocystosis[67]	*Sarcocystis*
Viruses	
Infectious canine hepatitis[56]	Canine adenovirus
Canine distemper[66]	Canine distemper virus
Aleutian disease[68]	Aleutian mink disease parvovirus
West Nile[69]	West Nile virus
Various cancers and tumors[70]	

Table 2
Serum chemistry and hematologic values[a] of striped skunks

	Mean	SD	Minimum	Maximum	N
Serum chemisty					
Albumin (g/dL)	3.4	0.7	2.3	4.5	17
ALP (IU/L)	62	48	7	168	21
ALT (IU/L)	99	79	29	303	25
AST (IU/L)	78	22	47	129	20
BUN (mg/dl)	26	12	9	58	24
Calcium (mg/dL)	10	1	7.7	12.3	21
Chloride (mEq/L)	112	8	99	135	16
Cholesterol (mg/dL)	178	85	0	314	19
CO_2 (mmol/L)	25.9	4.3	21.0	33.0	7
CPK (IU/L)	590	319	128	1235	11
Creatinine (mg/dL)	0.9	0.6	0.5	2.9	23
Direct bilirubin (mg/dL)	0.0	0	0	0.1	2
GGT (IU/L)	4	3	0	9	11
Globulin (g/dL)	3.4	1.0	1.2	4.8	16
Glucose (mg/dL)	113	51	45	259	25
LDH (IU/L)	734	590	303	1923	8
Mg (mg/dL)	1.93	0.64	0.65	2.6	7
Phosphorus (mg/dL)	5.9	2.2	2.7	10.8	19
Potassium (mEq/L)	5.1	0.7	3.8	6.3	20
Sodium (mEq/L)	148	9	127	169	19
Total bilirubin (mg/dL)	0.1	0.1	0.1	0.3	16
Total protein (g/dL)	6.4	1.0	4.4	8.2	23
Triglycerides (mg/dL)	100	77	24	303	10
Hematologic values					
Basophil ($*10^3/$ μL)	0.044	0.058	0	0.121	4
Eosinophil ($*10^3/$ μL)	0.374	0.443	0.098	1.7	18
HCT (%)	41	5.9	30.0	52.0	26
Hb (g/dL)	12.5	1.8	7.9	15.3	19
Lymphocytes ($*10^3/$μL)	3.105	1.678	0.594	6.71	22
MCH (pg)	15.6	1.8	13.3	18.7	14
MCHC (g/dL)	31.2	1.6	26.3	33.8	19
MCV (fL)	49.7	6.1	41.5	61.3	14
Monocytes ($*10^3/$μL)	0.193	0.093	0.056	0.375	21
Neutrophil ($*10^3/$μL)	3.97	2.063	1.31	7.65	22
Platelet count ($*10^3/$μL)	267	120	143	437	7
RBC ($*10^6/$mL)	8.21	1.22	6.0	10.2	14
WBC ($*10^3/$mL)	8.019	2.926	2.2	14.2	27

[a] ISIS reference values printed June 18, 2008.

20. Rosatte R, Sobey K, Dragoo JW, et al. Striped skunks and allies. In: Gehrt SD, Riley SPD, Cypher BL, editors. Urban carnivores: ecology, conflict, and conservation. Baltimore (MD): The Johns Hopkins University Press; in press.

21. Lariviere S, Messier F. Denning ecology of the striped skunk in the Canadian prairies: implications for waterfowl nest predation. J Appl Ecol 1998;35(2): 207–13.

22. Doty JB, Dowler RC. Denning ecology in sympatric populations of skunks (*Spilogale gracilis* and *Mephitis mephitis*) in west-central Texas. J Mammal 2006;87(1): 131–8.

23. Verts BJ. The biology of the striped skunk. Urbana (IL): University of Illinois Press; 1967.

24. Hamilton WJ. Winter activity of the skunk. Ecology 1937;18(2):326–7.

25. Houseknecht CR. Denning habits of the striped skunk and the exposure potential for disease. Bulletin of the Wildlife Disease Association 1969;5:302–6.

26. Davis WB. Texas skunks. Texas Game and Fish 1951;March:19–21,31.

27. Greenwood RJ, Newton WE, Pearson GL, et al. Population and movement characteristics of radio collared striped skunks in North Dakota during an epizootic of rabies. J Wildl Dis 1997;33(2):226–41.

28. Lariviere S, Messier F. Spatial organization of a prairie striped skunk population during the waterfowl nesting season. J Wildl Manage 1998;62(1):199–204.

29. Wade-Smith J, Richmond ME. Reproduction in captive striped skunks (*Mephitis mephitis*). American Midland Naturalist 1978;100(2):452–5.

30. Centers for Disease Control and Prevention. Compendium of animal rabies prevention and control. MMWR 2008;57(No. RR-2):1–9.

31. Wood W, Sollers B, Dragoo G, et al. Volatile components in defensive spray of the hooded skunk, *Mephitis macroura*. J Chem Ecol 2002;28(9):1865–70.

32. Reese KM. Lab method deodorizes a skunk-afflicted pet. Chem Eng News 1993; 72(18):90.

33. Baer GM. Rabies: an historical perspective. Infect Agents Dis 1994;3(4):168–80.

34. Meslin FX. Global review of human and animal rabies. In: Rabies: guidelines for medical professional. Trenton (NJ): Veterinary Learning Systems; 1999. p. 9–11.

35. Parker RL. Rabies in skunks. In: Baer GM, editor, The natural history of rabies, Vol. 2. New York: Academic Press; 1975. p. 41–51.

36. Krebs JW, Wilson ML, Childs JE. Rabies, epidemiology, prevention, and future research. J Mammal 1995;76(3):681–94.

37. Chomel BB. Rabies exposure and clinical disease in animals. In: Rabies guidelines for medical professionals. Trenton (NJ): Veterinary Learning Systems; 1999. p. 20–6.

38. Blanton JD, Hanlon CA, Rupprecht CE. Rabies surveillance in the United States during 2006. J Am Vet Med Assoc 2007;231(4):540–56.

39. Charlton KM, Webster WA, Casey GA. Skunk rabies. In: Baer GM, editor. The natural history of rabies. 2nd edition. Boca Raton (FL): CRC Press; 1991. p. 307–24.

40. Loza-Rubio E, Aguilar-Setien A, Bahloul C, et al. Discrimination between epidemiological cycles of rabies in Mexico. Arch Med Res 1999;30(2):144–9.

41. de Mattos CC, de Mattos CA, Loza-Rubio E, et al. Molecular characterization of rabies virus isolates from Mexico: implications for transmission dynamics and human risk. Am J Trop Med Hyg 1999;61:587–97.

42. Tolson ND, Charlton KM, Stewart RB, et al. Immune-response in skunks to a vaccinia virus recombinant expressing the rabies virus glycoprotein. Can J Vet Res 1987;51(3):363–6.

43. Hanlon CA, Niezgoda M, Morrill P, et al. Oral efficacy of an attenuated rabies virus vaccine in skunks and raccoons. J Wildl Dis 2002;38(2):420–7.
44. Jojola SM, Robinson SJ, VerCauteren KC. Oral rabies vaccine (ORV) bait uptake by captive striped skunks. J Wildl Dis 2007;43(1):97–106.
45. Rosatte RC, Power MJ, Macinnes CD, et al. Trap-vaccinate-release and oral vaccination for rabies control in urban skunks, raccoons, and foxes. J Wildl Dis 1992;28(4):562–71.
46. Krebs JW, Rupprecht CE, Childs JE. Rabies surveillance in the United States during 1999. J Am Vet Med Assoc 2000;217(12):1799–811.
47. Leslie MJ, Messenger S, Rohde RE, et al. Bat-associated rabies virus in skunks. Emerging Infect Dis 2006;12(8):1274–7.
48. Engeman RM, Christensen KL, Pipas MJ, et al. Population monitoring in support of a rabies vaccination program for skunks in Arizona. J Wildl Dis 2003;39(3): 746–50.
49. Hass CC, Dragoo JW. Rabies in hooded and striped skunks in Arizona. J Wildl Dis 2006;42:825–9.
50. Tinline RR. Persistence of rabies in wildlife. In: Campbell JB, Charlton KM, editors. Rabies. Boston: Kluwer Academic Publishers; 1988. p. 301–22.
51. Rosatte RC. Seasonal occurrence and habitat preference of rabid skunks in Southern Alberta. Can Vet J 1984;25(3):142–4.
52. Rosatte RC, Gunson JR. Dispersal and home range of striped skunks, *Mephitis mephitis*, in an area of population reduction in southern Alberta. Canadian Field-Naturalist 1984;98(3):315–9.
53. Rosatte RC, Gunson JR. Presence of neutralizing antibodies to rabies virus in striped skunks from areas free of skunk rabies in Alberta. J Wildl Dis 1984; 20(3):171–6.
54. Rosatte RC, Power MJ, MacInnes CD. Ecology of urban skunks, raccoons, and foxes in metropolitan Toronto. In: Adams LW, Leedy DL, editors. Wildlife conservation in metropolitan environments. Columbia (MD): National Institute for Urban Wildlife; 1991. p. 31–8.
55. Gunson JR, Dorward WJ, Schowalter DB. Evaluation of rabies control in skunks in Alberta. Can Vet J 1978;19(8):214–20.
56. Alexander AD, Flyger V, Herman YF, et al. Survey of wild mammals in a Chesapeake Bay area for selected zoonoses. J Wildl Dis 1972;8(2):119–26.
57. Richardson DJ, Gauthier JL. A serosurvey of leptospirosis in Connecticut peridomestic wildlife. Vector Borne Zoonotic Dis 2003;3(4):187–93.
58. Berrada ZL, Goethert HK, Telford SR. Raccoons and skunks as sentinels for enzootic tularemia. Emerging Infect Dis 2006;12(6):1019–21.
59. Matyas BI, Nieder HS, Telford SR. Pneumonic tularemia on Martha's Vineyard : clinical, epidemiologic, and ecological characteristics. In: Francisella tularensis: biology, pathogenicity, epidemiology, and biodefense. Oxford (England): Blackwell Publishing; 2007. p. 351–77.
60. Ganley-Leal LM, Brown C, Tulman ER, et al. Suppurative polyarthritis in striped skunks (*Mephitis mephitis*) from Cape Cod, Massachusetts: detection of mycoplasma DNA. J Zoo Wildl Med 2007;38(3):388–99.
61. Albassam MA, Bhatnagar R, Lillie LE, et al. Adiaspiromycosis in striped skunks in Alberta, Canada. J Wildl Dis 1986;22(1):13–8.
62. Woolf A, Gremillionsmith C, Sundberg JP, et al. Histoplasmosis in a striped skunk (*Mephitis mephitis* Schreber) from southern Illinois. J Wildl Dis 1985;21(4):441–3.
63. Saito EK, Little SE. Filarial dermatitis in a striped skunk. J Wildl Dis 1997;33(4): 873–6.

64. Neiswenter SA, Pence DB, Dowler RC. Helminths of sympatric striped, hognosed, and spotted skunks in west-central Texas. J Wildl Dis 2006;42(3): 511–7.
65. Ryan CP, Hughes PE, Howard EB. American trypanosomiasis (Chagas-disease) in a striped skunk. J Wildl Dis 1985;21(2):175–6.
66. Diters RW, Nielsen SW. Toxoplasmosis, distemper, and herpesvirus infection in a skunk (Mephitis mephitis). J Wildl Dis 1978;14(1):132–6.
67. Dubey JP, Hamir AN, Topper MJ. Sarcocystis mephitisi n. sp (Protozoa: Sarcocystidae), Sarcocystis neurona-like and Toxoplasma-like infections in striped skunks (Mephitis mephitis). J Parasitol 2002;88(1):113–7.
68. Pennick KE, Latimer KS, Brown CA, et al. Aleutian disease in two domestic striped skunks (Mephitis mephitis). Vet Pathol 2007;44(5):687–90.
69. Anderson JF, Vossbrinck CR, Andreadis TG, et al. A phylogenetic approach to following West Nile virus in Connecticut. Proc Natl Acad Sci USA 2001;98(23): 12885–9.
70. Smith DA, Barker IK. 4 Cases of Hodgkin's disease in striped skunks (Mephitis mephitis). Vet Pathol 1983;20(2):223–9.
71. Pion PD, Kittleson MD, Rogers QR, et al. Myocardial failure in cats associated with low plasma taurine: a reversible cardiomyopathy. Science 1987;237(14 August):764–8.

The Nutrition and Natural History of the Serval (*Felis serval*) and Caracal (*Caracal caracal*)

Shannon E. Livingston, MSc

KEYWORDS

- Nutrition • Behavior • Serval • Caracal • Natural history
- Diet • Hand rearing • Feeding

There exists a paucity of information with regards to the specific nutrient and dietary needs of many species of exotic cats, including those kept sporadically as house pets, such as the serval and the caracal. The diets of exotic cats kept in captivity are usually based on the nutrient requirements of the domestic cat, although there is some evidence that different cat species may not metabolize certain nutrients in the same manner as domestic species.[1–4] This article provides information on the natural diet and behavior of the serval and caracal and offers insight into some health issues that may arise in a domestic environment. Where there is a lack of more detailed information, the domestic cat should be used as the model for the serval and caracal.

SERVAL (*FELIS SERVAL*)

The serval is a medium-sized African cat. Taxonomically it is classified as both *Felis serval* and *Leptailurus serval*, depending on the source.[5,6] Adults stand approximately 60 cm at the shoulder.[5,6,7] Males are typically larger than the females and weigh on average approximately 14 kg, whereas females average 10 kg.[5,6] The average life expectancy in the wild is thought to be approximately 10 years,[6] although it can be significantly longer in captivity. They have typically been found in Sub-Saharan Africa, although they are likely no longer present in appreciable numbers in South Africa.[6,7] Their preferred habitat is open grassland areas near stable bodies of water, although occasionally they have been reported in various other habitat types.

Servals have the longest legs and ears in relation to body size of any of the cats.[6] The serval is a specialized hunter of rodents; they use their height and hearing to hunt for rodents in the grass.[5–7] They use a characteristic hunting technique wherein

Animal Nutrition Center, Disney's Animal Kingdom, 1180 N. Savannah Circle, Bay Lake, FL 32830, USA
E-mail address: shannon.e.livingston@disney.com

Vet Clin Exot Anim 12 (2009) 327–334
doi:10.1016/j.cvex.2009.01.017
1094-9194/09/$ – see front matter © 2009 Elsevier Inc. All rights reserved.

they may remain motionless for up to 15 minutes, using their hearing to pinpoint the location of prey. They then jump with all four feet in the air distances of 1 to 4 m and strike the prey with one or both front feet. They are able to jump straight up over 1 m in the air to catch prey such as birds and insects by clawing in midair or slapping the prey between their paws.[8] On occasion, they have been observed bounding three to four times in row to flush prey and then using their front paws to strike the prey down.[5–7,9] In addition to rodents, they are also known to hunt birds, reptiles, insects, and amphibians.[5,7] They have been recorded as having one of the better hunting success rates of the cats—up to 48%.[6,7] They tend to hunt smaller prey animals, such as mice and rats, but have been observed to hunt and catch prey as large as lesser flamingos (*Phoenicopterus minor*).[9] They have often been observed consuming vegetation as well.[5,7]

Servals are a solitary animals.[6,7] They are generally considered to be nocturnal, but are often observed hunting during the morning and late afternoon hours, especially in areas away from human activity.[6,7,9] Home range size depends on the habitat and prey density, but on average it is estimated to range from approximately 4 km^2 for females to 8 km^2 for males in the Ngorogora Crater in Tanzania.[7] Home range also has been calculated at double that size in less ideal habitats.[6,7]

THE CARACAL (*CARACAL CARACAL*)

The caracal is a sturdy, medium-sized cat found throughout many parts of Africa and the Middle East and through Asia into India and Pakistan.[6] As with the serval, there seems to be some disparity in nomenclature. Caracals are found in the literature referred to as both *Caracal caracal* and *Felis caracal*. In Africa, the caracal ranges in size from approximately 8 kg for females to close to 20 kg for males.[6] In India, caracals tend to be somewhat smaller, estimated at 6 kg.[10] Caracals in captivity have lived as long as 16 years.[6] The African population is listed on CITES II (not a species of concern); however, the Asian population is listed as CITES I (endangered).[10] The caracal can be found in most habitats other than deserts and the dense equatorial forests of Africa. It is rare in some parts of its range and so numerous in others that it is hunted as vermin.[8]

The main prey animals of caracals in the wild are reported to be mammalian,[11] most of which are rodents. Birds, reptiles, and invertebrates are also consumed.[12] Whereas the serval is a specialized hunter of rodents, the caracal is more diverse in its hunting preferences. Although rodents still make up a large portion of the diet, caracals are known to regularly hunt prey 2 to 2.5 times their own size.[6,12–14] The larger prey may include gazelles, duiker, springhares,[6] other small carnivores (eg, black-backed jackals, bat-eared fox, and African wild cat),[11] and various small livestock, such as sheep and goats.[6,11,12,14] There is some indication that caracals also consume vegetation.[11] Like the serval, caracals are noted for having impressive jumping abilities, reportedly more than 3 m.[6] In addition to their jumping abilities, caracals are reported to be excellent sprinters.[6] When killing prey, caracals seem to use a variety of methods, depending largely on the size of the prey. Small prey are killed with a bite to the nape. Mid-size prey are killed with a bite to the back of the neck; larger prey are killed with a bite to the throat.[6]

As with the serval, the caracal is mainly solitary.[6,13] Although it is normally thought of as nocturnal, caracals have been observed hunting during daylight hours in areas with little human activity.[6,11,12] They tend to have larger home ranges than the serval. A study in Africa recorded males with home ranges close to 27 km^2 and females with home ranges close to 7 km^2.[14] A study of home ranges in Israel showed territories of close to 220 km^2 for males and 57 km^2 for females,[6] whereas another study found even larger territories in Saudi Arabia.[13]

ISSUES IN CAPTIVITY

Some issues that may arise when servals and caracals are kept in a human home environment relate to their natural lifestyle. Both cat species are exceptionally gifted jumpers, and as such, there are few areas in a house that they would not be able to access. Their hunting abilities may be cause for concern when living in a house with smaller pets or children. As both species have been observed regularly eating vegetation,[9,11] care should be taken to ensure that there are no toxic plant species located within the cat's environment. Although unsubstantiated, Web sites devoted to keeping caracals and servals as pets have mentioned instances in which toxic house plants were consumed and medical intervention was required.

Both cat species are by nature active and intelligent. Care should be taken to ensure that their environment provides the opportunity for adequate exercise and mental stimulation. Many cat species kept in captivity are often observed exhibiting undesired behaviors, termed stereotypies. They can include—but are not limited to—pacing, excessive grooming, and inactivity. Studies have found that by offering food items in smaller meals hidden in various locations throughout the day as opposed to single larger meals can significantly increase more natural food-seeking behaviors and reduce undesired behaviors in other small felid species.[15]

Neither species has been observed covering their feces in the wild[6,7,9] and it may be difficult to completely litter train them. Both species are also reported to scent mark their territories regularly. Although males are recorded as scent marking more frequently than females, both sexes have been observed marking in the wild and in captivity.[16] One male serval was observed scent marking 95 times in 1 hour in the presence of a female.[7] Under other circumstances, male servals on average scent marked approximately 45 times per hour.[7]

NUTRITION

No recorded studies have looked specifically at the nutrient requirement of servals or caracals. Although a few studies have discovered some differences in metabolism between various species and the domestic cat,[1-4] the cat still remains the best model in terms of nutrient requirements. Most importantly, the cat is a strict carnivore.[17] Cats are unable to meet their requirements of vitamin A or niacin from plant-based diets.[18] It also seems that cats may be unable to meet their requirements for vitamin D through ultraviolet exposure and require a source of vitamin D in the diet.[19,20] Arachadonic acid also must be provided in the diet because cats lack the enzymes to convert linoleic acid to arachidonic acid. Taurine is required to prevent retinal degeneration and cardiomyopathy.[17]

All these criteria can be met if the cats are fed a complete diet. Commercial diets marketed for domestic cats also should provide the necessary requirements of the serval and caracal. Finding a diet that the serval and caracal will eat may be more challenging. Various complete meat-based diets are available on the market for exotic cats in zoos, such as those produced by the Toronto Zoo (Milliken Meats, Scarborough, Ontario Canada), Natural Balance (Pacoima, CA), and Nebraska Brand (North Platte, NE), although many of these products may not be practical for the home consumer to purchase because of minimum orders and shipping charges. Raw diets for cats and dogs are becoming more popular, as are dry diets formulated without grain and cereals, both of which may be more available at local area veterinarians and specialty pet stores. Quality of ingredients should be considered when choosing a diet, because lower quality ingredients can affect the digestibility and nutrient availability of the diet. With the variety of terms used in pet foods, it can become confusing trying to discern good products from those of poorer quality. According to the the Association of American Feed Control Officials, meat refers to any species of slaughtered mammal and includes just the meat portion of the animal. Poultry refers to a combination of flesh and skin with or without bones derived from part of or a whole carcass of poultry. Meat byproducts include secondary products such as lungs, heart, liver, and parts of the digestive system. It does not include hair, horns, hooves, or teeth. Poultry by-products also may contain bone, head, feet, and viscera but no feathers. Byproducts can vary greatly in the amount of indigestible material they contain.[21] Meal refers to any ingredient that is ground or otherwise has reduced particle size. Bone meal can be included in some diets and can affect the quality of the protein and the mineral balance of the diet. Although bone meal increases the calcium content of the diet, it often can increase the content of other minerals, leading to potential mineral imbalances.[21]

It is important to note that proper food handling procedures must be followed when dealing with raw meat diets (and any meat-based products) to avoid bacterial contamination. Potentially dangerous bacteria have been cultured from a variety of raw dog and cat foods, even when following manufacturer's guidelines for preparation. In addition to the dangers the bacteria pose for the pets, the danger can be passed on to the owner.[22,23] In addition to the risk of bacterial infection from the diet, these bacteria can be shed in the feces of the cats. Studies have shown that feeding diets produced with good quality meat sources reduced the occurrence of salmonella in the feces by more than 90%.[24] Care should be taken when using these diets to ensure that the appropriate nutrient levels are provided. Bones and whole animals (rats, mice, chicks, quail) also could be provided. Some people may choose to make their own diets. This works well for some people, but care needs to be taken to ensure that supplementation is done properly and that proper sanitation guidelines are followed.

Various studies have shown that many exotic cats are able to digest meat diets with similar digestive efficiency as domestic cats.[1–4] Studies looking at the digestibility of dry diets by exotic cats show a somewhat lower rate of digestibility than meat diets. One study examined the digestibility of meat and dry diets fed to sand cats, a small felid of Africa.[2] Digestibility of the meat-based diets was similar to those of other felid species fed a meat-based diet. The ability of the sand cats to digest the dry diet was less than that of the meat-based diet and less than domestic cats fed a dry diet. This may indicate a difference in the ability of exotic cat species to digest dry diets compared with domestic cats. The reduced digestibility of the dry diet by the sand cats also has implications in terms of amount of food needed. The cats may have to eat more of a dry food–based diet to obtain a similar amount of nutrients than could be digested from a more digestible meat-based diet. Another study found that there were some differences in the digestibility of beef-based diets for a variety of exotic cat species.[1]

There is no clear formula for predicting how much food servals or caracals require on a daily basis. Most food estimates are based on energy requirements, although there is no definitive method to determine energy requirements for exotic cats. The estimate for energy requirements of domestic cats is 70 to 80 kcal/kg body weight (BW)[25]; however, it seems that this calculation cannot be used to accurately predict the maintenance energy requirements of exotic species.[25] The differences observed in maintenance energy requirements are related not only to the large variation in body size but also to possible species-specific differences in metabolism.[25] An estimate of basal metabolic rate for animals is often determined using metabolic body size (BW $_{kg}$ 0·75).[26] The Nutrient Requirements of Cats lists the daily metabolizable energy requirements of exotic cats at maintenance as ranging from 55 to 260 kcal/kg BW 0·75.[27] Although diets differ greatly among zoologic institutions, servals receive approximately 200 g to 250 g of a meat-based diet or vertebrate prey daily with bones offered between one and three times weekly (personal communication). Caracals tend to receive between 400 g and 500 g daily of a similarly scheduled diet.

NUTRITION-RELATED DISEASE

Servals and caracals are subject to the same nutrition-related diseases as domestic cats. One of the most common problems observed in domestic and exotic cats is obesity. Captive cats lead a more sedentary lifestyle and lack the opportunity to expend the calories of their wild counterparts. Whenever possible, adequate exercise potential must be provided. Type II diabetes is increasingly diagnosed in cats and can be related to the consumption of excessive amounts of highly refined and easily digestible carbohydrates,[28] although activity level and obesity are contributing factors. Many commercially available diets for domestic cats include high levels of grains, which would provide higher levels of carbohydrates than would be encountered in wild diets.

Metabolic bone disease is also a concern for felines in captivity. Metabolic bone disease refers to issues regarding the health of the bones, and it can be attributed to many factors, most commonly excessive or inadequate amounts of calcium, phosphorus, and vitamin D.[20] When observed in captive carnivores, this disease is commonly caused by feeding improperly supplemented muscle meat. Although these nutrients are most likely to be of concern during the growth or reproductive phases, they can occur during maintenance as well.

Stone Formation

Either calcium oxalate or magnesium ammonium phosphate (MAP), although not well documented in caracals or servals, is a concern for domestic cats. There is a documented case of cysteine calculi in a captive caracal; however, it occurred in 1977 and dietary information was not provided.[29] As with domestic cats, certain dietary aspects should be considered to avoid stone formation. Feeding a diet that maintains a urine pH between 6.0 and 6.5 is ideal for preventing the formation of MAP crystals.[21] Cereal grains have a tendency to increase urine pH. Meat products tend to lower urine pH. Ensuring sufficient water intake also helps to maintain proper urine pH. In the event that the cat is not consuming sufficient moisture, water can be added directly to the food. The digestibility of the diet is also an important factor in maintaining sufficient urine volume. Diets that are poorly digested increase fecal volume, which increases the amount of water lost in the feces. Diets that are more energy dense and highly digestible lower the dry matter intake, decrease fecal volume/water loss, and help to maintain urine volume.[21] A feeding regimen also can affect urine pH. Cats fed "meals" tended to have a spike in urine pH after the meal, whereas cats fed "ad lib" throughout the day had a more constant pH.[21,29,30] Although it is important to keep feline urine pH on the acidic side to prevent the formation of MAP crystals, urine that is too acidic (< 6.0) can lead to the formation of calcium oxalate crystals[30,31] and metabolic acidosis.[21]

Although mostly anecdotal and poorly documented, there is some indication that servals, particularly juveniles, may have a tendency to consume non–food items that may require surgical removal.

HAND-REARING

In the event that a kitten cannot be raised by its mother, various milk replacers are available. Products such as KMR, Esbilac, Zoologic Milk Matrix 33/40, and Zoologic Milk Matrix 42/25 (PetAg, Hampshire, Illinois), Nurturall milk replacer (Veterinary Product Laboratories, Phoenix, Arizona), and Just Born (Farnam Pet Products, Phoenix, Arizona) have been used successfully to raise felid species.[32] KMR is designed for domestic cats, and Esbilac is designed for domestic dogs. Both products were reformulated in 1993 to contain butterfat for improved mixability. Some felid species, such as tigers and leopards, have had trouble digesting butterfat and have developed lactobezoars[32] as a result. Alternatives are the Zoologic Milk Matrix formulas 33/40 and 42/25, which are similar to KMR and Esbilac, respectively, in terms of nutrient content but contain vegetable oil instead of butter fat. According to one reference,[32] caracals have been successfully raised on 33/40 and KMR. Servals have been raised successfully on 33/40, 42/25, KMR, and Esbilac. Products designed for kittens are supplemented with taurine, and further supplementation should not be required. In the event that a non–kitten-designed formula is used, taurine should be supplemented to provide 400 mg/kg diet.[27] Most commercial milk replacers are also designed to provide the proper balance of minerals, such as calcium and phosphorus. During weaning, care should be taken to ensure that the proper ratio is maintained to prevent problems such as metabolic bone disease. An appropriate daily weight gain of 50 g should be expected for both caracals and servals. To start, small felids should be fed between 15% and 20% of body weight per day, split between six and eight feedings.[32]

The average litter size of the serval is three kittens. Gestation is somewhere between 66 and 79 days.[5,8,33] Kittens are typically weaned between 3 and 5 months. The average litter size for the caracal is two, but litters have ranged from one to six.[6] Gestation lasts between 68 and 81 days.[6] Kittens of both species weigh approximately 250 g at birth.[6,32]

SUMMARY

There is little information specifically regarding the nutrient requirements of the serval or caracal. Although not a perfect model, the domestic cat serves as the best estimation of nutrient needs and nutrition-related disease for both species. There is every indication that with proper diet and attention to the behavioral needs of each species, these cats can be kept in captivity with great success.

ACKNOWLEDGMENTS

The author would like to thank the people who helped to edit this article—Michelle Shaw, Kathleen Sullivan, and Eduardo Valdes—and the zoo nutrition departments that graciously provided diet information for servals and caracals in their collection.

REFERENCES

1. Vester B, Burke SL, Dikeman CL, et al. Nutrient digestibility and fecal characteristics are different among captive exotic felids fed a beef based diet. Z Biol 2008; 27:126–36.
2. Crissey SD, Swanson JA, Lintzenich BA, et al. Use of a raw meat based diet or a dry kibble for sand cats Felis margarita. J Anim Sci 1997;75:2154–60.
3. Wynne JE. Comparative digestibility values in 4 species of felidae. J Zoo Wildl Med 1989;20:53–6.

4. Barbiers RB, Vosburgh LM, Ku PK, et al. Digestive efficiencies and maintenance energy requirements of captive wild felidae: cougar (*Felis concolor*); leopard (*Panthera pardus*); and tiger (*Panthera tigris*). J Zoo Anim Med 1982;12:32–7.
5. Smithers RHN. The serval *Felis serval* Schreber 1776. S Afr J Wildl Res 1978;8: 29–37.
6. Sunquist M, Sunquist F. Wild cats of the world. Chicago: University of Chicago Press; 2002.
7. Geertsema AH. Aspects of the ecology of the serval in the Ngorogora Crater Tanzania. Neth J Zool 1985;35(4):527–610.
8. Visser J. The small cats. Afr Wildl 1977;31:26–8.
9. Geertsema AH. Impressions and observations on serval behaviour in Tanzania South Africa. Mammalia 1976;40(1):13–9.
10. Mukherjee S, Goyal SP, Johnsingh AJT, et al. The importance of rodents in the diet of jungle cat (*Felis chaus*), caracal (*Caracal caracal*) and golden jackal (*Canis aureus*) in Sariska Tiger Reserve, Rajasthan, India. J Zool London 2004; 262:405–11.
11. Melville HIAS, du P Bothma J, Mills MGL. Prey selection by caracal in the Kgalagadi Transfrontier Park. S Afr J Wildl Res 2004;34(1):67–75.
12. Avenant NL, Nel JAJ. Among habitat variation in prey availability and use by caracal (*Felis caracal*). Mamm Biol 2002;67:18–33.
13. VanHeezik YM, Seddon PJ. Range size and habitat use of an adult male caracal in Northern Saudi Arabia. J Arid Environ 1998;40:109–12.
14. Avenant NL, Nel JAJ. Home range use, activity and density of caracal in relation to prey density. African Journal of Ecology 1998;36:347–59.
15. Shepherdson DJ, Carlstead K, Mellen JD, et al. Influence of food presentation on the behaviour of small cats in confined environments. Z Biol 1993;12:203–16.
16. Mellen JD. A comparative analysis of scent-marking, social and reproductive behaviour in 20 species of small cats (*Felis*). Am Zool 1993;33(2):151–66.
17. MacDonald ML, Rogers QR, Morris JG. Nutrition of the domestic cat: a mammalian carnivore. Annu Rev Nutr 1984;4:521–62.
18. Morris JG, Rogers QR. Metabolic basis for form of the nutritional peculiarities of the cat. J Small Anim Pract 1982;23:599–611.
19. Morris JG, Earle KE, Anderson PA. Plasma 25-hydroxyvitamin D in growing kittens is related to dietary intake of cholecalciferol. J Nutr 1999;129:909–12.
20. Ullrey DE, Bernard JB. Vitamin D: metabolism, sources, unique problems in zoo animals, meeting needs. In: Fowler ME, Miller RE, editors. Zoo and wild animal medicine: current therapy 4. Philadelphia: WB Saunders Company; 1999. p. 63–78.
21. Case LP, Carey DP, Hirakawa DA, et al. Canine and feline nutrition. St. Louis (MO): Mosby; 2000.
22. Weese JS, Rousseau J, Arroyo J. Bacteriological evaluation of commercial canine and feline raw diets. Can Vet J 2005;46:513–6.
23. Strohmeyer RA, Morley PS, Hyatt DR, et al. Evaluation of bacterial and protozoal contamination of commercially available raw meat diets for dogs. J Am Vet Med Assoc 2006;228:537–42.
24. Lewis CE, Bemis DA, Ramsay EC. Positive effects of diet change on shedding of *Salmonella spp.* in the feces of captive felids. J Zoo Wildl Med 2002;33(1):83–4.
25. Allen ME, Oftedal OT, Earle KE, et al. Do maintenance energy requirements of felids reflect their feeding strategies? In: Proceedings of the 1st Annual Conference of the Nutrition Advisory Group. Toronto; 1995. p. 97–103.

26. Kleiber M. The fire of life: an introduction to animal energetics. Huntington (NY): Krieger Publishing; 1975.
27. National Research Council. Nutrient requirements of dogs and cats. Washington, DC: The National Academies Press; 2006. p. 366.
28. Rand JS, Fleeman LM, Farrow HA, et al. Canine and feline diabetes mellitus: nature or nuture? J Nutr 2004;134:2072S–80S.
29. Jackson OF, Jones DM. Cystine calculi in a caracal lynx (*Felis caracal*). J Comp Pathol 1979;89:39–42.
30. McNamara JP. Principles of companion animal nutrition. Upper Saddle River (NJ): Prentice Hall; 2006.
31. Lekcharoensuk C, Osborne CA, Lulich JP, et al. Association between dietary factors and calcium oxalate and magnesium ammonia phosphate urolithiasis in cats. J Am Vet Med Assoc 2001;219:1228–37.
32. Hedberg G. Exotic felids. In: Gage LJ, editor. Hand-rearing wild and domestic mammals. Ames (IA): Blackwell Publishing; 2002. p. 207–20.
33. Wackernagel H. A note on breeding the serval cat (*Felis serval*) at Basel Zoo. Int Zoo Yrbk 1968;8(1):46–7.

Feeding Behavior and Nutrition of the African Pygmy Hedgehog (*Atelerix albiventris*)

Ellen S. Dierenfeld, PhD, CNS

KEYWORDS

• Feeding • Hedgehog • Insectivore • Nutrition • Omnivore

At least four genera and 14 species of hedgehogs are widespread throughout Europe, Russia, China, and Africa. Adult hedgehogs weigh 400 to 1100 g.[1] African pygmy hedgehogs, *Atelerix albiventris*, are distributed from the southern Sahara through Central and East Africa. Weighing 250 to 700 g, pygmy hedgehogs are popular exotic pets in North America.

Hedgehogs are found in a variety of habitats, including deserts, steppes, and forests. They dig burrows; seek shelter under brush piles, logs, rocks, tree roots, and buildings; and need hiding places and nesting materials in captivity. European species hibernate during the coldest months of the year; African hedgehogs typically do not hibernate, but they can hibernate in cool environments.[2] Hibernation, however, is not recommended for captive hedgehogs, because the decrease in metabolism leaves them more susceptible to infection; thus, animals should be maintained at temperatures higher than 18°C.[2]

GENERAL FEEDING BEHAVIORS AND DIGESTIVE PHYSIOLOGY

Although classified as members of the order Insectivora, hedgehogs are quite omnivorous, eating a variety of invertebrates (eg, beetles, millipedes, worms, slugs, snails) in addition to small vertebrate prey (eg, frogs, snakes, lizards, eggs, young birds, mice) and plants.[1,3] Limited general information published on the dietary habits of African hedgehogs[4–6] suggests that they are also opportunistic omnivores, consuming a more varied diet based on food availability. Hedgehogs are nocturnal, starting to feed at dusk. Because they are good swimmers and active climbers, they have ample opportunities for exposure to varied food items.

Essentially no information is available on hedgehogs' specific nutrient requirements. They have a simple digestive tract, with no external distinction between small and

Sustainable Program Research, Novus International Inc., 20 Research Drive, St. Charles, MO 63304, USA
E-mail address: edierenfeld@aol.com

Vet Clin Exot Anim 12 (2009) 335–337
doi:10.1016/j.cvex.2009.01.006
1094-9194/09/$ – see front matter © 2009 Elsevier Inc. All rights reserved.

large intestine and no cecum.[7] Thus, they likely have limited ability to ferment plant cell wall constituents. Hedgehogs (at least *Erinaceous europaeus*) possess chitinase in their gastric mucosa and in their pancreas,[7] suggesting that they are able to digest the chitinous exoskeletons of insects. A preliminary study of fiber digestion in *A atelerix* confirmed that 64% to 68% of dietary fiber added as chitin (specifically, crab shell chitin) was digested, as compared with only 38% when fiber was added as cellulose.[8]

Captive hedgehogs tend to become obese;[2,6] thus, captive animals should be weighed regularly to monitor body condition. Obesity can lead to inactivity, metabolic changes, and other health issues. To combat this tendency toward obesity, because it is poorly digested, cellulose (plant matter) may be added to hedgehog diets to dilute nutrient density, thereby reducing overall dietary calories.[8] Hepatic lipidosis, which may be related to obesity, a high-fat diet, or too rapid weight loss, has been documented in African hedgehogs.[2] Therefore, weight-reduction diets containing not only decreased amounts of food but lower fat and caloric concentrations should be implemented gradually.

Specific nutritional problems, including taurine-deficiency cardiomyopathies or retinopathies and fatty acid insufficiencies, reported in obligate carnivores have not been reported in hedgehogs. The lack of these nutritional problems, in addition to hedgehogs' ability to utilize some dietary carbohydrates, suggests that hedgehog dietary requirements may be more similar to those of canids than of felids.

CAPTIVE DIETARY HUSBANDRY

Hedgehogs are easy to feed and are quite adaptable. As an example of diet flexibility, 300 to 700-g adult hedgehogs offered a canned feline diet (20–30 g) containing approximately 60% water were fed once daily during ad libitum intake feeding trials; leftover food always remained. Dry matter intake averaged 1.4% to 3% of body weight, or 3.5% to 7.5% of body weight on an as-fed basis; it did not vary by diet treatment, although dietary fiber concentration ranged from 3% to 27% of dry matter in that study.[8]

Thus, hedgehogs have been successfully maintained on a variety of moderately high-protein (30%–50%, dry matter basis) moderate-fat (10%–20%) diets, including canned and dry dog and cat foods; kitten foods; ferret foods; commercial products specific for hedgehogs; and dry and semimoist insectivore diets supplemented with earthworms, insects, and small quantities of chopped vegetable and fruit.[2,6,8] Treats include supplemented meat mixtures, hard-boiled or scrambled eggs, pinky mice, and vegetable or meat jarred human baby foods.[6] Dairy products, such as cottage cheese and milk, should be avoided, however, because of reports of lactose intolerance.[9] Insects offered should be from healthy colonies, fed gut-loaded diets, or dusted with a calcium supplement before feeding to hedgehogs. Insect-only diets are not recommended because of the potential for nutritional imbalances and to duplicate natural omnivorous feeding habits better.[2]

Dry foods or uncooked produce is suggested over soft dietary ingredients to maintain tooth and gum health. Fresh water should be provided ad libitum in a shallow dish; animals can also learn to drink from sipper bottles.

PREGANCY, LACTATION, AND HAND-REARING CONSIDERATIONS

Female hedgehogs that gain more than 50 g within 3 weeks after cohabiting with a male hedgehog are usually pregnant and should be isolated. Increased amounts of food can be offered during the 34- to 37-day gestation period and throughout lactation (4–6 weeks), with no need to alter dietary nutrient concentration.[2] Should supplemental feeding be required for young (termed *hoglets* or *urchins*), goat's milk and Esbilac (Pet Ag., Inc., Hampshire, Illinois) have been fed successfully.[10,11] An oral rehydration fluid, such as Pedialyte (Abbott Nutrition, Columbus, Ohio), is recommended initially, with consecutive feedings gradually decreasing rehydration fluid/formula concentrations.[10] Colostrum (preferably from goats, taken during the first 48 hours after kidding) should be added to hand-rearing formulas for at least 21 days (days 1 and 2, 50:50 colostrum/milk; next 21 days, 25:75 colostrum/milk).[11] Young can be fed with a plastic pipette or a 1-mL syringe fitted with a blunted 16-gauge needle covered with small-bore rubber tubing to be used as a teat. As with other species, weaning to an adult diet can be accomplished by gradually mixing a softened or blended solid diet into formula. Hand-reared hedgehogs should gain a minimum of 1.5 g/d but not more than 6 to 7 g/d when fully weaned.[10]

AREAS FOR FURTHER INVESTIGATION

1. Hedgehogs seem to be truly omnivorous. Studies still need to confirm that canid, rather than felid, digestive physiology underlies nutritional principles in captive feeding of hedgehogs, however.
2. Studies of the need for dietary taurine for protein metabolism, the role of δ-6 desaturase activity in fatty acid metabolism, and the ability to synthesize vitamin A from dietary carotenoids would improve our understanding of hedgehog nutritional physiology and might contribute to more optimal captive diet development.
3. Further investigation of dietary fiber nutrition in hedgehogs could be important in developing targeted life-stage or clinical diets for the species.

REFERENCES

1. Walker EP. Insectivora. In: Mammals of the world. Baltimore (MD): Johns Hopkins University Press; 1975. p. 103–79.
2. Larson RS, Carpenter JW. Husbandry and medical management of African hedgehogs. Vet Med 1999;94(10):877–88.
3. Reeve N. Hedgehogs. London: Poyser Natural History; 1994.
4. Merrit DA Jr. Husbandry, reproduction and behaviour of the West African hedgehog. Intern Zoo Yearbk 1981;21:128–31.
5. Okaeme AN, Oeakwe ME. Gastrointestinal helminthes and food of the African hedgehog *Atelerix albiventris* (Wagna) in the Kainji Lake area of Nigeria. Afr J Ecol 1988;26:239–41.
6. Smith AJ. Husbandry and medicine of African hedgehogs (*Atelerix albiventris*). J Small Exotic Anim Med 1992;2:21–8.
7. Stevens CE. The mammalian digestive tract. In: Comparative physiology of the vertebrate digestive system. Cambridge (UK): Cambridge University Press; 1990. p. 40–85.
8. Graffam WS, Fitzpatrick MP, Dierenfeld ES. Fiber digestion in the African white-bellied hedgehog (*Atelerix albiventris*): a preliminary evaluation. J Nutr 1998; 128:2671S–3S.
9. Stocker L. The St. Tiggywinkles hedgehog fact sheet. Haddenham (UK): The Wildlife Hospital Trust; 2003. p. 1–19.
10. Robinson I. Hedgehogs. In: Gage LJ, editor. Hand-rearing wild and domestic mammals. Ames (IA): Iowa State Press; 2002. p. 75–80.
11. Stocker L. Artificial rearing of orphaned hedgehogs. Haddenham (UK): The Wildlife Hospital Trust; 2003. p. 1–9.

Nutrition and Behavior of Lemurs

Randall E. Junge, MS, DVM, DACZM[a],*, Cathy V. Williams, DVM[b],
Jennifer Campbell, PhD[c]

KEYWORDS

• Lemur • Prosimian • Nutrition • Feeding • Behavior

The group of primates referred to as "lemurs" are classified in the suborder Prosimii. This suborder consists of six families, which include Lorisidae (lorises and pottos of Asia and Africa) and five families endemic to Madagascar: Cheirogaleidae (mouse lemurs, dwarf lemurs, and fork-marked lemurs), Megaladapidae (sportive lemurs), Lemuridae ("true lemurs" or black, brown, ring-tailed and ruffed lemurs, and bamboo lemurs), Indriidae (avahi, indri, and sifaka), and Daubentoniidae (aye-aye).[1] This article is limited to the Malagasy lemurs.

Lemurs are considered to be divergent from other primates taxonomically, and this uniqueness is reflected in anatomic, physiologic, behavioral, and health and nutritional parameters. The separation of Madagascar from the African continent 160 million years ago resulted in isolation that has allowed evolutionary radiation into a variety of niches, without competition from other primates. The unique flora and fauna are threatened by an expanding human population, forest cutting for agricultural use, bushmeat (eating wildlife), and introduced species.

Only a few lemur species are commonly held in captivity. Of species displayed in zoos, almost all are in the Lemuridae family, most commonly *Lemur catta* (ring-tailed lemur), *Eulemur* spp (black and brown lemurs), and *Varecia* (ruffed lemur). *Daubentonia* (aye-aye), *Hapalemur* (bamboo lemurs), and *Propithecus* (sifaka) have husbandry and nutritional requirements that restrict captive husbandry to specialists. Other species have not been established in captivity, often because of nutritional requirements that are difficult to mimic.

Keeping primates as pets should be discouraged. Many primate pets function as child substitutes for owners. Infant primates show similar behaviors to human infants and are completely dependent on their human caretakers. They are taken from their mothers very early in life to enhance bonding to human beings. However, as animals mature this misdirected affiliation causes abnormal behaviors. As the only primate

[a] St. Louis Zoo, 1 Government Drive, St. Louis, MO 63110, USA
[b] Duke Lemur Center, Duke University, 3705 Erwin Road, Durham, NC 27705, USA
[c] Department of Biology, Box 7617, North Carolina State University, Raleigh, NC, USA
* Corresponding author.
E-mail address: junge@stlzoo.org (R.E. Junge).

Vet Clin Exot Anim 12 (2009) 339–348
doi:10.1016/j.cvex.2009.01.011
1094-9194/09/$ – see front matter © 2009 Elsevier Inc. All rights reserved.

contact, human beings may become the focus of natural primate behaviors related to sexual maturity, social dominance, and territoriality. Once these behaviors become established, pet primates often must be securely confined for the owner's safety. These animals usually cannot be socialized with other primates, nor can they be integrated into display groups in zoos. Many species are relatively long-lived (20–30 years) and if sexual maturity at 3 to 4 years of age produces unacceptable behaviors, the animal may spend an extended life in an inappropriate setting.

UNIQUE ANATOMY AND PHYSIOLOGY

Lemurs share some characteristics that are considered primitive, including a tapetum lucidum (reflective layer of the cornea), a rhinarium (hairless glandular area around the nostrils), prominent scent glands, bicornuate uterus (typical of nonprimates), epitheliochorial placenta (typical of carnivores), small braincase, and open eye sockets.[2] Body size ranges from 25 g for the smallest mouse lemur to 7 kg for sifaka and indri.[3] Common captive species (Lemuridae) are medium-sized primates ranging from 1 kg to 4 kg. They move quadripedally through trees or on the ground and are diurnal or cathemeral (active day and night). Lemurids dental formula (except aye-aye) is 2/2, 1/1, 3/3, 3/3. Mandibular incisors and canines protrude forward and form a grooming comb, used for cleaning.[3]

The lemur gastrointestinal tract is generally characterized by a simple stomach, a small intestine of moderate length, and a cecum and colon of varied length, depending on the extent and mode of postgastric fermentation employed by the species. For example, the folivorous sifakas possess large salivary glands, extensible stomachs, a long small intestine, a well developed and haustrated cecum, and a spiral colon.[4] Ruffed lemurs, the most frugivorous lemur species, possess a comparatively simple gut, allowing for minimal fiber fermentation.[4] Members of the Lemuridae family (ring-tailed, black, and brown lemurs) all possess a gut designed for variable yet moderate consumption of fibrous feeds. The cecum is well developed and large and the colon is intermediate in length, allowing for a moderate fiber-fermentation capacity by microbes residing in the hind gut.[4]

A key characteristic of lemur physiology is a low basal-metabolic rate. Folivorous species minimize energy expenditures to use a diet marginal in energy. Low metabolic rate is also reflected in behavior of lemurs. Sportive lemurs spend up to 85% of their time eating or resting, with a resting metabolic rate that is among the lowest measured in mammals. The most extreme adaptation for energy conservation is seen in the fat-tailed dwarf lemurs (*Cheirogaleus medius*), which hibernate 6 to 8 months, a physiologic characteristic unique among primates.[5]

NUTRITION PHYSIOLOGY
Fiber Fermentation

Fibrous foods are those that contain a comparatively large portion of structural carbohydrates. Fermentation by bacteria is required in order break down these materials and produce short-chain fatty acids, which can be easily used by the host animal as a ready energy source. Cellulose and hemicellulose, commonly found in leaves, require lengthy processing times, thus the gastrointestinal tracts of sifaka and bamboo lemur are well designed to allow time for bacterial fermentation and absorption of short-chain fatty acids. Ruffed lemurs, on the other hand, consume diet items comparatively lower in fiber and higher in nonstructural carbohydrates, such as sugar and starch, items that require significantly less processing.

Secondary Plant Metabolites

Leaves often possess significant quantities of toxic compounds intended to act as feeding deterrents. Species that consume leaves in large quantities have evolved several adaptations for minimizing the impact of secondary plant compounds. Animals that consume large quantities of cyanide, such as some species of bamboo lemurs,[6] most likely possess a heightened ability to detoxify the compound. While some secondary plant compounds are clearly a part of these species wild diets, thus far there is no evidence for their necessity.

FEEDING ECOLOGY

Fairly extensive feeding-ecology studies are now available for most "true lemur" species. This group of lemurs has mainly been described as generalist feeders, meaning that their free-ranging diet typically consists of a variety of leaves and plant parts, wild fruits, and occasional animal matter. One difference between anthropoid and prosimian primates is that prosimians can generate vitamin C endogenously and do not require a dietary source of the nutrient.[7] In addition, it appears that lemurs do not accumulate carotenoids to the same extent as most other primates.[8,9]

The most common species of lemur in captivity (ring-tailed, ruffed, brown, and black lemurs) have been successfully maintained on commercially prepared, nutritionally complete primate biscuits. These biscuits have been used in combination with locally available produce for years without incident. These biscuits are designed to meet the minimum estimated requirements for primates as determined by the National Research Council[10] if consumed in adequate amounts. A variety of biscuit types are commonly fed to lemurs in captivity but the ideal biscuit type varies by species. Folivorous lemurs (sifakas and bamboo lemurs) should be fed a high-fiber biscuit designed for leaf-eating primates with acid detergent fiber (ADF) levels of at least 15%,[11] while the frugivorous ruffed lemurs tend to lose weight on high-fiber diets[12] and may maintain ideal weight better on biscuits designed for old-world monkeys with lower ADF levels. Ring-tailed, black, and brown lemurs can be maintained on biscuits with either moderate or high levels of fiber.

Although useful for providing variety in the diet, commercially available fruits and vegetables are not strictly necessary. Amounts fed should be limited and the types offered carefully selected. The nutrient composition of cultivated fruits and vegetables differ significantly from the fruits, leaves, and seeds available in wild diets in that cultivated varieties contain much higher levels of sugar and lower levels of fiber than wild-food items. For successful dietary management, the produce portion of the diet should never be overfed and should not be considered a significant contributor to the animals' nutritional needs. Over-consumption of produce that is high in sugar and starch can contribute to obesity, dental decay, diarrheal episodes, and diabetes.

Diets fed to lemurs in captivity vary by institution, but as a guideline, the total amount fed should be approximately 2.0% to 2.5% by dry weight of the animal's ideal body weight, with manufactured biscuit accounting for 80% to 85% of the dry matter, and the fruit and vegetable portion making up the remaining 15% to 20%. The total amount of food for a single animal can be approximated using the middle of the ideal weight range for the species[13] and feeding 25 g per day of primate biscuit per kilogram of ideal body weight plus 35 g per day of fruit-and-vegetable mix per kilogram of ideal body weight. Because foods high in simple sugars and starches can alter the microbe populations present in the gastrointestinal tract, fruits and starchy vegetables, such as white potatoes, sweet potatoes, and corn, should be strictly limited or avoided altogether in the diet of highly folivorous lemurs, such as sifakas and bamboo lemurs.

The addition of locally available fresh leaves and browse is beneficial for diurnal species as a means of increasing fiber in the diet, stimulating natural feeding behaviors, and providing enrichment. Browse plants should be selected carefully to avoid toxicity, pesticides, or contamination. Plant species commonly fed to primates in zoologic institutions include dogwood, mulberry, willow, ficus, sweetgum, shining leaf sumac, redbud, black locust, tulip poplar, and mimosa.[14] Cultivated bamboos found growing in the United States appear to be safe for consumption by bamboo lemurs.

SPECIAL NUTRITION
Pregnancy and Lactation

There is no evidence that dietary modifications are necessary during pregnancy when lemurs are consuming a well-balanced diet. However, moderate increases in the amount of food provided may be necessary during lactation, particularly if the dam is nursing multiple offspring. Adjustments are made by increasing both the biscuit and the fruit-and vegetable mix quantities by 25% of the standard diet amount and monitoring intake for 5 to 7 days.

Group diet amounts are increased as infants begin to eat solid foods. As a general guideline, a quarter of a standard adult diet ration is added to the group diet for each 500 g of body weight of the infant, with adjustments made as necessary if all the provided food is being consistently consumed. As infants tend to develop life-long taste preferences during the weaning period, it is important to offer a variety of healthy foods to youngsters to allow them the option of sampling new items. It is also crucial that infants begin consuming biscuit regularly before and during weaning to prevent the development of nutritional deficiencies during growth and later in life.

Obesity

Obesity is a major nutritional problem in captive lemurs and results from general overfeeding or overfeeding of highly palatable foods. Studies comparing body weights of wild and captive lemurs have found that animals are heavier in captivity than in the wild.[13] Providing excessive quantities of food, feeding inappropriate amounts of high-sugar and high-starch foods relative to primate biscuit, the overuse of food for enrichment, and the lack of exercise in captivity all contribute to obesity. Obesity is a result of calorie excess alone and does not eliminate the possibility that an animal may have an imbalance in one or more nutrients. Insufficient fiber intake can cause abnormally loose stool consistency, rapidly fluctuating blood-sugar levels, and the tendency for animals to feel hungry more rapidly after eating.

Diabetes Mellitus

Information on the prevalence of diabetes mellitus in lemurs is limited; however, occasional case reports and mention of diabetic lemurs can be found in the literature.[15–18] It is unknown if there is a species or genetic predilection in lemurs for developing the condition; however, obesity has been implicated as a predisposing factor in ring-tailed lemurs.[15]

Diagnosing diabetes in captive lemurs can be challenging as they readily develop hyperglycemia in response to stress, manipulation, or handling. Blood-glucose elevations associated with stress can be pronounced (300 mg/dL–500 mg/dL) and, in some cases, may be accompanied by transient glucosuria. Therefore, it is important to repeat fasting blood-glucose measurements when animals are minimally stressed to determine if the hyperglycemia is persistent. The measurement of serum fructosamine, glycosolated hemoglobin, or insulin-to-glucose ratios provides valuable information necessary for determining if a lemur is diabetic.[16,18]

Nutritional management of diabetic lemurs consists of limiting the consumption of simple sugars and starches, increasing dietary levels of fiber, fat, and protein, and spreading feedings throughout the day to minimize swings in blood glucose levels. Caloric restriction is necessary if animals are overweight. Practically, these goals can be achieved by eliminating all fruit and starchy vegetables in the diet, increasing the amount of green vegetables and fresh leafy browse, and by feeding a primate biscuit high in fiber. Check to make sure that the biscuit chosen does not contain sucrose or fructose. Cooked or unsweetened canned beans can also be added to the diet in small amounts. Depending on the species of lemur and individual taste preferences, small amounts of vegetable oil, nuts, or unsweetened peanut butter may be used to increase the fat and protein content while increasing palatability. In the early stages of diabetes, nutritional management alone may provide sufficient control; however, as diabetes progresses, medical management with oral hypoglycemic agents or insulin may be necessary in addition to dietary modifications and weight management to control the condition.[17,18]

Hemosiderosis and Iron Overload

Reports of hemosiderosis or excess iron accumulation in tissues of lemurs at necropsy initially appeared in the literature in the 1980s.[19–21] Recent studies suggest that different lemur species have varying propensities for developing iron-overload and that the prevalence of the condition is likely much lower than previously thought.[22,23]

Iron is an essential nutrient and is involved in many physiologic events, including oxygen transport, electron transport, and DNA synthesis. However, excessive accumulation of iron in tissues results in pathologic changes in tissues because of the ability of ferrous (Fe^{2+}) ion to catalyze reactions that generate toxic-free radicals.[24] Iron is absorbed from the intestinal tract in the upper duodenum and bound in the blood stream to the transport protein transferrin. Once combined to transferrin in the blood, it is transported to the bone marrow, muscles, and other sites for incorporation into hemoglobin, myoglobin, and a variety of metabolic enzymes involved in oxidative metabolism. Iron that is not immediately needed is stored either in combination with ferritin or deposited as hemosiderin in tissues. "Hemosiderosis" is the term used to describe iron accumulation in tissues in the absence of pathology, while the term "hemochromatosis" is reserved for conditions of iron-overload in which pathologic changes have occurred secondary to the excessive iron accumulation.

Initial reports of iron-overload in captive lemurs suggested that captive diets containing low levels of tannins and high levels of vitamin C were responsible for the high incidence of hemosiderosis observed.[21] However, the mechanisms contributing to excess iron absorption in captive lemurs are likely more complicated. While it has been well established in iron-deficient human beings that iron absorption increases when iron is consumed in conjunction with foods containing vitamin C,[25] absorption does not increase in individuals that have adequate iron stores.[26] No data is available regarding the effect of dietary vitamin C on iron absorption in lemurs. Levels of other trace minerals in the diet also influence iron absorption.[27–29] While some investigators have recommended adding tea, beans, or tannins to captive-lemur diets in an effort to reduce dietary iron absorption,[30] there is currently insufficient evidence to support these recommendations. Feeding a well-balanced plant-based diet containing species-appropriate fiber levels will likely minimize excessive iron absorption in diurnal lemurs.

NATURAL HISTORY FACTORS INFLUENCING BEHAVIOR

Daily activity patterns in lemurs vary greatly by species. The majority of lemurs kept in captivity are either diurnal or cathemeral (active day and night). Of the species described in this article, ring-tailed and ruffed lemurs are diurnal, while members of the *Eulemur* genus, brown and black lemurs, are cathemeral.[31] However, nocturnal or night-active lemurs, such as aye-ayes and mouse lemurs, are more commonly being kept in zoologic institutions as parts of nocturnal exhibits. Social structure and group size also varies by species. In general, diurnal and cathemeral species are social animals that live in groups of varying size.

Ring-tailed lemurs are the most terrestrial of the diurnal lemurs, spending 20% to 30% of their day on the ground.[5,32] In contrast, ruffed lemurs prefer to remain high in the canopy and rarely come down to the ground in the wild.[33] The average group size varies by species. Group size is largest for ring-tailed and ruffed lemurs, with the average size being between 13 and 15 individuals for ring-tailed lemurs and 5 and 31 individuals for ruffed lemurs. Groups include several adult males and females and related juvenile offspring. Most *Eulemur* species live in smaller multimale, multifemale groups, averaging 6 to 11 individuals, or in the case of mongoose lemurs (*Eulemur mongoz*) and red-bellied lemurs (*Eulemur rubriventer*), in monogamous pairs.[31]

Diurnal lemurs are seasonal in breeding receptivity, mating, and birthing, with reproductive activity occurring between October and February (varies with species) in North America. Gestation periods vary by species, from approximately 60 days in mouse lemurs and fat-tailed dwarf lemurs up to 157 to 172 days in the aye-aye. Gestation length in ruffed lemurs is 98 to 102 days, between 120 and 30 days in brown and black lemurs, 130 and 135 days in ring-tailed lemurs, and 155 and 165 days in sifakas.[5] Ring-tailed lemurs may have single births or twins and the young are precocial. Multiple births up to five infants are common in ruffed lemurs. Unlike other diurnal lemurs, ruffed lemurs practice absentee parenting, leaving altricial young in a nest.[34]

Among lemurs, several species are considered female-dominant, with characteristics of dominance patterns differing interspecifically.[35–37] Female dominance is pronounced in ring-tailed lemurs, with females having priority over males to all resources year round.[5,32,37] Female dominance is also characteristic of ruffed lemurs and black lemurs (*Eulemur macaco*), but is less pronounced or absent in the other brown lemur (*Eulemur*) species.[36]

The use of scent is an important form of communication in lemurs. Scent is used to mark territorial boundaries, advertise reproductive status, and establish dominance between members of a group. Scent glands are located in various sites on different species. Most diurnal lemurs have scent glands surrounding the anogenital region and deposit the scent by rubbing the anogenital area on the surface—or occasionally animal—being marked. Red-bellied lemurs have scent glands on the top of their head, bamboo and ring-tailed lemurs have pectoral glands (not to be confused with mammary glands), while ring-tailed lemurs have a third set of glands on the wrist (carpal glands).[2]

BEHAVIOR IN CAPTIVITY

Social interactions between primates make up much of the behavioral repertoire. These interactions include courtship, territoriality, infant rearing, and group dynamics. In captivity, many factors can affect behavior. Natural events, such as immigration, emigration, dispersal, and mate choice are controlled or restricted. It is important for psychological well being of captive primates that appropriate social situations are maintained. Single housing of animals should be avoided.

Competition and territoriality may become problems in inappropriate group compositions, size, or area of access. For most lemurs, pairs or family groups are appropriate; however, some species will expel juveniles as they mature. Lemurs are seasonal breeders, with reproductive activity occurring between October and February (varies with species) in North America. During this period, increased interest from males may occur, which may initiate aggression between males, and between females and males. While these interactions are usually not violent, bite and slash (by canine teeth) wounds may occur. Lemurs may scent-mark excessively during breeding season, which can result in abrasions and alopecia at scent-gland locations. Females with offspring may be protective, but maintenance of family groups encourages normal behaviors in juveniles.

Environments should provide complexity and stimulation for primates. Furniture in enclosures should encourage natural climbing behaviors. Novel objects introduced to enclosures stimulate investigation and exploration. In all cases, the environment and the objects within the environment should be evaluated for safety, such as toxicity, swallowing, trauma, or assistance with escape.

Feeding activity is one behavior that can be manipulated in captivity. Wild lemurs spend a great deal of time foraging. When maintained in captivity and fed a prepared diet, much of that behavior may be eliminated. Variable presentation of food will enhance normal behaviors. Food may be presented at different times of the day, in various locations, or in manners that require animal activity or manipulation. Spreading food within the enclosure encourages foraging. Food items may be placed into containers that require manipulation to get access to the food, even as simple as a paper bag. A variety of feeders can be devised for these purposes. Foraging activity increases time spent looking for food, mimicking behavior in the wild.[33]

Aggression is a normal part of the social repertoire of most lemur species. Cuffing, chasing, and biting are commonly employed when establishing and maintaining dominance, gaining access to food, mates, and other resources, and repelling intruders. Inter-male aggression peaks during the breeding season as competition for females becomes intense and levels of testosterone peak. Interfemale or male-female aggression also is common, and although levels may fluctuate, is less predictable. As lemurs enter puberty, both females and males become more aggressive. In captivity, interanimal aggression can become severe and even life threatening as animals have limited ability to avoid each other. Designing enclosures to include visual barriers allows subordinate animals to get out of sight of dominant animals and helps decrease tension and injuries when animals are housed in close confinement.

Stereotypic Behaviors and Self-Mutilation

In captivity, many factors can affect behavior. Natural events, such as immigration, emigration, dispersal, and mate choice are controlled or restricted. It is important for the psychologic well being of captive primates that appropriate social situations are maintained. Single housing of diurnal lemur species should be avoided. Keeping juveniles with their natal family group until they reach puberty (around 2 years of age) helps young lemurs learn species-appropriate behavior and parenting skills, and minimizes the development of atypical psychotic behaviors.

Even when care is taken to house lemurs in appropriate social groups and provide enriched environments, captive lemurs can exhibit an array of abnormal behaviors. These include stereotypic behavior, such as pacing, self-mutilation, and displaced aggression. Interestingly, some stereotypic behaviors appear to be coping mechanisms for animals to relieve stress in captivity.

Enrichment

Proper husbandry practices provide an enriched environment in captivity. This begins with appropriate social groupings housed in adequately complex and stimulating environments. Once these fundamental parameters are considered, food and activity enrichments may be added. Environments should provide complexity and stimulation. Lemurs use cage space in three dimensions, so the height of an enclosure is as important as the two-dimensional floor measurements. Cage furniture in enclosures should encourage natural climbing behaviors. In all cases, the environment and the objects contained therein should be evaluated for safety to ensure there are no sharp or pointed edges, hanging objects are well secured, there are no small objects that can be swallowed, and the external caging is secure and properly assembled to prevent animal escapes. Novel objects can be introduced into cages to stimulate investigation and exploration. Objects used in lemur cages should either be regularly sanitized or disposed of when they become soiled. Lemurs will explore and scent-mark large, empty cardboard boxes placed in their enclosures. They will also benefit from having cage furniture and branches moved around periodically to encourage variation in climbing patterns and use of space. Infants in particular should always be provided a surrogate stuffed animal to cling to if they need to be removed from their dam, even for short periods of time. Feeding and foraging activity is a behavior that can easily be manipulated in captivity, as previously described. Wild lemurs spend a great deal of time foraging. Food may be placed into containers that require manipulation to get access to the food. When food is used for enrichment, it is preferable to use portions of the standard diet rather than additional treat items to prevent obesity.

Training and Operant Conditioning

Lemurs respond well to operant training. Examples of behaviors that lemurs have learned successfully include stationing, following a target, sitting on a scale for weighing, taking oral medications, holding position for visual examinations, and remaining still for tactile examinations of the back, neck, and ventral abdomen. Training animals to actively participate in routine husbandry procedures decreases the need for manual or chemical restraint, decreases stress in both animals and husbandry staff, and provides mental stimulation for animals.

SUMMARY

Lemurs have nutritional requirements that are best met by feeding a balanced diet based on a nutritionally complete biscuit. This may be supplemented with browse, but high-starch and high-sugar food items should be limited. Common nutritionally related diseases including obesity, iron-overload, and diabetes can be avoided by adherence to appropriate diet. Behavioral needs are related to the social nature of primates. Housing in appropriate social groups in adequately complex environments, with added enrichment and operant conditioning, will reduce abnormal behaviors.

REFERENCES

1. Mittermeier RA, Konstant WR, Hawkins F, et al. Lemurs of Madagascar. Washington (DC): Conservation International; 2006.
2. Ankel-Simons F. Primate Anatomy—an introduction. Amsterdam: Academic Press; 2007.
3. Garbutt N. Mammals of Madagascar. New Haven (CT): Yale University Press; 1999.

4. Campbell JL, Eismann JH, Williams CV, et al. Description of the gastrointestinal tract of five lemur species: *Propithecus tattersalli*, *Propithecus verreauxi coquereli*, *Varecia variegata*, *Hapalemur griseus*, and *Lemur catta*. Am J Primatol 2000;52:133–42.
5. Sussman RW. Primate Ecology and Social Structure, vol. 1: Lorises, lemurs, and tarsiers. Needham Heights (MA): Pearson Custom Publishing: 1999.
6. Glander K, Wright PC, Seigler DS, et al. Consumption of cyanogenic bamboo by a newly discovered species of bamboo lemur. Am J Primatol 1989;19:119–24.
7. Nakajima Y, Shantha TR, Bourne GH. Histochemical detection of L-Gulonolactone: phenazine methosulfate oxidoreductase activity in several mammals with special reference to synthesis of vitamin C in primates. Histochemie 1969;18: 293–301.
8. Junge RE, Louis EE. Biomedical evaluation of black lemurs (*Eulemur macaco macaco*) in Lokobe Reserve, Madagascar. J Zoo Wildl Med 2007;38(1):67–76.
9. Slifka KA, Bowen PE, Sapuntzaksi M, et al. A survey of serum and dietary carotenoids in captive wild animals. J Nutr 1999;129:380–90.
10. National Research Council. Nutrient Requirements of Nonhuman Primates. Second revised edition. Washington (DC): National Academies Press; 2003.
11. Edwards MS. Leaf-eating primates: nutrition and dietary husbandry. Fact sheet 007, Nutrition Advisory Group Handbook. 1997. Available at: http://www.nagonline.net/technical_papers.htm. Accessed July 1, 2008.
12. Edwards MS, Ullrey ED. Effect of dietary fiber concentration on apparent digestibility and digest passage in non-human primates. I. Ruffed lemurs (*Varecia variegata variegata* and *V. v. rubra*). Z Biol 1999;18:529–36.
13. Terranova CJ, Coffman BS. Body weights of wild and captive lemurs. Z Biol 1997; 16:17–30.
14. Campbell JL, Glenn KM, Grossi B, et al. Use of local North Carolina browse species to supplement the diet of a captive colony of folivorous primates (*Propithecus* sp). Z Biol 2001;20:447–61.
15. Walzer C, Kuebber-Heiss A. Obesity in the development of diabetes mellitus in ring-tailed lemurs (*Lemur catta*): an obligatory component? Erkranjungen der Zootiere 1995;37:143–8.
16. Dutton CJ, Parvin CA, Gronowski AM. Measurement of glycated hemoglobin percentages for use in the diagnosis and management of diabetes mellitus in nonhuman primates. Am J Vet Res 2003;64(5):562–8.
17. Singleton C, Wack RF, Larsen RS. Use of oral hypoglycemic drugs for the management of diabetes mellitus in prosimians. In: Baer CK, editor. Proc Amer Assoc of Zoo Vet. Lawrence (KS): Allen Press; 2006. p. 379.
18. Walzer C. Diabetes in primates. In: Fowler ME, Miller RE, editors. Zoo and Wild Animal Medicine, Current Therapy 4. Philadelphia: WB Saunders; 1999. p. 397–400.
19. Gonzales J, Benirschke K, Saltman P, et al. Hemosiderosis in lemurs. Z Biol 1984; 3:255–65.
20. Benirschke K, Miller C, Ippen R, et al. The pathology of prosimians, especially lemurs. Adv Vet Sci Comp Med 1985;30:167–208.
21. Spelman LH, Osborn KG, Anerson MP. Pathogenesis of hemosiderosis in lemurs: Role of dietary iron, tannin, and ascorbic acid. Z Biol 1989;8:239–51.
22. Glenn KM, Campbell JB, Rotstein D, et al. Retrospective evaluation of the incidence and severity of hemsiderosis in a large captive lemur population. Am J Primatol 2006;68:369–81.
23. Williams CV, Junge RE, Stalis IH. Evaluation of iron status in lemurs by analysis of serum iron and ferritin concentrations, total iron-binding capacity, and transferrin saturation. J Am Vet Med Assoc 2008;232(4):578–85.

24. Crichton RR, Wilmet S, Legssyer R, et al. Molecular and cellular mechanisms of iron homeostasis and toxicity in mammalian cells. J Inorg Biochem 2002;91:9–18.
25. Ballot D, Baynes RD, Bothwell TH, et al. The effects of fruit juices and fruits on the absorption of iron from a rice meal. Br J Nutr 1987;57:331–43.
26. Cook JD, Watson SS, Simpson KM, et al. The effect of high ascorbic acid supplementation on body iron stores. Blood 1984;64(3):721–6.
27. Rossander-Hultén L, Brune M, Sandström B, et al. Competitive inhibition of iron absorption by manganse and zinc in humans. Am J Clin Nutr 1991;54:152–6.
28. Roughead ZKF, Zito CA, Hunt JR. Inhibitory effects of dietary calcium on the initial uptake and subsequent retention of heme and nonheme iron in humans: comparisons using an intestinal lavage method. Am J Clin Nutr 2005;82(3):589–97.
29. Olivares M, Pizarro R, Ruz M. Zinc inhibits nonheme iron bioavailability in humans. Biol Trace Elem Res 2007;117(1–3):7–14.
30. Wood C, Fang SG, Hunt A, et al. Increased iron absorption in lemurs: quantitative screening and assessment of dietary prevention. Am J Primatol 2003;61:101–10.
31. Freed BZ. An introduction to the ecology of daylight-active lemurs. In: Dolhinow P, Fuentes A, editors. The Nonhuman Primates. Mountain View (CA): Mayfield Publishing; 1999. p. 123–32.
32. Budnitz N, Dainis K. *Lemur catta*: ecology and behavior. In: Tattersall I, Sussman RW, editors. Lemur Biology. New York: Plenum; 1975. p. 219–35.
33. Britt A. Diet and feeding behavior of the black and white ruffed lemur (*Varecia variegata variegata*) in the Betampona Reserve, eastern Madagascar. Folia Primatol 2000;71:133–41.
34. Vasey N. Varecia, ruffed lemurs. In: Goodman SM, Benstead JP, editors. The Natural History of Madagascar. Chicago: University of Chicago Press; 2003. p. 1332–6.
35. Richard AF. Malagasy prosimians: female dominance. In: Smuts BB, Cheney DL, Seyfarth RM, et al, editors. Primate Societies. Chicago: University of Chicago Press; 1987. p. 25–33.
36. Pereira ME, Kaufman R, Kappeler PM, et al. Female dominance does not characterize all of the Lemuridae. Folia Primatol 1990;55:96–103.
37. Keppler PM. Female dominance in *Lemur catta*: more than just female feeding priority? Folia Primatol 1990;55:92–5.

Captive Invertebrate Nutrition

Ryan S. De Voe, DVM, MSpVM, DACZM, DABVP–Avian

KEYWORDS

- Invertebrate • Arthropod • Nutrition • Arachnid
- Insect • Food

Proper nutrition is paramount in maintaining healthy captive animals, be it a horse, dog, cat, or tarantula. Delivering appropriate nutrition is relatively easy in domestic animals, as excellent prepared diets are readily available. Providing acceptable diets for captive wildlife is more difficult, as commercially produced diets are often not available, and in many cases knowledge is lacking regarding the exact nutritional needs of a species. In addition, because of the limited market for diets specifically formulated for nondomestic species, few companies are willing or able to commit the resources necessary to research nutritional needs of a species and produce diets for sale. These issues with wildlife nutrition may seem daunting, but it is important to understand that great advances have been made over the last 20 to 30 years. These advances, enhanced by ongoing research, allow animal keepers greater success in feeding nondomestic animals in captivity than was possible in the past.

A large portion of the literature regarding nutrition of invertebrates is geared toward creating an animal that is appropriate for consumption by vertebrate species. Many dietary programs for invertebrate prey species are not intended to keep the invertebrate healthy for extended periods, but aim to fill the gastrointestinal tract with as much calcium and other nutrients as possible (ie, gut-loading). When fed many of the "gut-loading" diets, insects will often become terminally constipated and die within a few days.[1,2] This is not a concern when the invertebrate is intended as food, but is obviously undesirable when trying for long-term maintenance of a species.

Many invertebrate species are kept as pets by private individuals, as display or education animals by museums or zoos, as breeding stock by those producing food animals, or as agricultural animals (silk moths, honey bees). Proper nutrition for these animals is important to keep them healthy and make long-term maintenance, propagation, and production possible. Fortunately, the nutritional requirements of most invertebrate species kept in captivity are relatively easy to meet. There are some species that are dietary specialists (ie, silk moths), which feed exclusively on a particular species of plant or animal,[3] but most are fairly broad in their preferences and requirements. As with any nondomestic species it is important to have an understanding of the animal's natural history in an attempt to duplicate the wild diet in captivity.

North Carolina Zoological Park, 4401 Zoo Parkway, Asheboro, NC 27205, USA
E-mail address: ryan.devoe@nczoo.org

Vet Clin Exot Anim 12 (2009) 349–360
doi:10.1016/j.cvex.2009.01.016
1094-9194/09/$ – see front matter. Published by Elsevier Inc.

vetexotic.theclinics.com

This article focuses on terrestrial arthropods in the orders Insecta and Arachnida. For information regarding the nutrition and feeding of aquatic invertebrates, the clinician is advised to consult other references, such as any of the available invertebrate zoology texts and *Invertebrate Medicine* by Lewbart.[4]

WATER

Despite its undeniable importance, water is frequently overlooked when discussing nutrition. Inappropriate water quality, presentation, and availability are frequently implicated in captive invertebrate morbidity and mortality. Water requirements vary according to species, with desert-adapted species capable of efficiently conserving water, while those from rain forests or semi-aquatic environments will dehydrate quickly if not provided with enough water in the proper fashion. Some species, regardless of natural habitat or diet, can obtain all of the water they need from a proper diet. Nevertheless, most species will drink when water is available, so every effort should be made to provide appropriate access.

Water quality is important. It is probably safest to use water that would be appropriate for fish for maintenance of terrestrial invertebrates. Tap water can be used safely, but should either be allowed to de-gas overnight (for chlorine-treated water), or be treated with sodium thiosulfate (for chlorine- or chloramine-treated water). Offering chlorinated water to terrestrial invertebrates usually does not result in acute morbidity or mortality, but is thought to be associated with shortened life spans or ill-thrift syndromes by some keepers (Dan Dombrowski, personal communication, 2006).

Methods of presenting water can be problematic with invertebrates. Many species will drink from standing water sources; however, the risk of drowning is always a concern. For this reason, many pet stores and lay publications recommend providing water via a small sponge in the animal's enclosure. This is inappropriate for many reasons, not the least of which are the inability to keep a sponge clean and the possibility of toxic chemicals being present in commercially available sponges. A much more effective solution is to provide water in a shallow water dish with stones or gravel in the bottom, so the animal can easily escape if it falls in (**Fig. 1**). This type of set up can easily be removed and cleaned to maintain proper hygiene.

Many species will maintain adequate hydration by drinking water drops, following occasional misting of the enclosure. Terrestrial invertebrate species do not typically

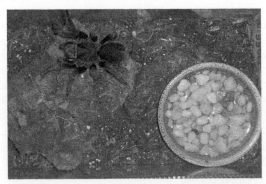

Fig.1. A layer of gravel on the bottom of a shallow water dish allows captive invertebrates to escape without drowning if they fall in.

enjoy being directly misted, so the mist stream should be aimed at the enclosure's furniture, walls, and substrate. The author employs this method of water presentation for maintenance of a variety of tarantula and scorpion species, including both desert-adapted and tropical species. The animals will usually approach droplets or pooled water and drink immediately following the misting.

Some keepers prefer the use of anionic polyacrylamide (PAM) gel for providing water to their invertebrates (**Fig. 2**). The primary use of PAM gel is to control irrigation-induced soil erosion at construction sites. It is sold at pet stores, either in gel cubes or as crystals that can be rehydrated by the keeper. Some PAM products have added calcium to improve the nutritional value to the invertebrate.[5] The PAM products seem safe and effective, but are not completely effort-free to use. The gel will dry out eventually, so it needs to be monitored and replaced when necessary. Another similar product is "cricket drink pillows" that are occasionally available. These drink pillows are composed of a durable polymer that will hold water when hydrated. The invertebrates suck water from the pillows, which can be rehydrated when dry. The author has not personally used these products, but suspects that some of the problems that exist with using sponges for water presentation may apply to the drink pillows as well.

Maintenance of an appropriate level of humidity in the environment is also extremely important for captive invertebrates. Some species are incapable of consuming enough water to keep up with losses if the environment is too dry. A good example of this are the myriapods (centipedes and millipedes), which need very humid conditions to thrive. The myriapods, especially centipedes, produce very wet droppings and lose a significant amount of water via evaporation through the respiratory system. This is because there is variable, but generally less ability to constrict the spiracles to conserve water.[6] Maintaining high-environmental humidity almost always creates issues with hygiene, as the warm and wet conditions promote the growth of bacteria and fungi. Therefore, those species requiring high humidity are much more labor intensive to keep than some of the desert-adapted species, as the keeper has to be vigilant with housekeeping.

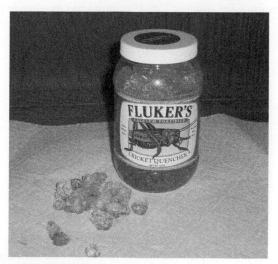

Fig. 2. Anionic PAM gel can be used to provide water to captive invertebrates without the risk of drowning. Many comparable products are commercially available.

FOOD PROCUREMENT, PREPARATION, AND PRESENTATION

Great care should be taken to avoid offering food contaminated with pesticides or other chemicals to captive invertebrates. Fruits and vegetables purchased at a grocery store should ideally be organic and washed thoroughly before feeding. If plant materials are collected from the wild, it should be from areas that are known to be free from pesticide and herbicide spraying or contamination by other chemicals. For instance, plant materials should not be collected from areas close to roads, as these plants can be heavily contaminated with heavy metals and chemicals from the automobile exhaust and other materials.[7]

The same basic principles apply when collecting wild-caught insects as food for captive invertebrates. In addition to the possibility of contamination with harmful chemicals, the risk of transmitting potential pathogens, such as parasites, bacteria, fungi, and viruses also exists. Although this is possible, the author feels that the benefit of receiving a healthy, varied diet far outweighs the risk of disease transmission in most cases.

Commercially produced diets are available for captive invertebrates and are usually focused on the creation of a nutritionally complete prey item (**Fig. 3**), and are not intended to support optimal health, growth, and reproduction. It is important to understand that some of the commercially available diets have not been scientifically evaluated. If one is considering use of a commercial diet, it is worthwhile doing some research, or even contacting the company that produces the product, to gather information regarding how it was evaluated for nutritional soundness.

There are many reports on the use of prepared diets for maintenance and reproduction of various arthropod species. Some of these diets are completely artificial and others are based on natural diets with various additives. In many cases, these artificial diets were administered to groups of invertebrates in an effort to identify essential nutrients for the species being studied.[8,9] With carnivorous invertebrates, there is usually no compelling reason for feeding an artificial diet when whole prey are readily available. Herbivorous and omnivorous species require a bit more effort to feed in captivity, often necessitating the creation of a mixture of items. **Box 1** outlines a number of diet mixtures that have proven useful in maintenance and rearing of a number of commonly kept species.[7] Various strategies for vitamin supplementation

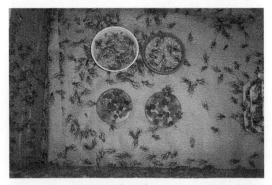

Fig. 3. Many companies produce pelleted diets for crickets. These diets are usually intended to produce animals that are nutritious for the vertebrate species that consume them and not for long-term maintenance.

Box 1
Diets for fruit flies

Dry mix

  14-oz potato flakes

  3.5-oz brewer's yeast

  1.5-cups confectioner's sugar

Mix together and refrigerate in sealed container.

Add 15 g (1 Tbs) of the dry mix to a 32-oz deli cup. Mix in 25 mLs of vinegar and 25 mLs of water. Allow to set before introduction of flies.

---

have been reported anecdotally by hobbyists and other keepers; however, there is little if any scientific support for these strategies.

NUTRITIONAL SUPPORT

Severely debilitated invertebrates are often presented for evaluation by veterinarians. These animals are often severely dehydrated and emaciated. As supportive care, all husbandry deficiencies should be corrected and efforts made to establish a normal level of hydratin and positive caloric balance. Hydration can be restored by increasing the ambient humidity, and encouraging the intake of oral fluids and administration of parenteral fluids. Because the respiratory openings in most invertebrate species are distant from the mouth, a very easy way to encourage drinking is simply to position the animal with its mouthparts immersed in water. Many arachnids suffering from severe dehydration because of prolonged holding in inadequate quarters during their transit through the pet trade respond very well to oral fluid replacement. The author simply uses dechlorinated water for oral fluid replacement. Electrolyte solutions may be beneficial; however, caution is recommended to avoid products with excessive artificial colors, preservatives, and heavily processed sugars.

With vertebrate species, the goals in feeding a sick animal in a negative-caloric balance are usually to provide a balanced diet that is complete, easy to ingest and digest, energy dense, and palatable. The goals should be the same with invertebrate species. It is common sense that a debilitated tarantula may have a difficult time capturing and consuming a large, healthy cricket. In addition to the inability to capture live prey, there is always a chance that the prey animal may turn the tables and injure or feed upon the debilitated captive. A simple way to avoid many of these problems is by offering pre-killed prey items. Some carnivorous invertebrates are not inclined to eat pre-killed prey, but most of the commonly kept species will readily do so. Debilitated carnivorous invertebrates can be offered pre-killed prey that may or may not have the body cavity opened to make ingestion easier. Wax worms are commonly used in this capacity, as this species in the larval form does not possess a chitinous exoskeleton.

For both carnivorous and herbivorous invertebrates, prepared diets, such as meat or vegetable baby foods, cat food, or slurries prepared from prey animals or vegetable matter can be offered. In cases where these types of foods are used, they can be offered in shallow dishes and the animal's mouth can be placed in the food as described to encourage drinking.

CARNIVORES

The vast majority of carnivorous invertebrates kept in captivity are either arachnids (spiders, tarantulas, and scorpions) or myriapods (centipedes). Fortunately, most species within these taxa are not terribly selective regarding what they will eat, making them easy captives. When feeding invertebrates to vertebrate species, great effort goes into making sure the feeder animals contain appropriate amounts of calcium and phosphorus. Because calcium is not typically an important component of the invertebrate exoskeleton, it does not seem to be a critical nutrient when feeding invertebrates. Therefore, specific supplementation with a calcium-laden product is not necessary. If offered well-fed prey items in appropriate amounts at appropriate intervals, most carnivorous arthropods do very well.

Most species will thrive feeding on the few insect species that are commercially produced in large numbers as feeders, such as crickets, mealworms, and waxworms (**Fig. 4**). Anecdotally, tarantulas seem to prefer appropriately sized crickets over mealworms or waxworms, though this has not been the personal experience of the author. Although many specimens have lived a long and healthy life feeding on a single species of insect, a varied diet is probably the best approach. A diet of commercially produced insects can be effectively supplemented with wild-caught insects as long as they are safely collected. Caution should be used to avoid offering wild-collected insects that may be toxic or otherwise dangerous to the captive.

A commonly encountered dilemma for keepers involved in propagation of various carnivorous arthropod species is finding prey species small enough for neonates. Tiny prey, such as small mealworm beetle larvae, pinhead crickets, fruit flies, and springtails are usually suitable, but can be difficult to work with and may not be readily available. Luckily, the neonates of most species will readily feed on pre-killed insects, or even parts of insects. If fed pre-killed adult insects, it is usually advantageous to open the body cavity of the prey item, as the neonate may have a difficult time penetrating the heavy chitinous exoskeleton. The author has raised many spiderlings on diets consisting primarily of cricket legs and mealworm pieces. Once the neonate has reached an appropriate size, it should be switched to whole-prey items.

Many captive carnivorous arthropods will go off feed for considerable lengths of time without ill effect. Physiologic reasons for anorexia include impending ecdysis, seasonal changes in temperature and light cycle, and reproductive activity. Most adult tarantulas and scorpions will not feed for 30 to 60 days before ecdysis.[10] If a concern exists regarding anorexia in a specimen, a careful history should be taken to rule out

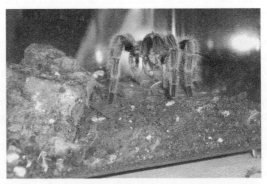

Fig. 4. A subadult Chilean rose-haired tarantula (*Grammostola rosea*) consuming a cricket (*Acheta domesticus*).

husbandry issues, followed by a thorough examination. If no problems are identified and the animal appears healthy, it should be weighed periodically, as a healthy arthropod will not typically lose more than 10% of its body weight during a fast. In the meantime, the specimen can be offered favored prey items and easily accessible food as described in the "Nutritional support" section.

It is important to understand that with many arthropods, once male animals reach sexual maturity they will stop feeding and eventually die of starvation or of complications of dysecdysis. This is true of male tarantulas in particular. Once the tarantula molts into an adult male (as indicated by the presence of palpal bulbs and tarsal hooks) in the wild, they become nomadic and go in search of females with which to mate.[10] In captivity, this is manifest as an animal that is constantly moving within its enclosure and trying to escape. Some keepers anecdotally report keeping these adult male animals alive for years with careful supportive care (Dan Dombrowski, personal communication, 2006). Supportive care consists of providing easily accessible water and food, as described above.

Certain carnivorous arthropods are formidable enough to prey on small vertebrate species. In fact, many species of tarantula are tagged with the name "bird-eater," which is probably more of a reference to their huge size rather than representative of a true dietary preference. Even so, small reptiles, amphibians, birds, and mammals will occasionally fall prey to the larger species of arachnids and centipedes in the wild. Many hobbyists are inclined to feed their captives vertebrate prey for the "thrill factor" involved with watching a large arthropod subdue and consume a mouse or other animal. This practice is quite dangerous for the captive invertebrate, as live vertebrate prey can be capable of injuring or killing the intended invertebrate predator. In addition, humane concerns exist, as the prey animals are sometimes not dispatched quickly and will struggle for extended periods of time. This is especially true when the prey animal is not a component of the natural diet or is larger than the arthropod would normally prey upon.

OMNIVORES

The omnivorous arthropods most frequently encountered in veterinary practice are those intended as food for various vertebrate species. This group includes the mealworm beetles (*Tenebrio molitor, Zophobus morio*), the crickets (*Acheta* sp, *Gryllus* sp), and various roaches (*Gromphadorhina* sp, *Blaberus* sp, and so forth). These species are incredibly adaptive, and will often survive on very questionable diets. However, if the intention is to propagate these animals in large numbers, a well-rounded diet is required to support reproduction. Breeding success and time of development will be directly affected by the diet offered.[7]

There are a variety of commercially available diets for crickets and mealworms. Although some of these diets are very good and will support good health and reproduction when used as directed, keep in mind that these diets are often not scientifically evaluated, and occasionally the quality control is questionable. Supplementing the commercially produced diets with fresh vegetables and fruits is probably the safest and healthiest approach for most species. With little effort, a conscientious keeper can provide an excellent, varied diet that will produce healthy (and subsequently nutritious, if that is the goal) invertebrates.

Another possibility for feeding omnivorous invertebrates is to base the diet around a commercially produced dry cat or dog food or other pelleted diet. Again, the prepared diet is supplemented with fresh fruits and vegetables. The exact makeup of the fresh portion of the diet is based on the species being kept. Most arthropod species do well receiving primarily vegetables as the fresh portion of the diet, though a number of cockroach species prefer fruits.[7]

There are many recommended diets for mealworm beetle larvae. Most can be used effectively, though some of the better diets will promote faster development times and higher average weight in the terminal larvae. A diet that has proven effective in the past is outlined in **Box 2**.[7] Usually, mealworm beetles will do well receiving the same diet as the larvae.

The author has had excellent success keeping and breeding the yellow mealworm (*Tenebrio molitor*), using a base diet of discarded high-quality parrot pellets (varying brands) and fish food, supplemented sparingly with fresh vegetables for moisture (**Fig. 5**). Development time seems to be variable according to the brand of pellet and temperature, but is usually adequate for production of 50 to 100 larvae a week from a 1-gallon container.

In recent years there has been increasing interest in propagation of invertebrates besides mealworms, waxworms, and crickets as food animals for captive vertebrates. The various fly species and their maggots are one of the more common species with which keepers are working. Unfortunately, the dietary requirements of these species make them somewhat repulsive captives. Diets for the adult flies are usually reasonable, with most mixtures described using honey as the base.[7] The diets for the maggots are a different story. The easiest and fastest way to rear maggots is to use raw meat as the diet. As people who have smelled a decaying, fly-blown carcass can attest, this is not an odor around which most would care to spend any significant amount of time. For this reason, a variety of less-odiferous mixtures have been tried over the years, with a few yielding positive results. A recipe for media to raise housefly maggots is outlined in **Box 3**.

HERBIVORES AND FRUGIVORES

It is extremely important that veterinarians working with invertebrate collections realize that herbivorous arthropods are potential agricultural pests and United States Department of Agriculture regulations exist regarding who can hold certain species, how they can be kept, and where they can be transported. Although they are often sold in ignorance in pet stores and through animal dealers, exotic herbivorous invertebrates are illegal to keep without a permit in the United States. It is also illegal to move potential agricultural pests that are native to North America between states.[11] The most commonly kept species that these laws pertain to are the large millipedes that are native to Africa and Madagascar. These millipedes are impressive, interesting, and easy to keep and breed. Unfortunately they are also illegal to keep without a permit. Be aware that these regulations exist so you don't inadvertently put yourself at risk.

Box 2
Diet for maggots
4 parts oats
4 parts soy flour
4 parts dried milk powder
1 part brewer's yeast
The dry ingredients are mixed together and enough water is added to produce a doughy consistency. The maggots can be kept in sawdust or hardwood shavings and balls of the diet can be added as needed.

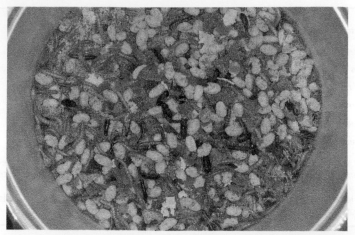

Fig. 5. The author's mealworm (*Tenebrio molitor*) colony using discarded parrot pellets and fish food as the base diet.

Because the millipedes have been so common in captivity for so many years, it is possible that the veterinarian may run into legally held specimens. In this case, it is important to be familiar with their nutrition. Millipedes feed primarily on rotting vegetable matter. In most cases, millipedes are kept on a substrate of soil and leaf litter. They will feed on the rotting leaf litter, but they should also be offered various fresh vegetables, greens, and occasionally fruits. All types of potatoes are favored by millipedes. As calcium is a significant component of the thick millipede exoskeleton, it is important to offer foods high in calcium, such as leafy green vegetables. Powdered calcium supplements can also be sprinkled onto the fresh foods that are introduced into the vivarium. Another strategy is to bury a piece of cuttlebone in the substrate.[6]

The majority of information in the literature regarding captive invertebrate nutrition focuses on silkworms. Sericulture, or the propagation of silkworms for silk production, is an extremely important industry in many Asian countries. Because of the economic importance of the silkworm, considerable effort has been invested in creating ways to enhance production. The silkworm is a specialized feeder, requiring an exclusive diet of mulberry (*Morus* sp) leaves to survive. Most of the nutritional research with this species has focused on adding supplements to mulberry leaves, many of which

---

Box 3
Diets for flies

200-g dried milk powder

750-mL water

90-mL honey

30-mL codfish oil

1-Tbs reptile or bird multivitamin powder

Mix in blender for 5 minutes. Resulting mixture can be refrigerated and used as needed.
Adapted from Friederich U, Volland W. Breeding Food Animals: live food for vivarium animals. Florida: Krieger Publishing Co; 2004. p. 133–42; with permission.

Box 4
Diets for mealworms

250-g wheat flour

250-g oats

100-g soy meal

70-g cornmeal

30-g brewer's yeast

300-g wheat bran

This diet can also be used as the substrate in which the beetle larvae burrow. Fresh vegetables, such as carrot, apple, potato, and leafy greens can be placed on top of the substrate to provide moisture. Adult beetles also do very well on this diet.
    From Friederich U, Volland W. Breeding food animals: live food for vivarium animals. Florida: Krieger Publishing Co; 2004. p. 110.

---

seem to improve production parameters. Formulated diets that do not contain mulberry leaves have not proven to be very effective.[11–15]

In a near tie with the silkworm in regards to literature pertaining to propagation and diet is the fruit fly (*Drosophila melanogaster*). The fruit fly remains a staple as a research animal and as a nutritional supply for small vertebrates. Many recipes exist for fruit fly food, and most are likely acceptable as long as they meet a few basic requirements. Diets must include a sugar, an acidifying agent, yeast, and a binding agent. The binding agent is necessary, as the maggots will do poorly in substrate that is too liquid.[7] The recipe for the fruit fly food used at the North Carolina Zoologic Park is presented in **Box 1**. The typical method for propagating fruit flies is to prepare the diet and cover the bottom of a sealable container with it (**Fig. 6**). The fruit flies are then placed into the container and require little attention as they feed and reproduce.

Another interesting species that is often kept in arthropod zoos are leafcutter ants from the genera *Acromymex* and *Atta*. These ants live in large complex nests where they compost vegetation collected by workers. The ants feed on the basidiomycete

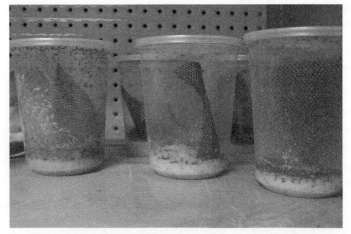

Fig. 6. Fruit fly (*Drosophila melanogaster*) cultures at the North Carolina Zoologic Park.

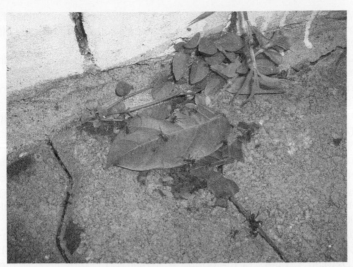

Fig. 7. Leafcutter ants of the genus *Atta*, collecting pieces of leaves for cultivation of basidiomycete fungi in their nest. (*Courtesy of* G. Lewbart, VMD, Raleigh, NC.)

fungi that grow on the composted plant material (**Fig. 7**). With most captive arthropods, it is recommended that moldy food material be removed from the enclosure as soon as possible. Leafcutter ants depend on fungus as a food source, so it must not be prematurely removed from the enclosure. The ants will remove all unnecessary or unsanitary material from the nest on their own.[3]

With other herbivorous invertebrates, appropriate diets should be based on knowledge of the natural history and should be as varied as possible. There are a few species of termite and beetles that also cultivate fungi for food.[3]

SUMMARY

The ability to maintain and propagate a species of animal in captivity is dependant on being able to provide adequate nutrition. Although the exact nutritional requirements of many invertebrate species are unknown, most commonly kept species are quite adaptable and seem to thrive on very basic diets. Veterinarians are often called upon to devise diets for captive invertebrates in research, display, and production facilities. A thorough knowledge of the natural history of the species is critical in developing dietary plans.

REFERENCES

1. Finke MD, Dunham SU, Kwabi CA. Evaluation of four dry commercial gut loading products for improving the calcium content of crickets, *Acheta domesticus*. J Herp Med Surg 2005;15(1):7–12.
2. Finke MD. Gut loading to enhance the nutrient content of insects as food for reptiles: a mathematical approach. Z Biol 2003;22(2):147–62.
3. Speight MR, Hunter MD, Watt AD. Ecology of Insects: concepts and applications. 2nd edition. Malden (MA): Wiley-Blackwell; 2008.
4. Lewbart GA, editor. Invertebrate Medicine. Ames (IA): Blackwell Publishing; 2006.

5. Finke MD, Dunham SU, Cole JS. Evaluation of various calcium-fortified high moisture commercial products for improving the calcium content of crickets, *Acheta domesticus*. J Herp Med Surg 2004;14(2):17–20.

6. Chitty JR. Myriapods (centipedes and millipedes). In: Lewbart GA, editor. Invertebrate Medicine. Ames (IA): Blackwell Publishing; 2006. p. 195–203.

7. Friederich U, Volland W. Breeding food animals: live food for vivarium animals. (FL): Krieger Publishing Co; 2004.

8. Amalin DM, Reiskind J, McSorley R, et al. Survival of the hunting spider *Hibana velox* (Araneae, Anyphaenidae) raised on different artificial diets. J Arachnol 1999;27:692–6.

9. Amalin DM, Pena JE, Reiskind J, et al. Comparison of the survival of three species of sac spiders on natural and artificial diets. J Arachnol 2001;29:253–62.

10. Murphy F. The care of spiders in captivity. London. In: Cooper JE, Pearce-Kelly P, Williams DL, editors. Arachnida: proceedings of a symposium on spiders and their allies. London: The Zoological Society of London; 1992.

11. Madhuri D, Prasad R. Effect of phyto-extract based medicines on the development of silkworm *Bombyx mori* L. nistari race. Environ Ecol 1999;17(3):717–20.

12. Bharti D, Miao Y. Effect of methoprene, MH-III and combination of methoprene and MH-III on larval adult moth characters, cocoon quality and silk proteins of silkworm, *Bombyx mori* fed on mulberry leaf and artificial diet. Phillipine J Sci 2001;130(1):45–52.

13. Goyal SK, Tenguria RK, Saxena RC. Nutritional management of *Morus alba* for good quality cocoon production. Int J Chem Sci 2003;1(4):440–5.

14. Devi P, Borkotoki A. Efficacy of som *Machilus bombycina* King and soalu *Litsea polyantha* Juss on hemolyph, silk gland protein and cocoon structure in muga silkworm *Antheraea assama* WW under indoor rearing condition. Environ Ecol 2006;24(1):66–70.

15. Rahmathulla VK, Nayak P, Vindya GS, et al. Influence of antibiotic on feed conversion efficiency of mulberry silkworm (*Bombyx mori* L). Anim Biol 2006;56(1): 13–22.

Nutrition, Feeding, and Behavior of Fish

Santosh P. Lall, PhD*, Sean M. Tibbetts, MSc

KEYWORDS

• Fish • Nutrition • Feeding • Behavior • Feeds • Diet

Nutrition and feeding influence growth, reproduction, and health of fish and their response to physiologic and environmental stressors and pathogens. The basics of fish metabolism are similar to those of warm-blooded animals in that they involve food intake, digestion, absorption, and transport of nutrients to the various tissues. Fish, however, being the most primitive form of vertebrates, possess some distinguishing features, such as the absence of a stomach in certain species, lack of mandibular teeth, and nondifferentiated small and large intestines. Some major physiologic and metabolic differences between other vertebrates and fish include the mechanisms involved in intestinal cell wall absorption by pinocytosis, metamorphosis in larval fish development, and the shift in osmoregulation in salmonids during sea water adaptation, carbohydrate metabolism, nitrogen excretion, and skeletal development. Unlike warm-blooded animals, which are homoeothermic, fish are poikilothermic, so their body temperature and metabolic rate depends on the water temperature. Environmental temperature influences energy expenditure and nutrient intake. At low temperatures, the cell membranes of fish remain fluid because of the incorporation of high amounts of polyunsaturated fatty acids from dietary fish oils and other lipid sources. Many fish efficiently use protein and lipid for energy rather than carbohydrates. Fish are also unique among vertebrates in their ability to absorb minerals not only from their diets but also from water through their gills and skin.

NUTRIENT REQUIREMENTS OF FISH

All the essential nutrients for other animals, including amino acids, fatty acids, vitamins, minerals, and energy-yielding macronutrients (protein, lipid, and carbohydrate), are important for fish also. A diet must supply all the essential nutrients and energy required to meet the physiologic needs of growing animals or for successful reproduction of broodstock. The rapid growth of global aquaculture has resulted in the production of more than 123 finfish species in intensive and extensive culture systems. Despite considerable advances reported over the past 5 decades, the quantitative

Institute for Marine Biosciences, National Research Council of Canada, 1411 Oxford Street, Halifax, Nova Scotia, Canada B3H 3Z1
* Corresponding author.
E-mail address: santosh.lall@nrc-cnrc.gc.ca (S.P. Lall).

Vet Clin Exot Anim 12 (2009) 361–372
doi:10.1016/j.cvex.2009.01.005
1094-9194/09/$ – see front matter. Crown Copyright © 2009 Published by Elsevier Inc. All rights reserved.

requirements for all essential nutrients for most farmed fish species are not well established. The criteria of nutrient adequacy for approximately 40 specific nutrients and their quantitative nutrient requirements have been made for rainbow trout, Pacific salmon, channel catfish, tilapia, and common carp, while partial nutrient requirements have been established more recently for numerous other fish species.[1,2] Although the minimum nutrient requirements established promote growth and prevent deficiency signs, higher intakes of vitamins, minerals, amino acids, and essential fatty acids increase buildup of their reserves in the tissues. The continued intake of certain nutrients in excess amounts causes saturation of various coenzymes. Certain fat-soluble vitamins (eg, vitamin A) and trace elements (eg, copper, selenium) are toxic when taken in excess. Deficiencies or excesses of each of the major dietary components, including proteins, fats, total calories, vitamins, and trace elements may have profound effects on disease development and the survival of the fish, largely through their effects on host defense mechanisms. Nutritional deficiencies may influence the integrity of skin and epithelial tissues, alter the composition of tissues and body fluids, and reduce mucus secretions, consequently predisposing the fish to infections. Major nutrient deficiency and toxicity signs are summarized in **Table 1**.

Macronutrients

Protein is an important component of fish diets, and to satisfy this dietary requirement a well-balanced mixture of amino acids from various animal and plant protein sources is critical to ensure proper growth and health of the fish. Protein is the most expensive component of the diet and levels greater than that needed to satisfy requirements result in elevated nitrogenous waste excretion into the surrounding waters. Excessive levels of protein in the diet are thus economically and environmentally undesirable. Most herbivorous and omnivorous fish require 25% to 35% protein in their diet but

Table 1
Major nutrient deficiency and toxicity signs in fish

Symptom	Nutrient Deficiency	Nutrient Toxicity
Fin erosion	Riboflavin, niacin, vitamin C, inositol, lysine, tryptophan, zinc	Vitamin A, leucine, cadmium
Fin and skin hemorrhage	Vitamin A, vitamin K, vitamin C, thiamin, riboflavin, pantothenic acid, niacin, inositol	Oxidized fish oil
Scoliosis and/or lordosis	Vitamin C, tryptophan, magnesium, phosphorus, essential fatty acids	Vitamin A, lead, cadmium, oxidized fish oil
Exophthalmia	Vitamin A, vitamin E, pantothenic acid, folic acid, niacin	Oxidized fish oil
Fatty liver	Choline, inositol, essential fatty acids, excessive dietary fat (mainly gadoids)	Oxidized fish oil
Cataracts	Vitamin A, riboflavin, methionine, histidine (mainly salmon smolts), tryptophan, zinc	Choline, oxidized fish oil
Skeletal deformity	Phosphorus, manganese, zinc	Vitamin A, oxidized fish oil
Anemia	Folic acid, iron	Oxidized fish oil
Nephrocalcinosis	Magnesium	Selenium
Convulsions	Thiamin, magnesium	—

carnivorous species require higher levels of protein ranging from 40% to 55% of diet.[1] This difference seems to be related to the limited use of carbohydrate as an energy source by carnivorous fish, which in turn use dietary protein for energy purposes. The efficient use of dietary protein in these fish is also attributable to the mechanism by which ammonia, produced by deaminated protein, is excreted by way of the gills with limited expenditure of energy. Energy density of the diet and the ratio of energy to protein in the diet also influence dietary protein requirements. The dietary requirement for protein is essentially a requirement for the amino acids contained within the protein. Ten amino acids, namely arginine, histidine, isoleucine, leucine, lysine, methionine, phenylalanine, threonine, tryptophan, and valine, are considered indispensable (essential) for most fish species studied to date. Among the dispensable (nonessential) amino acids that commonly make up protein, two are particularly important for their ability to partially replace or spare indispensable amino acids. Tyrosine can spare approximately 50% of phenylalanine in meeting the total aromatic amino acid requirement of fish and cystine can replace a similar amount of methionine as part of the total sulfur amino acid requirement.

No dietary requirement for carbohydrates has been demonstrated in fish; however, if carbohydrates are not provided in the diet, a higher percentage of protein and lipid are catabolized for energy. The ability of fish to use dietary carbohydrate for energy varies considerably, with most carnivorous species having more limited ability than herbivorous or omnivorous species. The amount of soluble carbohydrate included in prepared diets for carnivorous species is generally less than 20%, whereas diets for omnivorous species generally contain between 25% and 40% soluble carbohydrate. Non-starch polysaccharides, such as cellulose, hemicellulose, and chitin, are essentially indigestible by most fish species.

Lipids supply essential fatty acids (EFAs) and energy in the diet of fish and the EFA requirement of most fish can only be met by supplying the long-chain unsaturated fatty acids of linolenic (18:3 n-3) and linoleic (18:2 n-6) series. Salmonid and marine fish tissues contain eicosapentaenoic acid, 20:5 n-3 and/or docosahexaenoic acid, 22:6 n-3, particularly in cell membranes. This finding reflects a high dietary requirement for these fatty acids (20:5 n-3 and/or 22:6 n-3). These fish seem to have limited ability to chain elongate and desaturate 18:3 n-3 and 18:2 n-6 to meet their requirement, unlike many freshwater fish that have been shown to meet their requirements for these essential fatty acids.[3] Dietary lipids also serve as precursors of steroid hormones and prostaglandins in fish and provide a vehicle for intestinal absorption of fat-soluble vitamins. Lipid from the diet deposited in the flesh may affect the flavor and storage quality of edible products derived from the fish, particularly when the dietary oils are oxidized.

Micronutrients

Fish have unique physiologic mechanisms to absorb and retain minerals from their diets and from the surrounding water.[4] The knowledge of trace element requirements and their physiologic functions and bioavailability from feed ingredients is limited. Although the main functions of minerals involve skeletal structure maintenance, cellular respiration, oxygen transport, immune function, and regulation of acid–base equilibrium, they are also important components of hormones, enzymes, and enzyme activators. An excessive intake of minerals either from the diet or from gill uptake causes toxicity, and therefore maintaining a fine balance between mineral deficiency and surplus is vital for aquatic organisms to maintain their homeostasis either through increased absorption or excretion. Quantitative dietary requirements have been reported for phosphorus, magnesium, zinc, iron, copper, manganese, iodine, and selenium for selected fish species. Dissolved minerals in the aquatic environment may contribute to satisfying the metabolic requirements of fish and interact with dietary sources. In particular, fresh water of moderate hardness (~50 mg/L as $CaCO_3$) has been shown to provide fish with adequate calcium to sustain metabolic functions in the presence of low levels of dietary calcium. Chloride, potassium, and sodium are other minerals that may be present in fresh water at concentrations sufficient to partially meet the metabolic requirements of fish. Dietary deficiencies of most of the macrominerals generally have been difficult to produce in fish because of the presence of these minerals in the surrounding water. Supplementation of phosphorus in fish diets, however, is often critical because its presence in the water is limited and the availability from common plant feed ingredients is low. Although supplementation of practical diets with other microminerals has not been shown to be necessary in most fish species, a mineral premix is typically added to most nutritionally complete diets to ensure adequacy.

Most vitamins that are considered essential for terrestrial animals are also required by fish. Quantitative dietary requirements for fat-soluble (vitamin A, D, E, and K) and water-soluble (thiamine, riboflavin, pyridoxine, pantothenic acid, folic acid, niacin, biotin, vitamin B_{12}, vitamin C, and choline) vitamins have been determined for channel catfish, tilapia, common carp, rainbow trout, and Pacific salmon, while partial vitamin requirements have been established for some other fish species as well. The functions and dietary deficiencies of many of these vitamins are well documented[1,2] (see **Table 1**). These requirement values have been used to provide guidelines for vitamin supplementation for those fish species for which such information is not available.

FEEDING BEHAVIOR

The feeding behavior of fish is complex and has been studied extensively in cultured fish and wild fish from ecological perspectives.[5,6] Several behavioral responses have been linked to methods of feeding, feeding habits, frequency of feeding, mechanisms of food detection, and food preferences. The food organisms consumed by fish in natural environments may range from algae, plants, and detritus to small prey, such as crustaceans, mollusks, polychaetes, and other fish. It is well recognized that various combinations of sensory systems during the different phases of gustation and feeding are required to achieve desired food consumption; however, the acceptance or rejection of feed is physiologically dependent on inputs from chemoreception.[7] Fish possess several chemosensory systems, which include gustation (taste), olfaction (smell), and chemical sensory and chemoreceptor cells. The role of each system is often difficult to distinguish because each system responds to aqueous chemical stimuli, some of which may be common in these different systems. It seems that the gustatory system is the most important in acquisition and ingestion of food and with the rejection of potentially harmful and toxic substances.[8] The gustatory system, which is highly developed in several fish species, also consists of taste buds in the epithelia of the oropharynx **Fig. 1**, **Table 2**.

Like all animals, food intake in fish is controlled by a central feeding system in combination with a peripheral satiation system regulated by various key neuropeptides and hormones.[9–11] Various endocrine and metabolic factors convey information regarding nutritional status to the fish's brain, either directly or indirectly by way of the vagus nerve.[12] The information is then processed by the brain and neuropeptide signaling systems are triggered to secrete factors that either initiate or terminate feeding.[13–15] Although most neuropeptides down-regulate feeding behavior, a smaller number have a stimulatory effect.[10,11] Certain biochemical factors that control food intake to some extent in fish are cholecystokinin, gastrin-releasing peptide, ghrelin, glucagon-like peptides, insulin, amylin, and leptin; these have been discussed in detail elsewhere[9]

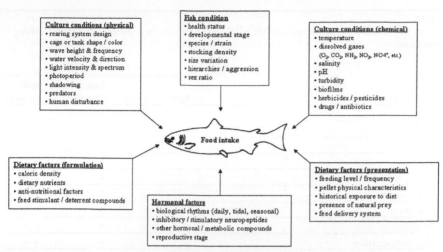

Fig. 1. The complexity of factors affecting feeding behavior in fish.

and are beyond the scope of this section. With the exception of the gastric factor ghrelin, all of these factors serve as satiety signals to reduce food intake and feeding behavior. Certain nutrients or related compounds, such as carbohydrates, peptides, amino acids, and lipids, may also affect food intake. For example, glucose administration induces hyperglycemia in fish and intraperitoneal injections of glucose cause a decrease of food intake and increase in food latency time in carp and tilapia.[16]

FEEDING RHYTHMS

The major factors that can influence feeding behavior of fish, such as stocking density, sex ratio, reproductive status, and biologic rhythms, have been subject to limited investigation and results often conflict between and within species.[17] Endogenous clock mechanisms may control some of these rhythms, but environmental factors, such as day length or temperature, may either control others or act as time setters or synchronizers. Rhythmic feeding activity, whether based on days, weeks, or months, is generated within the fish and the extent to which the external factors can influence feeding rhythms is complex. The anticipatory behavior seems to persist in fasting animals; thus it seems that there are internal timing mechanisms in fish similar to birds and mammals. The practical implications are that fish may adjust to the feeding of meals at set times, and there are likely optimum feeding times for each species. One important topic is whether the presence of rhythms can influence not only the amount of food consumed but also the efficiency with which food is converted into somatic growth. Recent developments in improving the understanding of the physiologic rhythms in farmed fish are providing useful information that allows selection of proper times for feeding fish to maximize growth, improve feed efficiency, and reduce feed wastage and fecal output to minimize the environmental impacts of aquaculture.

The three predominant feeding rhythms that affect food consumption in fish are diel (daily), annual (seasonal), and tidal (lunar) rhythms. Most fish in culture systems have diel feeding rhythms whereby they are either diurnal feeders (eat during the day) or nocturnal feeders (eat at night). Many fish species change their preferred time of feeding throughout the day based on the influences of biotic factors[18] (such as threat of predation) and abiotic factors[19] (such as lighting conditions). In a culture situation, it

Table 2
Factors that affect feeding behavior of fish as related to the culture system used and their relative controllability

| | Culture System | | | |
Influencing Factor	Pond	Cage	Tank (Outdoor)	Tank (Indoor)
Rearing system characteristics				
Shape	+	+	+	+
Color	−	−	+	+
Light				
Intensity	−	−	+	+ +
Photoperiod	−	−	+	+ +
Spectrum	−	−	+	+ +
Shadowing	+	+	+	+ +
Water temperature	−	−	+	+ +
Waves				
Height	−	−	+	n
Frequency	−	−	+	n
Water flow				
Velocity	+	−	+ +	+ +
Direction	+	−	+ +	+ +
Water chemistry				
Dissolved oxygen	+	+	+ +	+ +
Nitrogenous compounds (NH_3, NO_3, NO_4^+, and so forth)	−	−	+	+
Other dissolved gases	−	−	+	+
pH	−	−	−	−
Salinity	−	−	+	+
Toxicants or pollutants (drugs, antibiotics, biofilms, pesticides, herbicides, and so forth)	−	−	+	+
Turbidity	−	−	+	+
Stocking density	+ +	+ +	+ +	+ +
Social structure				
Size variability	+ +	+ +	+ +	+ +
Sex ratio	−	−	−	−
Dominance hierarchy (aggression)	+	+	+	+
Predators	−	−	+	+ +
Human disturbances				
Acute (weighing, sampling, cleaning, disease treatment, transferring, and so forth)	+	+	+	+
Chronic (prolonged noise or vibration, and so forth)	+	+	+	+
Feeding rhythms				
Diel (diurnal or nocturnal)	+	+	+ +	+ +
Tidal and lunar	−	−	+	n
Annual (seasonal)	−	−	−	n

(continued on next page)

Table 2 (continued)				
		Culture System		
Influencing Factor	Pond	Cage	Tank (Outdoor)	Tank (Indoor)
Nutritional factors				
Pellet physical characteristics	+ +	+ +	+ +	+ +
Dietary nutrients	+	+	+	+
Caloric density	+	+	+	+
Feeding stimulants	+	+	+	+
Deterrent compounds	+	+	+	+
Antinutritional factors	+	+	+	+
Access to natural prey	−	−	+	+ +
Feed delivery system	+ +	+ +	+ +	+ +
Historical exposure (adaptation)	+ +	+ +	+ +	+ +
Feeding level/frequency	+ +	+	+ +	+ +
Neurologic factors				
Inhibitory neuropeptides	−	−	−	−
Stimulatory neuropeptides	−	−	−	−
Hormones	−	−	−	−
Species/strain	+ +	+ +	+ +	+ +
Health status	+	+	+ +	+ +
Age				
Developmental stage	+ +	+ +	+ +	+ +
Reproductive stage	+	+	+	+

Factor is easily controllable (+ +), controllable (+), difficult to control (−) or not a factor (n).

is important to know the optimum time of day to feed the fish when their appetite is highest to promote high growth rates and minimize feed wastage.

The feeding preference of fish can also be affected by other environmental rhythms, such as annual (seasonal) changes and tidal (lunar) rhythms.[17] Annual or seasonal changes are often predictable because they are closely correlated with other environmental factors, namely water temperature and day length. Most cold-water fish (eg, Arctic char, rainbow trout, Atlantic salmon, and turbot)[19–23] and warm-water fish (eg, European sea bass, catfish, and goldfish)[24–27] cultured under ambient water temperatures with access to natural light and photoperiods typically increase their feeding behavior in the spring and throughout the summer months when the days are longer and water temperatures higher. They gradually reduce feeding in the autumn and into the winter months as water temperatures fall and day length decreases. This cycle generally holds true for most fish in the growth phase before sexual maturation, but is often broken by the onset of sexual maturity and preparation for spawning, at which time feeding activity may diminish or completely cease.[28–31] Tidal or lunar rhythms have little or no effect on fish cultured in indoor or outdoor tank systems with artificial lighting and sufficient filtration to minimize natural prey items from entering the culture water. In open surface outdoor tank systems and in ponds and cage/net pen systems, however, the daily tidal and lunar cycles can significantly affect feeding behavior of fish.[17] The mechanism is most frequently associated with the abundance of natural prey items present in seawater during incoming and high tides. This phenomenon is illustrated in killfish, wherein stomach fullness has been directly correlated with the high-tide cycle.[32] Similar observations have been made with other fish species also,[33–35] although it is not always clear whether the effect is due to the high-tide abundance of food or the lunar effects of increased light for foraging during a full moon. It is likely that during periods of full moon and high tides both factors are working together synergistically.

FEEDING STIMULANTS AND DETERRENTS

Fish primarily detect food in the natural aquatic environment through olfaction (smell) and sight; however, appearance, feel, and taste of the diet are key factors in determining whether food will be swallowed or rejected by fish held in captivity.[36] A well-defined and species-specific tuning of the taste receptors of fish for particular cues is known to be present in their food items. Generally, various substances are added to fish feeds in an effort to enhance palatability and feed acceptance. The use of feeding stimulants is particularly important in the production of larval and starter feeds, wherein feed acceptability is a major concern. Four major chemical characteristics of feeding stimulants for fish have been identified: (a) low molecular weight (<1000), (b) nitrogen- containing, (c) nonvolatile and water soluble, and (d) simultaneous acid and base properties or amphoteric.[37] Several compounds are known to act as feeding stimulants in carnivorous and omnivorous species, including betaine and amino acids, notably glycine and alanine or mixtures of L-amino acids, and the nucleotides inosine or inosine 5'-monophosphate. Some dipeptides elicit a greater feeding response in combination than either of the constituent amino acids presented alone.[38] Limited data exist on feeding stimulants for herbivorous species; however, organic acids along with certain amino acids and dimethyl-β-propiothetin were found to be stimulatory for carp and tilapia.[39] In general, the following patterns related to feeding stimulants have emerged from laboratory studies: (1) carnivores show a positive response to alkaline and neutral nitrogenous substances (such as glycine, proline, taurine, valine, and betaine) and (2) herbivores respond more to acidic substances (such as aspartic acid and glutamic acid). Studies conducted on common feed ingredients used to produce fish feeds for cold-water fish show that certain high-quality fish, crustacean, krill, and squid meals or their hydrolysates stimulate feeding behavior in salmonids and marine fish.

Fish have the ability to discriminate between high-quality and poor-quality feeds and refuse to ingest the latter. Certain compounds present in feeds are known as feeding deterrents. Trimethylamine (or its oxidation products), produced in decaying fish flesh, is known to cause a decrease in food consumption when added to the diet. Highly oxidized oils and fish meals in salmonid and marine fish feeds are also known to cause food aversion. Improper storage and use of poor-quality feed ingredients in feed manufacture are the common cause of rancidity in commercial feeds. The presence of aflatoxins, produced by molds growing on improperly stored feed, depress feed intake and can result in death if consumed by the fish in significant amounts. In addition, the presence of adventitious toxins (antinutritional factors) such as gossypol in cottonseed meal, protease inhibitors in soybean meal, glucosinolates in canola/rapeseed meals, and numerous others results in anorexia due to inactivation of digestive proteases and reductions in digestion, absorption and physiological utilization of dietary nutrients.

FEED INTAKE

Generally, hunger stimulates feeding behavior in fish. When feed is offered, fish may initially feed at a faster rate and slowly decrease or stop with a gradual decline of appetite. Environmental factors, such as light, temperature, water velocity, social factors, predators, and disturbance by humans, may also influence fish feeding behavior.

Feeding practices, such as the even distribution of the feed into the water, can also affect the fish's chances of gaining access to food. There may thus be numerous combinations of biotic and abiotic factors that can have an important influence on feeding behavior of fish. Often, fish suddenly stop feeding for no apparent reason and the rates of feeding can either decrease or increase over a period of days. A better understanding of the factors that can influence feeding may allow for better feed management and the allocation of food, and reduce the variability in feeding and growth rates that are usually evident among individuals and among groups of fish.

It is generally accepted that fish feed to satisfy their energy requirements. Fish fed a diet low in energy content are forced to increase their consumption rate and gastric evacuation rate to compensate for the lower caloric diet. Other nutrients also impact feed intake, however, with anorexia being a common symptom of nearly all nutrient deficiencies.[1] Particle size is closely related to feed intake and the correct feed particle size induces a positive behavioral response. Feed particles must be sufficiently small to be ingested, while being large enough to be consumed without expending too much energy in the process.

To increase the efficiency of farming systems through proper feed management, the prediction of feed intake and growth under a wide range of environmental and culture conditions is necessary. Several environmental, genetic, and physiologic factors have been identified that correlate with feed intake and are considered as regulators of feed intake. When food availability is unlimited, the amount of food eaten is referred to as the voluntary feed intake (VFI). One key feature of VFI is the description of regulatory feedback mechanisms, which are not clearly identified for most fish. In particular, the identification of multiple feedback signals and their integration into specific responses may ultimately control the feeding behavior. Biologic factors, including fish size, physiologic stage, and genotype, are known to influence VFI. Among the environmental factors, both water temperature and photoperiod control feed intake. Feed intake is also under close metabolic, endocrine, and neuronal control, all of which are intimately related to the nutritional status of the animal. Several techniques are available to monitor individual feed intakes and the passage of feed through the digestive tract. They include radiography and analysis of gut contents.[40,41]

Like higher vertebrates, when there is an increase in the energy density of the feed, the VFI is reduced at any given production level. If the feed provides a lower ratio of protein to energy than required, fish may increase feed intake to obtain sufficient protein. There is growing evidence that fish are capable of adjusting their VFI depending on the quality of the diets and especially on the dietary digestible energy (DE) content.[42,43] Excessive DE in the diet may affect VFI and cause lower intake of other nutrients, which may cause metabolic imbalance and accentuate marginal nutrient deficiencies. Knowledge of nutrient and energy balance in diets is therefore considered important to better understand the mechanisms involved in the control of feed intake. Feeding tables have been developed for the major farmed fish species that take into account the water temperature, fish size, genotype, growth rate, dietary energy density, and nutrient concentration, but few take into account the principles of nutritional bioenergetics in fish.[44]

FEEDS AND FEEDING

Feeds and feeding of fish depend on the type of culture system used: extensive, semi-intensive, or intensive. In the first two systems, fish derive all or a substantial part of their nutrients from natural food organisms in culture ponds. Fish maintained in intensive fish culture systems (tanks, raceways, and cages) are totally dependent on the provision of nutritionally complete diets produced in dry, semi-moist, or moist forms. Diets fed to fish are subject to leaching of nutrients while they remain in the water column or at the bottom of the culture system. This leaching creates a challenge for feed manufacturers, particularly when small-sized granules or flakes are used to feed larval and small fish, often referred to as fry or fingerlings. Formulated dry feeds are more common and produced either by steam or cold compression pelleting or by a cooking extrusion process to produce feed in various physical forms and shapes, and of different buoyancy (floating, slow sinking, or fast sinking). Catfish, salmon, and shrimp, for example, require floating, slow-sinking, or fast-sinking feeds, respectively, because of their different preferred feeding habits in the water column. Extrusion technology is widely used to produce feeds of cold-water salmonids and marine fish. Application of extrusion technology allows for the production of feeds with high energy contents based on high levels of lipid (~20%–40% of the diet). The heat processing associated with extrusion also inactivates antinutritional components that can be present in plant ingredients and increases the digestibility of protein, carbohydrate, and other nutrients. Gelatinization of starch during extrusion processing also increases feed stability and allows for higher absorption of lipid into the pellets.

Proper feed distribution is necessary to achieve good feed efficiency. The amount of feed offered to fish per day has been based on feeding tables developed on the basis of a percentage of body weight and water temperature. Young fish require feed at a greater percentage of their body weight per day (>5%) than older fish. Demand or *ad libitum* feeding is commonly used in hatcheries where demand feeders dispense small quantities of feed when activated by the fish. Automatic feeders or hand feeding are used to feed fish in tanks or sea cages where fish feeding behavior can be monitored manually or on video camera. Frequency of feeding is important, with larval fish and fry offered a small amount of feed more than 12 times per day and the frequency is gradually decreased to 1 to 4 times per day. Additional time is required to feed fish at cold temperatures when their metabolic rate and appetite are lower.

Because fish live in aquatic environments, water quality affects their feed consumption, growth, survival, and health. Overfeeding results in feed wastage and deterioration in water quality, particularly when there is an increase in suspended particles and lower dissolved oxygen levels. Generally, undigested protein or carbohydrate produces suspended solids and this increases biologic oxygen demand, which should be kept minimized. The principal excretory end products of protein catabolism, an ionized and a nonionized form of ammonia, are excreted through the gills and the latter is toxic to fish. Fat not properly retained in the feed may leach out producing a thin film on the surface water causing respiration problems.

Feeding of larval fish requires special consideration because their digestive systems are not fully developed after hatching. Currently, larviculture depends on feeding live food organisms (eg, brine shrimp [*Artemia*], rotifers, and other planktonic organisms) that have been enriched with specific nutrients (essential fatty acids, vitamins, amino acids) to improve their nutritional value. Manufactured dry feeds are becoming increasingly important in hatcheries because diets can be tailored to provide optimum levels of nutrients and incorporate ingredients that adapt to larval digestive and metabolic needs (eg, hydrolyzed protein). Visual and chemical stimuli are important considerations for capture and acceptance of artificial food by larvae. Larvae are gradually weaned onto highly digestible, water-stable microparticulate dry feeds of appropriate particle size (~100–600 μm) or flakes and attractive color and organoleptic properties.

REFERENCES

1. National Research Council. Nutrient requirements of fish. Washington, DC: National Academy Press; 1993. p. 114.

2. Halver JE, Hardy RW. Fish nutrition. San Diego (CA): Academic Press; 2002. p. 824.
3. Bell JG. Current aspects of lipid nutrition in fish farming. In: Black KD, Pickering AD, editors. Biology of farmed fish. Sheffield (UK): Sheffield Academic; 1998. p. 114–45.
4. Lall SP. Minerals. In: Halver JE, Hardy RW, editors. Fish nutrition. San Diego (CA): Academic Press; 2002. p. 260–308.
5. Gerking SD. Feeding ecology of fish. New York: Academic Press; 1994. p. 416.
6. Houlihan D, Boujard T, Jobling M. Food intake in fish. Oxford (UK): Blackwell Science Ltd; 2001. p. 418.
7. Hara TJ. Olfaction and gustation in fish: an overview. Acta Physiol Scand 1994; 152:207–96.
8. Lamb CF. Gustation and feeding behaviour. In: Houlihan D, Boujard T, Jobling M, editors. Food intake in fish. Oxford (UK): Blackwell Science Ltd; 2001. p. 130–56.
9. Pedro N, Björnsson BT. Regulation of food intake by neuropeptides and hormones. In: Houlihan D, Boujard T, Jobling M, editors. Food intake in fish. Oxford (UK): Blackwell Science Ltd.; 2001. p. 269–96.
10. Morley JE. Neuropeptide regulation of appetite and weight. Endocr Rev 1987;8: 256–87.
11. Morley JE. The role of peptides in appetite regulation across species. Am Zool 1995;35:437–45.
12. Volkoff H, Peter RE. Feeding behavior of fish and its control. Zebrafish 2006;3:131–40.
13. Wynne K, Stanley S, McGowan B, et al. Appetite control. J Endocrinol 2005;184: 291–318.
14. Stanley S, Wynne K, McGowan B, et al. Hormonal regulation of food intake. Physiol Rev 2005;85:1131–58.
15. Broberger C. Brain regulation of food intake and appetite: molecules and networks. J Intern Med 2005;258:301–27.
16. Kuz'mina VV, Garina DV, Gerasimov YV. The role of glucose in regulation of feeding behavior of fish. J Ichthyl 2002;42:210–5.
17. Madrid JA, Boujard T, Sánchez-Vázquez FJ. Feeding rhythms. In: Houlihan D, Boujard T, Jobling M, editors. Food intake in fish. Oxford (UK): Blackwell Science Ltd; 2001. p. 189–215.
18. Daan S. Adaptive daily strategies in behavior. In: Aschoff J, editor. Handbook of behavioral neurobiology 4, biological rhythms. New York: Plenum Press; 1981. p. 275–98.
19. Boujard T, Leatherland JF. Demand-feeding behavioural and diel pattern activity in Oncorhynchus mykiss held under different photoperiod regimes. J Fish Biol 1992;40:535–44.
20. Saether BS, Johnsen HK, Jobling M. Seasonal changes in food consumption and growth of Arctic char exposed to either simulated natural or a 12:12 LD photoperiod at constant water temperature. J Fish Biol 1996;48:1113–22.
21. Smith IP, Metcalfe NB, Huntingford FA, et al. Daily and seasonal patterns in the feeding behaviour of Atlantic salmon (Salmo salar) in a sea cage. Aquaculture 1993;117:165–78.
22. Blanchet S, Loot G, Bernatchez L, et al. The effects of abiotic factors and intraspecific versus interspecific competition on the diel activity patterns of Atlantic salmon (Salmo salar) fry. Can J Fish Aquat Sci 2008;65:1545–53.
23. Mallekh R, Lagardère JP, Bégout-Anras ML, et al. Variability in appetite of turbot, Scophthalmus maximus under intensive rearing conditions: the role of environmental factors. Aquaculture 1998;165:123–38.
24. Anthouard M, Divanach P, Kentouri M. An analysis of feeding activities of sea bass (Dicentrarchus labrax, Moronidae) raised under different lighting conditions. Ichtyophysiologica Acta 1993;16:59–73.

25. Aranda A, Sánchez-Vázquez FJ, Madrid JA. Influence of temperature on demand-feeding rhythms in sea bass. J Fish Biol 1999;55:1029–39.
26. Boujard T. Diel rhythms of feeding activity in the European catfish, *Silurus glanis*. Physiol Behav 1995;58:641–5.
27. Hirata H. Diurnal rhythms of the feeding activity of goldfish in winter and early spring. Bulletin of the Faculty of Fisheries Hokkaido University 1957;7:72–84.
28. Metcalfe NB, Huntingford FA, Thorpe JE. Feeding intensity, growth rates, and the establishment of life-history patterns in juvenile Atlantic salmon, Salmo salar. J Anim Ecol 1988;57:463–74.
29. Kadri S, Mitchell DF, Metcalfe NB, et al. Differential patterns of feeding and resource accumulation in maturing and immature Atlantic salmon, Salmo salar. Aquaculture 1996;142:245–57.
30. Kadri S, Thorpe JE, Metcalfe NB. Anorexia in one-sea-winter Atlantic salmon (Salmo salar) during summer, associated with sexual maturation. Aquaculture 1997;151:405–9.
31. Tveiten H, Johnsen HK, Jobling M. Influence of maturity status on the annual cycles of feeding and growth in Arctic char reared at constant water temperature. J Fish Biol 1996;48:910–24.
32. Weisberg SB, Whalen R, Lotrich VA. Tidal and diurnal influence on food consumption of a salt marsh killfish, Fundulus heteroclitus. Mar Biol 1981;61:243–6.
33. Farbridge KJ, Leatherland JF. Lunar cycles of coho salmon, Oncorhynchus kisutch. I. Growth and feeding. J Exp Biol 1987;128:165–78.
34. Gibson RN. Tidally-synchronised behaviour in marine fish. In: Ali MA, editor. Rhythms in fishes. New York: Plenum Press; 1992. p. 63–81.
35. Leatherland JF, Farbridge KJ, Boujard T. Lunar and semi-lunar rhythms in fishes. In: Ali MA, editor. Rhythms in fishes. New York: Plenum Press; 1992. p. 83–107.
36. Adron MA, Mackie AM. Studies on chemical nature of feeding stimulants in rainbow trout, Salmo gairdneri Richardson. J Fish Biol 1978;12:303–10.
37. Carr WES. Chemical stimulation of feeding behaviour. In: Hara TJ, editor. Chemoreception in fishes. Amsterdam: Elsevier; 1982. p. 259–73.
38. Harada K. Feeding attraction activities of L-dipeptides for abalone, oriental watherfish and yellowtail. Bull Jap Soc Sci Fish 1989;55:1629–34.
39. Nakajima KA, Uchida A, Ishida Y. A new feeding attractant dimethyl-β-propiothetin, for freshwater fish. Nippon Suisan Gakk Shi 1989;55:689–95.
40. Jobling M, Baardvik BM, Jørgensen EH. Investigations of feed-growth relationships of Arctic charr, *Salvelinus alpinus* L., using radiography. Aquaculture 1989;81:367–72.
41. McCarthy ID, Carter CG, Houlihan DF. Individual variation in consumption in rainbow trout measured using radiography. In: Kaushik SJ, Luquet P, editors. Fish nutrition in practice. Paris: INRA Editions; 1993. p. 85–8.
42. Boujard T, Médale F. Regulation of voluntary feed intake in juvenile rainbow trout fed by hand or by self-feeders with diets containing two different protein to energy ratios. Aquat Living Resour 1994;7:211–5.
43. Kaushik SJ, Médale F. Energy requirements, utilization and supply to salmonids. Aquaculture 1994;124:81–97.
44. Thorpe JA, Cho CY. Minimising waste through bioenergetically and behaviourally based feeding strategies. Water Sci Technol 1995;31:29–40.

Index

Note: Page numbers of article titles are in **boldface** type.

A

Abandonment, of opossum infants, supportive care for, 221–222
Abiotic factors, of nutrition, for degus, 250
Abscesses, nutrition and, in squirrels, 295
Acidophilus additive, for squirrels, 293–294
Acute pain response, in opossum, 223
Adult nutrition, for coatis, 191
    for degus, 244–246
    for kinkajou, 173–177, 180
    for opossum, 229
    for raccoons, 192
African Pygmy hedgehog, nutrition of, **335–337**
    captive husbandry and, 336
    digestive physiology and, 335–336
    environmental factors of, 335
    feeding behavior and, 335
    hand-rearing and, 337
    lactation and, 337
    pregnancy and, 336
    species background and, 335
Aggressive behavior, of cavies, 269
    of kinkajou, 180
    of lemurs, 345
    of opossum, 219–220
    of skunks, 319
Agoutis, captive, diet determinants for, **279–286**
    apparent requirements as, 282
    as frugivores, 279–281
    as omnivores, 280–281, 283–284
    ascorbic acid and, 281–282
    average body weights in, 279–280
    catching behavior and, 281, 284
    classification of, 283–284
    dentition and, 279–280
    diabetes and, 283–284
    energy requirements as, 282
    feeding behavior and, 282
    fiber intake and, 282
    for dental caries prevention, 283–284
    for gestation, 283–284
    for lactation, 283–284

Vet Clin Exot Anim 12 (2009) 373–399
doi:10.1016/S1094-9194(09)00027-9
1094-9194/09/$ – see front matter © 2009 Elsevier Inc. All rights reserved.

vetexotic.theclinics.com

Agoutis (*continued*)
    for obesity prevention, 284
    gastrointestinal tract and, 281
    meat and, 282
    metabolic rate and, 282
    preference as, 282
    recommendations for, 283–284
    reproductive stage and, 282–284
    scatter-hoarding behavior and, 281, 284
    sexuality maturity and, 282
    species background and, 279–280
Amino acids, essential, for degus, 243
    for exotic cats, 329
    for fish, 361–363, 368
    for hedgehogs, 336
    for kinkajou, 174, 176–177
    for skunks, 322
    for squirrels, 289
    for sugar glider, 211, 214
Anesthesia, for restraint, of cavies, 273
    of opossum, 219–220
Antibiotics, for cavies, 274–275
    for squirrels, 295
Antifungal agents, for cavies, 275–276
Antiparasitic drugs, for cavies, 274–275
Arachidonic acid, for exotic cats, 329
Arachnids, diets for, 354–355
Arthropods, consumption of. See *Insectivores.*
    nutrition for. See *Invertebrates.*
Ascorbic acid, endogenous synthesis of, by agoutis, 281
    intake of. See *Vitamin C intake.*

B

Bacterial contamination, of raw meat diets, 330
Bacterial flora, in macropod stomach, 201–202
    fermentation role of, 197, 203–204
Bacterial infections, in cavies, 274–275
    in kinkajou, 174
    in opossum, 219, 228
    in skunks, 320
    in squirrels, 294–295
Basal metabolic rate (BMR), calculation of, for agoutis, 282
    for exotic cats, 330–331
    for kinkajou, 173
    for lemurs, 340
    for macropods, 202
    for raccoons, 192
    for sugar glider, 211
Behavioral considerations, of nutrition, for opossum, as pets, 224–226
    disease manifestations and, 221–224

of captive and owned opossum, 217–221
social. See *Social behavior.*
Biochemical factors, of feeding behavior, in fish, 364–365
Birth weight, of degus, 247
of exotic cats, 332
of fennec fox, 301
of kinkajou, 179
of opossum, 219–220, 222, 228
of raccoons, 190
of squirrels, 289, 292–293
Body condition scoring, for kinkajou, 180–182
Body temperature, hand-rearing and, of fennec foxes, 306
of squirrels, 292
nutrition and, of fish, 361
of kinkajou, 173
of opossum, 219, 221
Body weight, nutrition and, at birth. See *Birth weight.*
of agoutis, 279–280
of coatis, 188
of degus, 238–239, 242, 247–248
of exotic cats, 330–331
of fennec foxes, 303
tracking during hand-rearing, 309–310
of invertebrates, 355
of kinkajou, 173, 175, 179–180
in body condition scoring, 180–182
of lemurs, 340–341
of macropods, 204
of opossum, 219–222, 228
of prairie dogs, 257, 261
of raccoons, 188
of skunks, 316
of squirrels, 289, 292–293
of sugar glider, 212–213
Bone disease, nutrition and. See *Metabolic bone disease.*
Breeding behavior, in degus, 250
in fennec fox, 300
in skunks, 315
nutrition for. See *Gestation; Reproductive stage.*

C

Calcium intake, of exotic cats, 331–332
of invertebrates, 354
of kinkajou, 175–176, 183
of opossum, 228, 230–232
of skunks, 322
of squirrels, 289, 295
of sugar glider, 212–214
Calcium oxalate calculi, in exotic cats, 331
Calories. See *Energy expenditure/requirements.*

Cannibalism, by opossum, 220
   by prairie dogs, 260–261
Captive agoutis, diet determinants for, **279–286**. See also *Agoutis.*
Captive invertebrates, nutrition of, **349–360**. See also *Invertebrates.*
Caracal, nutrition of, **327–334**
      body weight and, 330–331
      captivity issues with, 329
      disease related to, 331
      feeding behavior and, 328–329
      hand-rearing and, 332
      requirements for, 329–331
      species background and, 328
      stone formation and, 331
      summary overview of, 327, 332
Caracal caracal, nutrition of, **327–334**. See also *Caracal.*
Carbohydrate intake, of degus, structural vs. nonstructural, 239, 243
   of fish, 361, 363, 365, 370
   of kinkajou, 174, 176
   of sugar glider, 210–211
Cardiomyopathy, nutrition and, hypertrophic, in cavies, 275
      in skunks, 322
Cardiopulmonary disease, nutrition and, in cavies, 275
Cardiovascular collapse, trauma-related, in opossum, 222
Carnivores, agoutis as, 282
   coatis and raccoons as, 187–188, 191–192
   exotic cats as, 327–331
   fennec foxes as, 301
   fish as, 363, 368
   invertebrates as, 352–355
   kinkajou as, 171–172, 174, 183
   plant consumption by. See *Omnivores.*
   prairie dogs as, 260–261
   skunks as, 313, 316
Case management, for nutrition, of opossum, 221
Castration, of cavies, 269
   of opossum, 226
   of prairie dogs, 264
Cataracts, nutrition and, in degus, 249
Catching behavior, diet and, of agoutis, 281, 284
      of raccoons, 192
Cats, exotic, nutrition of, **327–334**. See also *Caracal; Serval.*
Cavies, nutrition of, **267–278**. See also *Patagonian cavies.*
Cecum, of macropods, 201–202
Chemistry values, normal, for cavies, 273–274
      for skunks, 321–322
Chemoreception, feeding behavior and, in fish, 364–365
      in kinkajou, 178
Chlorinated water, preparation of, for invertebrates, 350
Chronic pain response, in opossum, 223
Clinical pathology, nutrition and, in cavies, 273–274
Clock mechanisms, endogenous. See *Daily activity patterns.*

Coatis, nutrition of, **187–195**
    adult requirements for, 191
    average body weights in, 188
    feeding behavior and, 188–189
    functional anatomy and physiology in, 188–189
    neonatal requirements for, 190–191
    reproductive stage and, 190–191
    species background and, 187
    summary overview of, 192
Colon, digestion in, of degus, 238
    of macropods, 201–202
Colony sites, of prairie dogs, 256–257
Colostrum, hand-rearing vs., for fennec foxes, 306
    for hedgehogs, 337
Commercial formulas, for hand-rearing, of cavies, 272
    of exotic cats, 332
    of fennec foxes, 306
    of hedgehogs, 337
    of kinkajou, 179
    of macropod joeys, 206
    of opossum, 228
    of squirrels, 290–292
Communication mechanisms, of degus, 249–250
Confinement response, nutrition and, of opossum, 221
Coprophagy, by degus, 238
Copulation behavior. See *Breeding behavior.*
Courtship behavior, of cavies, 268–269
    of degus, 250
    of lemurs, 344–345
    of prairie dogs, 256–257
Cowpoxvirus, in cavies, 276
Cow's milk, for squirrels, 290–291
Crickets, diets for, 351–352, 355–356
Culture systems, nutrition and, of fish, 361, 365–366, 368–370
Cushing's-like syndrome, in opossum, 226

D

Daily activity patterns, feeding behavior and, in African Pygmy hedgehog, 335
    in agoutis, 282
    in caracal, 328–329
    in coatis, 188–189
    in degus, 258
    in exotic cats, 327–328
    in fish, 365–368
    in kinkajou, 178
    in lemurs, 344
    in opossum, 221
    in raccoons, 189–190
    in serval, 327–328

Daily activity (*continued*)
    in skunks, 315
    in sugar glider, 209–210
Dasyprocta spp., diet determinants for, **279–286**. See also *Agoutis.*
Defecation. See *Fecal output.*
Degus, nutrition of, **237–253**
    abiotic factors in, 250
    adult, example foods, quantities, and metabolism for, 244–246
    assessment criteria for, 248–249
    body weight and, 238–239, 242, 247–248
    breeding and, 246, 248
    carbohydrate intake in, structural vs. nonstructural, 239, 243
    cataracts and, 249
    dentition and, 237–238, 246
    diabetes and, 249
    digestibility of sample foods, 238, 242
    dry matter intake and, 238, 242, 246
    energy requirements in, 239
    fecal output in, 248–249
    feeding ecology in, 258
    fiber intake in, 239, 242
    gastrointestinal tract and, 237–238
    geriatric, 248
    gestation and, 248
    gross energy intake and, 242
    lactation and, 243, 248
    lens lesions and, 249
    lipid intake in, 243
    metabolizable energy of sample foods, 246
    mineral intake in, 243–245
    morphometrics in, 248
    neonatal requirements, 246
    nutrient composition of foods for, 240–241
    protein intake in, 243
    reproductive stage and, 246–248
    social behavior and, 249–250
    species background and, 237
    species description and, 237
    starch intake in, 239, 243
    sugar intake in, 239, 243
    summary overview of, 250–251
    vitamin intake in, 243, 246
    water intake and, 246
Dehydration, trauma-related, in opossum, 221–222
Dental caries/disease, prevention of, in agoutis, 283–284
    in hedgehogs, 336
    in kinkajou, 183–184
    in opossum, 233–234
Dentition, as diet determinant, of agoutis, 279–280
    of cavies, 272
    of coatis, 190

of degus, 237–238, 246
of fennec foxes, 301
of kinkajou, 180–181
of macropods, 197–199
of raccoons, 190
Diabetes mellitus, nutrition and, in agoutis, 283–284
in cats, 331
in degus, 249
in kinkajou, 174, 182–183
in lemurs, 342–343
Diarrhea, nutrition and, in squirrels, 292–295
Didelphis virginiana, nutrition of, **217–236**. See also Virginian opossum.
Diet. See Nutrition.
Dietary energy, for degus, 242, 246
for kinkajou, 175–178
for sugar glider, 210
Digestibility, of fiber, in cavies, 270
of raw meat, in exotic cats, 330–331
of sample foods, for degus, 238, 242
Digestive system. See also Gastrointestinal tract.
morphology of, in fennec foxes, 301
in opossum, 226–227
physiology of, in African Pygmy hedgehog, 335–336
in fish, 361, 364
in macropods, 197–202
in sugar glider, 211
Disease manifestations, nutrition and, dental. See Dental caries/disease.
in caracal, 331
in cavies, 274–276
in kinkajou, 173, 175, 180, 183–184
in opossum, 221–224
in prairie dogs, 261–263
in serval, 331
in skunks, 318–322
in squirrels, 294–295
integumentary. See Skin disease.
nutritional disorders as. See Iron storage disease; Metabolic bone disease.
Dog kibble, for kinkajou, 174–175, 178, 180, 182
Dolichotis patagonum, nutrition of, **267–278**. See also Patagonian cavies.
Dry matter intake, of degus, 238, 242, 246
of fennec fox, 302
of hedgehogs, 336
of kinkajou, 175–178
of sugar glider, 213

E

Ecosystem, grassland, prairie dogs impact on, 256, 260
Electrolyte intake/solutions, for fish, 362, 364
for hand-rearing, of fennec foxes, 308

Ecosystem (*continued*)
    of hedgehogs, 337
    of squirrels, 292
  for invertebrates, 353–354
  for kinkajou, 176, 362
  for macropods, 205
Elimination habits. See also *Fecal output*.
  of prairie dogs, 260
Endometritis, in opossum, 226
Energy expenditure/requirements, daily, of agoutis, 282
    of degus, 239
    of exotic cats, 330–331
    of fennec foxes, 303
    of fish, 361, 369
    of invertebrates, 350
    of kinkajou, 173–174
    of lemurs, 340
    of macropods, 202–203
    of opossum, 233
    of raccoons, 192
    of sugar glider, 211, 213–214
Energy intake. See *Dietary energy.*
Enteritis, nutrition and, in squirrels, 290, 294–295
Environmental factors, of nutrition, for cavies, 269–270
    for degus, 250
    for exotic cats, 329
    for fennec fox, 301
    for fish, 361, 365–366, 368–369
    for hedgehogs, 335
    for invertebrates, 350–351
    for kinkajou, 172–173
    for lemurs, 345–346
    for macropods, 203–204
    for skunks, 314–317
    for squirrels, 287–289
    for sugar glider, 209–210
Esbilac powder, for hand-rearing, of cavies, 272
    of exotic cats, 332
    of fennec foxes, 307–308
    of hedgehogs, 337
    of opossum, 228
    of squirrels, 291
Esophagus, of macropods, 200–201
Estrus cycle, of cavies, 269
  of fennec foxes, 300
  of kinkajou, 180
  of skunks, 3
Ethics, of prairie dogs, as pets, 263
Euthanasia, of opossum, vs. return to wild, 223–224
Evaluation/examination, of cavies, 273
    of opossum, 218–220

for trauma, 222–223
    healthy appearance in, 220–221
Exotic cats, nutrition of, **327–334**. See also *Caracal; Serval.*

F

Fat/fatty acid intake. See *Lipid intake.*
Fecal output, in nutrition assessment, of degus, 248–249
    of prairie dogs, 260
    of sugar glider, 209, 211
Feces, reingestion of, by degus, 238
Feed intake, of fish, 368–369
Feeding behavior, of African Pygmy hedgehog, 335
    of agoutis, 282
    of caracal, 328–329
    of coatis, 188–189
    of degus, 258
    of exotic cats, 327–328
    of fish, 364–367
    of lemurs, 344
    of macropods, 203–204
    of raccoons, 189–190
    of serval, 327–328
    of skunks, 316
    of sugar glider, 209–210
Feeding deterrents, for fish, 368
Feeding ecology, of cavies, 270
    of degus, 258
    of fennec foxes, 301
    of lemurs, 341–342
    of sugar glider, 209–210
Feeding regimen, for fennec foxes, 303
    with hand-rearing, 308–309
    for fish, 369–370
    for hedgehogs, 336
    with hand-rearing, 337
    for opossum, 227
    with hand-rearing, 228
    for squirrels, with hand-rearing, 292–293
    for sugar glider, 213–214
Feeding rhythms, daily. See *Daily activity patterns.*
    seasonal, of fish, 367–368
    tidal/lunar, of fish, 367–368
Feeding stimulants, for fish, 368–369
Felis serval, nutrition of, **327–334**. See also *Serval.*
Fennec foxes, nutrition of, **299–312**
    digestive morphology and, 301
    feeding ecology in, 301
    food availability and, 302
    hand-rearing and, 306–311
        body temperature in, 306

Fennec foxes (*continued*)
    body weight tracking in, 309–310
    colostrum vs., 306
    feeding quantities in, 309
    feeding regimen for, 308–309
    formula selection for, 306, 308
    indications for, 303, 306
    milk composition in, 306–307
    weaning from, 309–311
  husbandry for, 301–303
  nutrient content of natural diet, 301–302
  nutrient content of sample diets, 302, 304–305
  nutrient requirements in, 302
  parental care and, 301
  practical captive diets in, 302–305
  reproductive stage and, 300–301
  social behavior and, 300
  species background and, 299
  summary overview of, 299–300
  water intake and, 301
Fermentation, microbial, in macropods, 197, 274
  of fiber, in lemurs, 340
Fiber digestibility, in cavies, 270
  in macropods, 203
Fiber fermentation, in lemurs, 340
Fiber intake, of agoutis, 282
  of cavies, 270–271
  of degus, 239, 242
  of hedgehogs, 336
  of kinkajou, 174–175
  of sugar glider, 210, 214
Fish, nutrition of, **361–372**
  feed intake and, 368–369
  feeding behavior and, 364–367
  feeding rhythms and, 365, 367–368
  feeding stimulants and deterrents in, 368
  feeds and feeding recommendations for, 369–370
  larval, 370
  nutrient deficiency and toxicity signs in, 362, 364, 369
  nutrient requirements in, 361–364
    essential, 361–362
    macronutrients, 362–363
    micronutrients, 363–364
  summary overview of, 361
Fish larvae, feeding of, 370
Flesh, consumption of. See *Carnivores.*
Flies, diets for, 353, 356–358
Flying squirrels, wild diets of, 289. See also *Tree-dwelling squirrels.*
Food chain, prairie dogs role in, 256
Food preferences, of agoutis, 282
  of coatis, 191

of fish, 364, 369
of hedgehogs, 336
of opossum, 229
of prairie dogs, 260–261
of raccoons, 192
of squirrels, 287–289
of sugar glider, 209–211
Food presentation, for invertebrates, 352–353
  for kinkajou, 178, 182
Food-dousing behavior, of raccoons, 189–190
Forestomach, digestion in, of macropods, 197, 200–201, 203–204
Formula, milk replacement. See *Commercial formulas.*
Foxes, nutrition of, **299–312**. See also *Fennec foxes.*
Frugivores, agoutis as, 280–282
  invertebrates as, 358–359
  kinkajou as, 171–174
  macropods as, 198
Fruit flies, diets for, 353, 358
Fungal infections, in cavies, 274–276
  in skunks, 320

G

Gastrointestinal disease, nutrition and, in cavies, 274–276
    in squirrels, 290, 294–295
Gastrointestinal tract, nutrition and, in African Pygmy hedgehog, 335–336
    in agoutis, 281
    in cavies, anatomy and, 272–273
      disease of, 274–276
      morphology of, 270–271
    in degus, 237–238
    in fennec fox, 301
    in kinkajou, 172
    in lemurs, 340
    in macropods, 197–202
    in opossum, 226–227
      trauma to, 233
    in squirrels, infections with, 290, 294–295
Geophagy, in squirrels, 287–289
Geriatric nutrition, for degus, 248
  for kinkajou, 174, 180
Gestation, nutrition for, in agoutis, 283–284
    in cavies, 269
    in coatis, 190
    in degus, 246, 248
    in exotic cats, 332
    in fennec fox, 300
    in hedgehogs, 336
    in kinkajou, 175, 177, 180
    in lemurs, 342, 344
    in macropods, 205

Gestation (*continued*)
    in prairie dogs, 257
    in raccoons, 190
    in skunks, 315
Glucose metabolism. See *Insulin response.*
Goat's milk, for squirrels, 291
Grassland ecosystem, prairie dogs impact on, 256, 260
Grooming behavior, of opossum, 225
Gross energy intake, of degus, 242
Ground squirrels, wild diets of, 289
Gumivores, sugar glider as, 210–211, 214

H

Handling, for veterinary care. See also *Restraint/restraining.*
    of Patagonian cavies, 273
Hand-rearing, nutrition for, of cavies, 272
    of exotic cats, 332
    of fennec foxes, 306–311
        body temperature and, 306
        body weight tracking in, 309–310
        colostrum vs., 306
        feeding quantities in, 309
        feeding regimen in, 308–309
        formula selection for, 306, 308
        indications for, 303, 306
        milk composition in, 306–307
        weaning from, 309–311
    of hedgehogs, 337
    of kinkajou, 179–180
    of macropods, 205–206
    of opossum, 228
        weaning from, 229
    of squirrels, 290–295
        feeding regimen for, 292–293
        indications for, 290
        milk additives for, 293–294
        milk formulas for, 290–292
        weaning from, 294
Head trauma, nutrition and, in squirrels, 296
Hedgehog, nutrition of, **335–337**. See also *African Pygmy hedgehog.*
Helminth infestations, in skunks, 320
Hematologic values, normal, for cavies, 273–274
    for skunks, 321–322
Hemosiderosis. See *Iron storage disease.*
Herbivores, cavies as, 268, 270
   degus as, 238–239, 250
   fish as, 368
   flesh consumption by. See *Omnivores.*
   invertebrates as, 352–353, 356–359
   kinkajou as, 174

macropods as, 197–198, 204–205
　prairie dogs as, 256, 260–261
　skunks as, 316
　squirrels as, 289
Histoplasmosis, in cavies, 274–275
History taking, in opossum evaluation, 218
Housing, as nutrition factor, for cavies, 269–270
　　for degus, 250
　　for lemurs, 345–346
　　for opossum, 220–221
　　for prairie dogs, 259–260, 264
Humidity, as nutrition factor, for degus, 250
　　for invertebrates, 351
Hunger, as feeding stimulus, in fish, 368–369
Hunting techniques, of exotic cats, 327–328
Husbandry, captive nutritional, for African Pygmy hedgehog, 336
　　for cavies, 269–270
　　for degus, 250
　　for fennec fox, 301
　　for fish, 365–366, 368–369
　　for invertebrates, 350–351, 354
　　for kinkajou, 174–178, 182
　　for lemurs, 345–346
　　for macropods, 202–203
　　for prairie dogs, 259–260
Hydration. See *Water intake.*
Hyperparathyroidism, nutritional secondary, in opossum, 226, 230–232

I

Infections, in cavies, 274–276
　in kinkajou, 174
　in macropods, 204
　in opossum, 219–220, 228
　　trauma and, 222–223
　in prairie dogs, 262
　in skunks, 318–320, 322
　in squirrels, 294–295
　wild-caught insects transmission of, 352
Insectivores, coatis and raccoons as, 191–192
　hedgehogs as, 335–336
　opossum as, 229
　skunks as, 316
　squirrels as, 287
　sugar glider as, 209–212, 214
Insulin response, in agoutis, 283–284
　in degus, 249
　in macropods, 203
Integumentary disease. See *Skin disease.*
Internet sources. See *Web sites.*

Invertebrates, captive, nutrition of, **349–360**
    carnivorous, 352–355
    food preparation and presentation in, 352–353
    food procurement for, 352
    frugivorous, 358–359
    herbivorous, 352–353, 356–359
    omnivorous, 352, 355–356
    reproductive stage and, 4, 355
    species background and, 349–350, 359
    summary overview of, 349–350, 359
    supportive, 353
    water intake and, 350–351, 353
  consumption of. See *Insectivores.*
Iron intake, of sugar glider, 213
Iron overload, in lemurs, 343
Iron storage disease, diet and, in coatis, 191
    in lemurs, 343
    in sugar glider, 213, 215

J

Joeys, macropod, nutrition of, 205
    hand-rearing and, 205–206
Jump-yip, of prairie dogs, 257–259
Juvenile nutrition, for kinkajou, 173, 179–180
  for opossum, 229
  for prairie dogs, 261

K

Kangaroos, nutrition of, **197–208**. See also *Macropods.*
Kinkajou, nutrition of, **171–185**
    adult, 173–175, 180
    body condition scores and, 180–182
    energy requirements and, 173–174
    enrichment for captivity, 182–183
    final thoughts on, 184
    food presentation and, 178, 182
    gastrointestinal anatomy and, 172
    geriatric, 174, 180
    hand-rearing and, 179–180
    juvenile, 173, 179–180
    life span/stage and, 173–174, 179–180
    natural history of, 171–172
    neonatal, 179–180
    nutrient content of sample foods, 175–178
    nutrient requirements and, 172–174
    nutritional disorders and, 183–184
    practical captive diets in, 174–178
    reproductive stage and, 174–175, 177, 180
    species background and, 171–172

KMR formula, for hand-rearing, of cavies, 272
        of exotic cats, 332
        of kinkajou, 179

L

Laboratory tests, blood, for cavies, 273–274
        for skunks, 321–322
Lactaid, for squirrels, 293–294
Lactase activity, in macropods, 202
    in squirrels, 291, 293
Lactation, nutrition for, in agoutis, 283–284
        in cavies, 269, 272
        in coatis, 190–191
        in degus, 243, 248
        in fennec foxes, 306, 308
        in hedgehogs, 336–337
        in kinkajou, 175, 177, 179
        in lemurs, 342
        in macropods, 205
        in opossum, 228
        in raccoons, 190
        in squirrels, 290–291
Lactobacillus additive, for squirrels, 293
Larvae, fish, feeding of, 370
Leafcutter ants, diets for, 358–359
Lemurs, nutrition of, **339–348**
        anatomy and physiology in, 340
        body weight and, 340–341
        captive behavior and, 344–345
        enrichment for captivity, 346
        feeding behavior and, 344
        feeding ecology in, 341–342
        fiber fermentation and, 340
        hemosiderosis and iron overload in, 343
        lactation and, 342
        obesity and, 342–343
        operant training and, 346
        pregnancy and, 342, 344
        secondary plant metabolites in, 341
        self-mutilation and, 345
        social behavior and, 344–345
        species background and, 339
        summary overview of, 339–340, 346
Lens lesions, nutrition and, in degus, 249
Lifespan, nutrition for, of coatis, 191
        of degus, 244–246, 248
        of kinkajou, 173–174
        of opossum, 225, 229
        of prairie dogs, 261, 263
        of raccoons, 192

Lighting, as nutrition factor, for degus, 250
    for fish, 365–366
Lipid intake, of cavies, 271
  of degus, 243
  of fennec foxes, 303–304
  of fish, 361–363, 368, 370
  of hedgehogs, 336
  of kinkajou, 175, 178
  of macropods, 202–203
  of squirrels, 291
Litter training, of exotic cats, 329
  of opossum, 225
Longevity. See *Geriatric nutrition; Lifespan.*

M

Macropods, nutrition of, **197–208**
    captive diet in, 204–205
    energy metabolism and, 202–204
    feeding behavior and, 203–204
    for joeys, 205
      hand-rearing and, 205–206
    gastrointestinal anatomy and physiology in, 197–202
    reproductive stage and, 205–206
    species background and, 197
    summary overview of, 197, 206
    water intake and, 204
Maggots, diets for, 356
Magnesium ammonium phosphate (MAP) calculi, in exotic cats, 331
Malocclusion, nutrition and, in cavies, 273–274
Mange, nutrition and, in squirrels, 295
Manna intake, of sugar glider, 210
Mating behavior. See *Breeding behavior; Courtship behavior.*
Mealworm beetle, diets for, 355–357
Meat, consumption of. See *Carnivores.*
Mephitis mephitis, nutrition of, **313–326**. See also *Striped skunks.*
Merycism, in macropods, 203–204
Metabolic bone disease, in coatis, 191
  in exotic cats, 331–332
  in kinkajou, 180
  in skunks, 322
  in squirrels, 289
Metabolic disorders, in skunks, 322
Metabolic rate, diet and, of agoutis, 282
    of exotic cats, 330–331
    of lemurs, 340
    of macropods, 202, 204
    of raccoons, 192
    of sugar glider, 211
Metabolizable energy. See *Dietary energy.*

Milk, commercial replacements for. See *Commercial formulas.*
　　cow/goat, for squirrels, 290–291
　　natural gestational. See *Lactation.*
Milk additives, for macropod joeys, 206
　　for squirrels, 293–294
Milk Matrix formulas, Zoologic, for cavies, 272
　　　　for exotic cats, 332
　　　　for opossum, 228
　　　　for squirrels, 291–292
Millipedes, diets for, 356–357
Mineral intake, of cavies, 271
　　of degus, 243–245
　　of exotic cats, 330–332
　　of fennec foxes, 303, 305
　　　　hand-rearing and, 307–308
　　of fish, 361–364
　　of kinkajou, 175–177
　　of macropods, 205
　　of sugar glider, 211–212
Monkeypox virus, in prairie dogs, 262–263
Morphometrics, in nutrition assessment, of degus, 248
Musculoskeletal disease, nutrition and, in cavies, 275–276
Myriapods, diets for, 354–355

N

Nectar intake, of sugar glider, 210, 212
Neonatal nutrition, for agoutis, 283–284
　　for coatis, 190–191
　　for degus, 246
　　for exotic cats, 332
　　for fennec foxes, 303, 306–311
　　for invertebrates, 354
　　for kinkajou, 179–180
　　for opossum, 228
　　　　abandoned infants and, 221–222
　　for raccoons, 190–191
　　for squirrels, 290–295
Neurologic disease, trauma-related, in opossum, 222
Neutering, of opossum, 226
　　of prairie dogs, 264
Nitrogen requirements, for macropods, 203
　　for sugar glider, 211
Nutrient composition, of sample foods, for degus, 240–241
　　　　for fennec fox, 301–302, 304–305
　　　　for invertebrates, 352–353
　　　　for kinkajou, 175–178
　　　　for sugar glider, 210–211
Nutrient requirements, for cavies, 271
　　for exotic cats, 329–331
　　for fennec fox, 302

Nutrient requirements (*continued*)
    for fish, 361–364, 369
        essential, 361–362
        macronutrients, 362–363
        micronutrients, 363–364
    for hedgehogs, 335–336
    for kinkajou, 172–174
Nutrition, of agoutis, **279–286**. See also *Agoutis.*
    of caracal, **327–334**. See also *Caracal.*
    of cavies, **267–278**. See also *Patagonian cavies.*
    of coatis and raccoons, **187–195**. See also *Coatis; Raccoons.*
    of degus, **237–253**. See also *Degus.*
    of fish, **361–372**. See also *Fish.*
    of foxes, **299–312**. See also *Fennec foxes.*
    of hedgehogs, **335–337**. See also *African Pygmy hedgehog.*
    of invertebrates, **349–360**. See also *Invertebrates.*
    of kinkajou, **171–185**. See also *Kinkajou.*
    of lemurs, **339–348**. See also *Lemurs.*
    of macropods, **197–208**. See also *Macropods.*
    of opossum, **217–236**. See also *Virginian opossum.*
    of prairie dogs, **255–266**. See also *Prairie dogs.*
    of serval, **327–334**. See also *Serval.*
    of skunks, **313–326**. See also *Striped skunks.*
    of squirrels, **287–297**. See also *Tree-dwelling squirrels.*
    of sugar glider, **209–215**. See also *Sugar glider.*
Nutritional assessment, of degus, 248–249
    of prairie dogs, 260
    of sugar glider, 209, 211
Nutritional disorders, bone disease as. See *Metabolic bone disease.*
    diabetes as. See *Diabetes mellitus.*
    hemosiderosis as. See *Iron storage disease.*
    hyperparathyroidism as. See *Secondary hyperparathyroidism.*
    in hedgehogs, 336
    in kinkajou, 183–184
    in skunks, 322
    overweight as. See *Obesity.*

O

Obesity, nutrition and, in agoutis, 284
        in cats, 331
        in coatis, 191
        in fennec foxes, 303
        in hedgehogs, 336
        in kinkajou, 183–184
        in lemurs, 342–343
        in opossum, 232–233
        in prairie dogs, 261
        in raccoons, 192
        in sugar glider, 214
Octodon degus, nutrition for, **237–253**. See also *Degus.*

Odontoma, in prairie dogs, 262
Omnivores, agoutis as, 279–284
   coatis and raccoons as, 188, 191–192
   exotic cats as, 328–330
   fennec foxes as, 303, 310
   fish as, 368
   hedgehogs as, 335–336
   invertebrates as, 352, 355–356
   kinkajou as, 174
   lemurs as, 341–342
   opossum as, 226, 229
   skunks as, 316
   sugar gliders as, 209–210
Operant training, nutrition and, of cavies, 270
     of lemurs, 346
     of prairie dogs, 260
Opossum, nutrition of, **217–236**. See also *Virginian opossum.*
Oral morphology, nutrition and, of opossum, 226
Oral rehydration fluid, for hedgehogs, 337
   for invertebrates, 353

P

Pain response, in opossum, 223
Pancreatitis, in kinkajou, 183
Parasitic infections, in cavies, 274–275
   in kinkajou, 174
   in macropods, 204
   in opossum, 219–220
     trauma and, 222–223
   in prairie dogs, 262–263
   in skunks, 320
   in squirrels, 294–295
Parental care, nutrition and, in fennec foxes, 301
     in lemurs, 344–345
Patagonian cavies, nutrition of, **267–278**
     behavior in wild and, 268–269
     captive management and, 269–270
     cardiopulmonary diseases and, 275
     gastrointestinal diseases and, 274–276
     gastrointestinal tract anatomy and, 272–273
     gastrointestinal tract morphology and, 270–271
     hand-rearing and, 272
     integumentary diseases and, 275–276
     malocclusion and, 273–274
     musculoskeletal diseases and, 275–276
     natural foraging ecology and, 270
     reproductive stage and, 269
     social behavior and, 268–269
     species background and, 267–268
     target nutrient values for, 271

Patagonian cavies (*continued*)
    veterinary care and, 272–276
        anatomy in, 272–273
        anesthesia in, 273
        clinical pathology in, 273–274
        for diseases and health concerns, 273–276
        handling in, 273
        venipuncture in, 273
    zoo settings and, 269, 271–272
Peanuts, for squirrels, 289
Pedialyte, for hand-rearing, of fennec foxes, 308
    of hedgehogs, 337
    of squirrels, 292
Pelleted diets, for invertebrates, 352, 356–357
    for macropods, 204–205
Personalities, of prairie dogs, 258–259
Pet Ag formula, for hand-rearing, of squirrels, 291
Petaurus breviceps, nutrition of, **209–215**. See also *Sugar glider.*
Phosphorus intake, of exotic cats, 331–332
    of invertebrates, 354
    of kinkajou, 175–176, 183
    of opossum, 230–232
    of squirrels, 289, 295
    of sugar glider, 212–214
Physical assessment. See *Evaluation/examination.*
Plague, in prairie dogs, 262
Plant exudates, in sugar glider diet, 210, 214
Plant metabolites, secondary, in lemurs, 341
Plants, consumption of. See *Herbivores.*
Pollen, as protein intake, for sugar glider, 210–211
    kinkajou and, 172–173
Polyacrylamide (PAM) gel, in water preparation, for invertebrates, 351
Postoperative pain response, in opossum, 223
Potos flavus, nutrition of, **171–185**. See also *Kinkajou.*
Prairie dogs, nutrition of, **255–266**
    as pets, 258–259, 264
        age choice for, 260
        sex choice for, 260
        where to obtain, 263
    body mass and, 257, 261
    diseases and, 261–263
        miscellaneous infections as, 262
        odontoma as, 262
        parasites as, 262–263
        plague as, 262
        tularemia as, 261–262
    elimination habits of, 260
    grassland ecosystem and, 256, 260
    housing and, 259–260
    injuries and, 263
    juvenile, 261

        longevity of, 263
        neutering of, 264
        personalities and, 258–259
        predators and, 256–258
        recommended foods for, 260–261
        reproductive stage and, 257
        return to wild and, 264
        social behavior and, as pets, 258–259
            colony sites in, 256–258
        species background and, 255
        veterinary checkups and, 264
Predators, of prairie dogs, 256–258
Pregnancy, nutrition for. See *Gestation.*
Probiotics, for squirrels, 293–295
Protein intake, of cavies, 271
    of degus, 243
    of exotic cats, 329–330
    of fennec foxes, 303–304
    of fish, 361–363, 370
    of hedgehogs, 336
    of kinkajou, 174–175
    of macropods, 203
    of squirrels, 289–291
    of sugar glider, 209–214
Protozoan infestations, in skunks, 320

    R

Rabies virus, in prairie dogs, 262
    in skunks, 318–319
Raccoons, nutrition of, **187–195**
        adult requirements for, 192
        average body weights in, 188
        energy requirements in, 192
        feeding behavior and, 189–190
        functional anatomy and physiology in, 189
        metabolic rate and, 192
        neonatal requirements for, 190–191
        reproductive stage and, 190–191
        species background and, 187–188
        summary overview of, 192
Radiographs, of opossum, for nutritional secondary hyperparathyroidism, 231–232
        for trauma evaluation, 221–223
Reproductive stage, nutrition for, in agoutis, 282–284
        in cavies, 269
        in coatis, 190–191
        in degus, 246–248
        in exotic cats, 331
        in fennec foxes, 300–301
        in hedgehogs, 336–337

Reproductive stage (*continued*)
    in invertebrates, 352, 355
    in kinkajou, 174–175, 177, 180
    in lemurs, 342, 344
    in macropods, 205–206
    in raccoons, 190–191
    in skunks, 315
    in sugar glider, 209–210, 213
Respiratory disease, in cavies, 275
  trauma-related, in opossum, 222
Restraint/restraining, of cavies, 273
  of opossum, 219–220
Return to wild, of opossum, vs. euthanasia, 223–224
  of prairie dogs, 264
Rodents, terrestrial, diet determinants for, **279–286**. See also *Agoutis.*

S

Salivary glands, of macropods, 199
Satiation system, in fish, 364–365
  in kinkajou, 178
Scatter-hoarding behavior, diet and, of agoutis, 281, 284
Scent elimination, for skunk scent, 317–318
Secondary hyperparathyroidism, nutritional, in kinkajou, 183
    in opossum, 226, 230–232
Sedatives, for restraint, of cavies, 273
Seed/nut intake, of agoutis, 282
  of macropods, 198
  of opossum, 229
  of squirrels, 287–289
Seizures, nutrition and, in squirrels, 295–296
Self-mutilation, nutrition and, in lemurs, 345
Serval, nutrition of, **327–334**
    body weight and, 330–331
    captivity issues with, 329
    disease related to, 331
    feeding behavior and, 327–328
    hand-rearing and, 332
    requirements for, 329–331
    species background and, 327
    stone formation and, 331
    summary overview of, 327, 332
Sexuality maturity, nutrition and, of agoutis, 282
    of degus, 246, 248
    of invertebrates, 355
    of kinkajou, 180
    of prairie dogs, 257
Shock, trauma-related, in opossum, 222
Silkworms, diets for, 357–358
Skin disease, nutrition and, in cavies, 275–276
    in opossum, 222–223

Skunks, nutrition of, **313–326**. See also *Striped skunks.*
SMA Gold formula, for cavies, 272
Small intestine, of macropods, 201–202
Social behavior, of cavies, 268–269
    of degus, 249–250
    of exotic cats, 329
    of fennec foxes, 300
    of kinkajou, 183
    of lemurs, 344–345
    of prairie dogs, as pets, 258–259
        colony sites and, 256–258
Socialization, of opossum, 225
Spaying, of opossum, 226
    of prairie dogs, 264
Spinal trauma, nutrition and, in squirrels, 296
Squirrels, nutrition of, **287–297**. See also *Tree-dwelling squirrels.*
Starch intake, of degus, 239, 243
    of fish, 370
    of kinkajou, 174
    of lemurs, 341–343
    of macropods, 204
Stereotypies, of exotic cats, 329
Stomach, digestion in, of cavies, 270–271
    of degus, 238
    of fennec fox, 301
    of macropods, 200–202
    of opossum, 226–227
Stone formation, urinary, in exotic cats, 331
Striped skunks, nutrition of, **313–326**
    as problem for humans, 316–318
    diseases and, 318–322
        metabolic disorders as, 322
        other infections as, 320, 322
        rabies as, 318–319
    feeding behavior and, 316
    health issues and, 318–322
        laboratory values in, 321–322
    natural history and, 314–315
    physical description and, 314
    reproductive stage and, 315
    species background and, 313–314
    summary overview of, 313, 322
Sugar glider, nutrition of, **209–215**
    areas for further investigation, 214–215
    common diets for captive, 212–213
    digestive physiology and, 211
    feeding behavior and, 209–210
    native constituents in, 210–211
    recommendations for, 213–214
    reproductive stage and, 209–210, 213
    species background and, 209

Sugar intake, of degus, 239, 243
    of fish, 365
    of kinkajou, 174, 178, 182–183
    of lemurs, 341–343
    of macropods, 203
    of squirrels, 290, 293
Sunflower seeds, for squirrels, 289
Supportive nutrition. See also *Hand-rearing.*
    for abandonment opossum infants, 221–222
    for captive invertebrates, 353

T

Tannins, in natural foods, 288, 343
Tap water, preparation of, for invertebrates, 350
Tarantula, diets for, 349, 354–355
Target nutrient values. See *Nutrient requirements.*
Temperature, as nutrition factor, for degus, 250
    body. See *Body temperature.*
Terrestrial rodents, diet determinants for, **279–286**. See also *Agoutis.*
Transit time, gastrointestinal tract, of degus, 238
Trapped response, of opossum, 218–219
    considerations with treating, 217–218
Trauma, nutrition and, to opossum, 220–223
    behavioral manifestations in, 221–223
    euthanasia in, 223–224
    pain treatment in, 223
    to prairie dogs, 263
    to squirrels, 296
Tree-dwelling squirrels, nutrition of, **287–297**
    body weight and, 289, 292–293
    captive diets in, 289–290
    hand-rearing and, 290–295
        feeding quantities in, 292
        feeding regimen for, 292–293
        indications for, 290
        milk additives for, 293–294
        milk formulas for, 290–292
        weaning from, 294
    health problems associated with, 289, 294–296
        abscesses as, 295
        diarrhea as, 292–295
        head trauma as, 296
        mange as, 295
        seizures as, 295–296
        spinal trauma as, 296
      species background and, 287
      summary overview of, 287, 296
      wild diets in, 287–289
Tube feeding, of opossum joeys, 228
Tularemia, in prairie dogs, 261–262

U

Urban diets, adjustment to, by raccoons, 192
Urinary calculi, formation of, in exotic cats, 331
Urination, by prairie dogs, 260
Urine pH, nutrition and, in exotic cats, 331

V

Venipuncture, for cavies, 273
Vertebrates, consumption of. See *Carnivores; Omnivores.*
Veterinary care, for cavies, 272–276
    anatomy in, 272–273
    anesthesia in, 273
    clinical pathology in, 273–274
    for diseases and health concerns, 273–276
    handling in, 273
    venipuncture in, 273
  for opossum, restraint techniques in, 219–220
  for prairie dogs, 264
Viral infections, in cavies, 276
  in prairie dogs, 262
  in skunks, 318–320, 322
Virginian opossum, nutrition of, **217–236**
    adult, 229
    as pets, 224–226
        behavior in, 224–225
        diseases in, 226
        grooming in, 225
        lifespan in, 225
        litter training in, 225
        socialization in, 225
        spaying and neutering n, 226
    behavioral considerations in, as pets, 224–226
        disease manifestations and, 221–224
        of captive and owned opossum, 217–221
    body weight and, 219–222, 228
    Cushing's-like syndrome in, 226
    dental disease and, 233–234
    disease manifestations and, 221–224
        euthanasia in, 223–224
        of captive and hospitalized opossum, 230–234
        of pets, 226
        pain response in, 223
        trauma in, 220–223
    feeding schedule for, 227
    for captive and hospitalized opossum, 226–234
        diseases in, 230–234
        gastrointestinal aspects in, 226–227
        general diet information in, 227–230
    for captive and owned opossum, 217–221

Virginian opossum (*continued*)
  case management of, 221
  confinement response and, 221
  evaluating and, 218
  examining and, 219–220
  healthy appearance of, 220–221
  housing and, 220–221
  restraining and, 219–220
  trapped response and, 218–219
  treating and, 217–218
 gastrointestinal morphology and, 226–227
 in clinical setting, behavioral considerations for, 217–221
  captive and hospitalized opossum, 226–234
 juvenile, 229
 neonatal, 228
 obesity and, 232–233
 oral morphology and, 226
 return to wild and, 223–224
 secondary hyperparathyroidism related to, 226, 230–232
 summary overview of, 234
 vitamins in, 229–230
Vitamin A intake, of kinkajou, 175–177
 of opossum, 230
Vitamin B intake, of opossum, 230
Vitamin C intake, of agoutis, diet requirements for, 282
  endogenous synthesis vs., 281
 of cavies, 271
 of degus, 243, 246
 of lemurs, 343
 of sugar glider, 213
Vitamin D intake, of exotic cats, 329, 331
 of kinkajou, 183
 of opossum, 229–230
 of skunks, 322
 of sugar glider, 213–215
Vitamin E supplementation, for macropods, 205
Vitamin intake, of cavies, 271
 of degus, 243, 246
 of fennec foxes, 303–305
 of fish, 361–362, 364
 of kinkajou, 176–177, 180
 of opossum, 229–230
 of skunks, 316
 of sugar glider, 211–212
Vulpes zerda, nutrition of, **299–312**. See also *Fennec foxes.*

  W

Wallabies, nutrition of, **197–208**. See also *Macropods.*
Water intake, of degus, 246
 of exotic cats, 331

of fennec foxes, 301, 308
of hedgehogs, 336
of invertebrates, 350–351, 353
of kinkajou, 172
of macropods, 204
of sugar glider, 213–214
Weaning, from hand-rearing, of cavies, 272
    of exotic cats, 332
    of fennec foxes, 309–311
    of opossum, 229
    of squirrels, 294
Web sites, for exotic cats, 329
    for sugar glider diets, 212, 214
Weight-reduction diets, for hedgehogs, 336
    for opossum, 233

Z

Zoo settings, nutrition and, for cavies, 269, 271–272
    for kinkajou, 174, 184
Zoonotic diseases, in skunks, 320

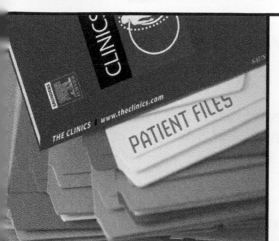
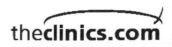

Moving?

Make sure your subscription moves with you!

To notify us of your new address, find your **Clinics Account Number** (located on your mailing label above your name), and contact customer service at:

E-mail: elspcs@elsevier.com

800-654-2452 (subscribers in the U.S. & Canada)
314-453-7041 (subscribers outside of the U.S. & Canada)

Fax number: 314-523-5170

Elsevier Periodicals Customer Service
11830 Westline Industrial Drive
St. Louis, MO 63146

*To ensure uninterrupted delivery of your subscription, please notify us at least 4 weeks in advance of move.

Printed and bound by CPI Group (UK) Ltd, Croydon, CR0 4YY

03/10/2024

01040462-0005